IMMUNOLOGY
for Life Scientists

SECOND EDITION

LESLEY-JANE EALES

University of Surrey, Guildford, UK

WILEY

Other Wiley Editorial Offices

John Wiley & Sons Inc., 111 River Street, Hoboken, NJ 07030, USA

Jossey-Bass, 989 Market Street, San Francisco, CA 94103-1741, USA

Wiley-VCH Verlag GmbH, Boschstr. 12, D-69469 Weinheim, Germany

John Wiley & Sons Australia Ltd, 33 Park Road, Milton, Queensland 4064, Australia

John Wiley & Sons (Asia) Pte Ltd, 2 Clementi Loop #02-01, Jin Xing Distripark, Singapore 129809

John Wiley & Sons Canada Ltd, 22 Worcester Road, Etobicoke, Ontario, Canada M9W 1L1

Wiley also publishes its books in a variety of electronic formats. Some content that appears in print may not be available in electronic books.

Library of Congress Cataloging-in-Publication Data

Eales, Lesley-Jane.
    Immunology for life scientists / Lesley-Jane Eales. – 2nd ed.
        p. cm.
    Includes bibliographical references and index.
    ISBN 0-470-84523-6 (cloth : alk. paper) – ISBN 0-470-84524-4 (pbk. : alk. paper)
    1. Immunology.   2. Immunopathology.   3. Immunity.   I. Title.
QR181.E24 2003
616.07'9–dc21   2003050184

British Library Cataloguing in Publication Data

A catalogue record for this book is available from the British Library

ISBN 0 470 84523 6
ISBN 0 470 84524 4 (pbk)

Typeset in Times 11/13pt by Dobbie Typesetting Ltd, Tavistock, Devon
Printed and bound in Great Britain by T J International, Padstow, Cornwall
This book is printed on acid-free paper responsibly manufactured from sustainable forestry in which at least two trees are planted for each one used for paper production.

b
2.1.07

IMMUNOLOGY
for Life Scientists

DEDICATION

For my dad who gave me patience and for Scott who
taught me the skills

CONTENTS

PREFACE TO THE 2ND EDITION

It is hard to believe how much our understanding of immunology has progressed in the few short years since the first edition of this book was produced. Like its predecessor, this edition is very much aimed at students who have no clinical background and no prior knowledge of immunology. It is for students who are doing immunology as part of another discipline such as biomedical scientists and is strictly designed to help students help themselves to learn. It introduces each concept at the most basic level and then guides students, either by recommended reading or through the dedicated web site, to where they can gain more knowledge or solve comprehension problems.

This edition is not accompanied by a self-assessment diskette (too many readers found that theirs went missing!), but the database will be downloadable from the web site for the book. In addition, a lecturer's version will be available to help you expand and/or build your own question databases. In addition the web site will provide all the figures from the book as downloadable files. You are encouraged to visit the site on a regular basis as it will be constantly updated with new information and useful material.

L.-J. E.

Supplementary material can be obtained from
www.wiley.co.uk/ealesimmunology

PREFACE TO THE 1ST EDITION

Immunology for Life Scientists is, as its title suggests, a textbook for students who are studying immunology as part of another degree course. If you consider how we first begin to learn as children, we do so through repeated exposure to words and examples. It is only once we have obtained a working vocabulary and an understanding of what those words mean that we are taught the grammar of the language. Learning a new science may be treated in a similar way. Thus in *Immunology for Life Scientists*, unlike other texts, I have tried to introduce you to immunological terms and concepts (and to explain them fully) using everyday language. I have avoided detailed practical descriptions since, unless you are familiar with the techniques and terminology, they may lead to confusion. This book aims to give students a thorough grounding in the concepts of both basic and clinical immunology and to give them the ability and (I hope) enthusiasm to read review articles and seminal papers which do describe exactly how the work was performed. It is important to learn to walk before you run, and by having a firm grounding and thorough understanding of the concepts of immunology, you should be able to go on to more complex texts without becoming confused or disheartened.

This book is designed as a starting point. For students who wish to learn more or require a fuller understanding of immunology, annotated lists of references and review articles have been included.

Finally, with increasing student numbers there is a move towards self-assessed and self-directed learning. This text is also designed to meet these requirements. It comes with a self-assessment program which can help students to learn and can provide information to tutors about areas of difficulty which may then be addressed in tutorial sessions. Perhaps, most importantly, I hope it will make learning fun!

L.-J. E.

GLOSSARY

Accessory cell: Term used for a cell (often an antigen presenting cell), which plays a vital role in a specific immune response but cannot by itself mediate the same.

Affinity: A measure of the strength of binding (the binding constant) between a single, monovalent antigenic determinant and a single antigen combining site.

Agglutination: The aggregation of cells or particulate antigens as a result of antibody binding to antigenic determinants on the cells or antigens.

Allele: One of two or more different forms of the same gene, which occupy the same position (locus) on a particular chromosome.

Allelic: Relating to an allele.

Allelic exclusion: The expression of only one form of a particular antigen receptor (e.g. TCRα/β or TCRγ/δ) despite having the genetic material to produce both.

Allergen: An antigen that has the capability of inducing IgE rather than IgG or A production in an individual, resulting in an allergic response.

Allergy: A largely IgE-mediated, inflammatory response to non-pathogenic antigens resulting in pathological changes that may be damaging to the host.

Allogeneic: Term referring to genetically different members of the same species.

Allograft: A tissue graft between two members of the same species who are not genetically identical.

Allotypes: Usually used in relation to antibodies, this term refers to the antigenic differences between antibodies of the same class caused by transcription of different alleles at the same locus.

Alternative pathway: Activation of complement via C3 which does not involve the activation of C1, C4 and C2 by immune complexes.

Anaphylatoxin: A pro-inflammatory substance, which causes the release of histamine from mast cells.

Anaphylaxis: A response to challenge by an allergen that is largely IgE and mast cell mediated. It is an extreme form of immediate hypersensitivity where a range of pharmacologically active mediators are released. In anaphylaxis these chemicals are released in very high quantities and have rapid effects on smooth muscle cells and vascular permeability. The results can be life-threatening.

Antibody: A globular, serum protein formed in response to stimulation with an immunogen. They are capable of highly specific discrimination between antigens and perform a variety of biological functions. They may also be found on the surface of B cells as part of the B cell antigen receptor (see BCR).

Antibody-dependent cellular cytotoxicity (ADCC): Cells expressing foreign antigen (e.g. viral antigens) become the target of antigen-specific antibodies. These antibody-labelled target cells may then be destroyed by specialised killer cells (including some large granular lymphocytes and macrophages) which have receptors for the Fc part of the antibody (Fc receptors, FcR) and bind to the target cell.

Antigen: A molecule or group of molecules that bind to specific receptors on lymphocytes. If an antigen is capable of stimulating an immune response alone, it is also known as an immunogen. If it cannot, it is known as a hapten.

Antigen-binding site: That part of an antibody or a T cell antigen receptor that binds to antigen.

Antigen-presenting cell (APC): Cells that express molecules coded for by the Class II genes of the major histocompatibility complex (MHC). They are capable of processing and presenting antigen to T cells. APC include dendritic cells, macrophages and B lymphocytes.

Antigenic determinant: That part of an antigen which binds to antigen-binding sites on the T or B cell antigen receptors. Also known as an epitope. Complex antigens may have many different antigenic determinants or epitopes, each of which can be recognised by different T or B cells.

Antigen processing: The pathways (endogenous or exogenous) by which large molecules are broken down within antigen presenting cells so that they can associate with the products of the major histocompatibility complex genes and be presented on the surface of the antigen-presenting cell.

Anti-idiotype: An antibody that recognises the antigenic nature of the variable region (or idiotype) of another antibody.

Atopy: Usually used synonymously with allergy. It is used to describe IgE-mediated hypersensitivity responses.

Autograft: Transplantation of tissue from one area to another on the same individual.

Autoimmunity: An immune response to self antigens which may be confined to a particular tissue or may be expressed systemically or throughout the body. Such a response may have a range of pathological effects resulting in autoimmune disease.

Avidity: A measure of the strength of binding between antigen and antibody when one or both are polyvalent (i.e. have more than one binding site).

BCR (B cell antigen receptor): The complex of molecules on the surface of a B cell responsible for recognising antigen and signalling to the B cell after binding the antigen. It comprises a membrane anchored immunoglobulin and two molecules responsible for the signalling namely CD79a (Igα) and CD79b (Igβ)

B lymphocyte (B cell): Mature products of the lymphoid progenitor cell that when stimulated by antigen may proliferate and differentiate into memory cells or terminally differentiated plasma cells, which secrete antibody of the same specificity as that on the originally activated parent cell.

Basophil: A polymorphonuclear leukocyte or granulocyte with cytoplasmic granules that stain intensely blue with basic dyes. These granules contain histamine, heparin and other vasoactive amines and are important in hypersensitivity responses.

Bursa of Fabricius: The primary lymphoid tissue in birds responsible for the development of B lymphocytes.

Carcinoembryonic antigen (CEA): An antigen expressed during embryonic development often expressed by malignant tissues.

Carrier: A large molecule, which when attached to a smaller, non-immunogenic molecule (hapten) allows the latter to stimulate an immune response.

Cell-mediated cytotoxicity: The killing of another cell by an effector cell (e.g. cytotoxic T cell, natural killer cell, macrophage).

Cell-mediated immunity (CMI): All those immune responses in which antibody plays little or no part. Largely mediated by T cells, macrophages and NK cells.

Chemotaxin: A chemical capable of attracting cells through binding of specific receptors on the cell surface and promoting their chemotaxis.

Chemotaxis: The directed migration of cells up a concentration gradient of an attractive chemical.

Class I, II and III MHC genes: See Major histocompatibility complex.

Class switching: When B cells are stimulated during the response to a T-dependent antigen, cytokines are produced, which encourage the B cell to switch from producing antibody of one class (usually IgM in a primary response) to another (e.g. IgG or IgA in a secondary response or IgE in an allergic response).

Classical pathway: Activation of the serum complement proteins usually via immune complexes (antibody bound to antigen) and involving the activation of C1, C4 and C2.

Clonal deletion: The elimination of lymphocytes that recognise a particular antigenic epitope either due to contact with self (e.g. thymic selection) or an artificially introduced antigen (desensitisation).

Clonal selection theory: The proliferation and expansion of specific lymphocytes with receptors that recognise part of a particular antigen.

Cluster determinant (CD): The nomenclature used to identify specific antigens on the surface of cells (also known as surface markers). Such markers may have several different epitopes each recognised by a different antibody. In order to regularise the process, any antibody which recognises a particular surface marker (regardless of the epitope) is given the same CD designation e.g. anti-CD3.

Combinatorial joining: This occurs during the development of variable regions in antibody and the TCR. It involves the joining of DNA segments to create new genetic information.

Complement: A group of serum and cell surface proteins involved in inflammation and immunity. They exist in an inactive form but may be triggered by the classical, alternative or lectin pathways to form an enzyme cascade, the products of which have highly pro-inflammatory and lytic activities.

Complement components: The proteins that comprise the complement cascade. They are designated as either C1, C2 etc or Factor B, Factor D etc.

Complement receptor: Molecules capable of binding C3 and its degradation products found on the surface of a range of cells including red cells, lymphocytes, neutrophils, monocytes and macrophages.

Constant regions (C region): The region of a molecule (e.g. antibody, TCR) usually the carboxyl terminus, the chemical structure of which is relatively invariant.

Cross-reactivity: When one epitope or antigenic determinant shares similarity with another, both may bind to the same antigen receptor but with different affinities. This is known as cross-reactivity. It is a measure of relatedness between two antigens.

Cytokines: Soluble chemicals secreted by cells, which have a range of effects on the cells which produced them or on other cells within the vicinity e.g. tumour necrosis factor, interleukin-1.

Cytotoxic T cell: See Cell-mediated cytotoxicity.

D(iversity) region: A small region associated with the variable region of the antigen binding site of both the BCR and TCR. It codes for the third hypervariable region of most receptors.

Delayed type hypersensitivity (DTH): A cell-mediated immune response that develops over 24–48 hours that results in a variable degree of tissue damage depending on the extremity of the response. Characterised by the infiltration of monocytes and macrophages into the area of the lesion.

Determinant: See Antigenic determinant.

Domain: A region found in molecules coded for by members of the immunoglobulin supergene family, which comprises approximately 110 amino acids held together in a globular-type form by disulphide bonds.

DR antigens: See Major histocompatibility complex.

Eosinophil: A polymorphonuclear leukocyte or granulocyte with distinct cytoplasmic granules that stain red with eosin. The granules contain important proteins (e.g. eosinophil basic protein), which are toxic to parasitic organisms.

Epitope: See Antigenic determinant.

Exon: The region of a gene coding for a protein or part of a protein.

Fab: (Fragment antigen binding) That part of an antibody, which contains the antigen binding site of the molecule composed of the variable regions of one light chain and one heavy chain.

F(ab)2: A fragment of antibody formed by cleavage at the hinge region (e.g. by pepsin) giving a fragment that contains both antigen binding sites of the molecules.

Fc: (Fragment crystallisable) A fragment of an antibody molecule lacking the antigen binding sites caused by papain digestion. The Fc fragment contains the constant regions of both the heavy chains from the hinge region to the carboxyl terminus of the molecules.

Fc receptors (FcRs): Molecules found on the surface of a range of cells which bind to the Fc region of antibodies. Each antibody class has its own receptor i.e. FcγR for IgG, FcεR for IgE etc.

HLA (Human leukocyte antigen) complex: Cell surface and soluble antigens coded for by the genes of the major histocompatibility complex.

Hapten: See Antigen.

Heavy chains (H chains): Pairs of molecules found in antibodies, which are larger than the other pair and dictate the class of an antibody molecule i.e. an antibody with μ (mu) heavy chains is IgM.

Helper T cells: A subpopulation of T cells, which help in the generation of effector T and B cells usually through the production of cytokines. Previously identified by the expression of cell surface molecule CD4 (although this molecule is not unique to T helper cells).

Hinge region: That area of an antibody between the first and second constant regions of the heavy chain, which confers flexibility upon the molecule. It is highly susceptible to enzymatic cleavage.

Histocompatibility: (Histo referring to cells and tissues) Refers to the degree of identity between two tissues with regard to their cell surface antigens coded for by the major histocompatibility complex genes (see MHC).

Humoral immunity: Any immune response in which antibody plays the principal or sole role.

Hybridoma: A cell and its progeny that result from the fusion of a continuously replicating (malignant) cell and an antibody-secreting cell. Hybridomas replicate indefinitely and secrete antibody without the need for stimulation by specific antigen.

Hypersensitivity: An immune response, which in one individual results in a greater degree of tissue damage than would occur normally in others. This includes allergy (type I hypersensitivity) and delayed type hypersensitivity (type IV hypersensitivity).

Hypervariable regions: This refers to sequences in proteins such as the immunoglobulins and the T cell antigen receptor which show a high degree of genetic variability and are found in the antigen binding regions of these molecules.

Idiotope: The variable region of an antibody which, when introduced into a foreign host may act as an antigen. An idiotope is a single antigenic epitope within that variable region.

Idiotype: The antigenic nature of all the idiotopes of an antibody.

Immediate-type hypersensitivity: A hypersensitivity response that occurs within minutes after exposure to antigen. This is usually a type I response involving IgE but may also be type II (IgG bound to a cellular antigen) or type III (IgG bound to soluble antigen).

Immune complex: Antigen bound to antibody. The antigen may be soluble, particulate or cell-associated.

Immunogen: An antigen capable of inducing an immune response.

Immunoglobulin (Ig): A globular protein involved in the immune response. Used interchangeably with the term antibody. Each Ig unit has at least two heavy chains, two light chains and two antigen-binding sites.

Interferon: A group of proteins, members of which have a range of anti-viral activities and variable capabilities of moderating the immune response.

Interleukins (ILs): A large group of glycoproteins secreted by a wide variety of cells, which may affect the cells that produce them or other cells in the vicinity. Often collectively referred to as cytokines.

Intron: That part of a genetic sequence that does not code for a protein.

Isotypes: Minor differences in the constant region of a particular class of antibody may lead to altered epitopes, which can stimulate the production of antibodies when it is introduced into another species. These antibodies can be used to identify the different isotypes, which may have distinct biological properties.

Isotype switch: See Class switch.

J chain (joining chain): A polypeptide that stabilises the polymeric IgA and IgM molecules.

J gene: Codes for the J or joining segment involved in the formation of the variable region in the BCR and TCR.

K cell: Killer cells bind antibody-coated target cells through their FcR and destroy them by antibody-dependent cellular cytotoxicity. K cells include some large granular lymphocytes, macrophages and some T cells.

Killer T cells: Also called cytotoxic T cells. The cell recognises antigen on the surface of a target cell through its antigen specific receptor (TCR). This and subsequent events trigger the T cell to destroy the target cell. Previously identified by the expression of CD8, it is now known that not all T cells with cytotoxic activity express this antigen.

Light chain (L chain): The smaller of the two molecules that comprise an antibody. Light chains may be either kappa or lambda.

Lymphocyte: A small cell (6–8 μm in diameter) found in the blood and in specialised lymphoid tissues. They have little cytoplasm but when activated can become enlarged (blast cells) and highly metabolically active. They are the key cells in a specific immune response having the capability to recognise antigen through their antigen-specific receptors.

Lymphokines: Soluble substances produced by lymphocytes which have a range of effects on the cells that produce them and other cells. Often also referred to as cytokines.

Macrophage: A large cell found in the tissues derived from the blood-borne monocyte. It may have a range of characteristics and functions depending upon the tissue in which it is found. It plays a key role in both the innate and specific immune responses.

Major histocompatibility complex: Genes encoding proteins expressed on cell surfaces. Class I genes code for the human leukocyte antigens (HLA) A, B and C found on all nucleated cells. Class II genes code for the HLA DP, DQ and DR expressed on antigen presenting cells. Class III genes code for molecules such as some complement components and some heat shock proteins which do not appear to truly be part of the MHC.

Mast cell: A large cell with extremely large cytoplasmic granules found particularly in the connective and mucosal tissues. The key cells in IgE-mediated allergic responses.

Memory: Exposure to an antigen usually results in the formation of memory cells, which upon subsequent exposure to the same antigen are able to respond more rapidly and (in the case of B cells) produce highly specific antibodies.

MHC class I gene products: Molecules expressed on the surface of all nucleated blood cells and platelets, which participate in the recognition of virally infected cells by CD8 positive T cells. They are also involved in graft rejection by the immune system in poorly matched donors and recipients.

MHC class II gene products: Molecules expressed on the surface of cells involved in antigen presentation to CD4 positive T cells (e.g. macrophages, dendritic cells, B cells and activated T cells).

MHC restriction: T cells can only respond to antigen presented to them in association with self-MHC antigens on antigen presenting cells.

Mitogen: A molecule or group of molecules, which stimulate the proliferation of a number of different lymphocytes, regardless of their antigen specificity. The responding cells may recognise a range of different epitopes and the response is therefore known as polyclonal.

Mixed lymphocyte response (or reaction, MLR): Lymphocyte proliferation, which occurs when lymphocytes from two different donors are mixed together *in vitro*.

Monoclonal: A response that occurs when all the responding cells are the progeny (daughter cells) of a single cell.

Monocyte: The blood borne form of the tissue macrophage. A large cell capable of phagocytosis.

Monokines: Cytokines secreted by monocytes that have an effect on a range of other cells.

NK (Natural killer) cell: A large granular lymphocyte capable of killing a limited range of tumour or virally infected cells and of a restricted type of antigen recognition.

Opsonin: A substance which enhances phagocytosis of particulate material such as bacteria by binding to surface receptors on cells. Opsonins include antibodies, complement components and acute phase proteins.

Opsonisation: The coating of a particulate antigen by an opsonin, which results in enhanced phagocytosis.

Paratope: That part of an antibody, which binds to an antigenic epitope. It is therefore complementary to the epitope.

Phagocytosis: The active formation of extrusions of the cellular membrane to enclose material within an intracellular vesicle known as a phagosome.

Phenotype: The physical expression of the genotype.

Pinocytosis: Ingestion of extracellular fluid and soluble particles by small invaginations of the cellular membrane to form a membrane bound intracellular vesicle.

Plasma cell: A terminally differentiated, antigen-stimulated B cell, which produces large quantities of antibody.

Polyclonal activator: See Mitogen.

Polymorphonuclear leukocytes: White blood cells (leukocytes) possessing nuclei with many varied shapes. They include the neutrophils, basophils and eosinophils.

Primary lymphoid tissues (organs): Tissues or organs in which lymphocytes differentiate and first acquire their antigen-specific receptors.

Primary responses: Those specific immune responses that occur upon first exposure to an antigen. They are usually characterised by the production of antigen-specific IgM. They usually have a long lag phase (before any specific antibody is detected) and result in the formation of memory cells.

Respiratory burst: An increase in metabolic activity, which is dependent upon oxygen and occurs in phagocytic cells as a result of phagocytosis or other stimuli. The resulting radicals of oxygen are highly reactive and either directly, or indirectly, microbicidal.

Reticuloendothelial cells: Now known as the mononuclear phagocyte system comprising the network of monocytes and tissue-based macrophages.

Rheumatoid factor: An antibody, (usually IgM or IgG) that reacts with the non-variable regions of self immunoglobulin (usually IgG). Found in sero-positive rheumatoid arthritis.

Secondary lymphoid organs: Organised tissues in which the interaction between antigen presenting cells and antigen-specific lymphocytes is facilitated and lymphocyte activation and differentiation occurs.

Secretory component: A protein produced by mucosal epithelial cells, which binds to dimeric IgA and facilitates its transport into the lumen of the gut.

Syngeneic: Genetically identical.

T cells: A subpopulation of lymphocytes that undergoes development and maturation within the thymus.

T cell antigen receptor (TCR): The complex of molecules on the surface of a T cell responsible for binding antigen and signalling the fact to the T cell. It comprises a bimolecular complex the $\alpha\beta$TCR or the $\gamma\delta$TCR, which binds antigen and the CD3 molecular complex, which is responsible for the intracellular signalling.

T-dependent antigen: An antigen that depends upon the activation of effector T cells for the production of cytokines required for B cell activation, proliferation and differentiation.

T-independent antigens: Antigen that can by themselves directly activate B cells leading to their proliferation and differentiation. T-independent antigens generally only stimulate an IgM response.

Tolerance: The inability (or severely reduced ability) to respond to a specific antigen. Usually caused by exposure to a non-immunising dose of antigen.

Vaccination: Also known as immunisation. Involves the stimulation of an immune response to a non-toxic, non-infectious agent that will subsequently protect the host when exposed to the toxic or infectious agent.

1

CELLS AND TISSUES OF THE IMMUNE SYSTEM

The immune system comprises a range of cells, tissues and chemicals that interact to overcome infection, repair tissue damage and maintain the integrity of the body. The immune response is affected by the food we eat, environmental, genetic, neurological and psychological influences. To understand how the immune system fights infection, you must be able to identify the cells involved and to associate the correct physical (**phenotypic**) and functional characteristics with them. These attributes (and many other aspects of the immune response) are described using specific terms that have precise meanings. So learning immunology is like learning a new language, once you have mastered the terminology and the basic structure, the rest falls into place quite easily!

The cells and tissues of the immune system provide part of the basic structure of immunology and these sections place special emphasis on introducing a number of relevant terms that you will come across again and again throughout this book. The purpose of this chapter is to introduce you to the terminology used to describe the cells involved in the immune response and to describe the physical organisation of the tissues within the body that comprise the immune system.

When you have completed a section, try the self-assessment programme that you can download from the web site. Do not try and cover too much new ground at one go!

1.1 CELLS INVOLVED IN THE IMMUNE RESPONSE

For many years, the immune response has been described as comprising the non-specific or **innate** response and the acquired or **specific** response. The innate

Immunology for Life Scientists, Second Edition. Lesley-Jane Eales.
© 2003 John Wiley & Sons, Ltd: ISBN 0 470 84523 6 (HB); 0 470 84524 4 (PB)

Table 1.1 Standard adult white blood cell count	
Cell	Number ($\times 10^{-9}$/L)
Neutrophils	2.0–7.5
Eosinophils	0.04–0.4
Basophils	<0.1
Monocytes	0.2–0.8
Lymphocytes	1.5–4.0

response occurs as a result of tissue damage caused by trauma or infections. It is a generalised response irrespective of the precipitating agent. By contrast, the specific immune response involves the precise recognition of particles that are foreign to the host's body (i.e. they are not normally present in the healthy body and are called **non-self**). These may be molecules on host cells, which have been altered in some way, or invading microorganisms. The cells involved in mediating these responses are found in the blood and in specialised tissues throughout the body (the **lymphoid tissues**). Although different types of cells tend to be associated with either the innate or specific immune response, the reality is that these responses are not discrete and some cells are key to both reactions. Thus, it is important to understand the characteristics and functions of the different cell types and how they may contribute to the immune response in general. The cells involved in immunity are the white blood cells, collectively known as **leukocytes** (Greek: leuko = white; cytes = cells). Table 1.1 introduces you to the different white blood cells by providing a summary of standard counts in the blood of a normal adult.

1.1.1 CELLULAR ORIGINS – THE PLURIPOTENT STEM CELL

The mature cells of the immune system have a limited life span and therefore must be replaced continuously by new ones that arise from immature precursor cells in the bone marrow. These multiply and the daughter cells go through a series of changes and further divisions that result in cells with particular physical, chemical and functional characteristics, which are typical of the mature cells found in the blood or tissues. This process of arriving at the mature cell phenotype is known as **differentiation**.

The immature precursor cells themselves develop from **progenitor cells** that are thought to have a common origin – the pluripotent or common haemopoietic **stem cell** – found in the bone marrow. These cells are able to renew themselves by proliferation and are able to differentiate into progenitor cells. Thus, the process of blood cell production – **haematopoiesis** – comprises a complex sequence of events (including cell proliferation, differentiation and

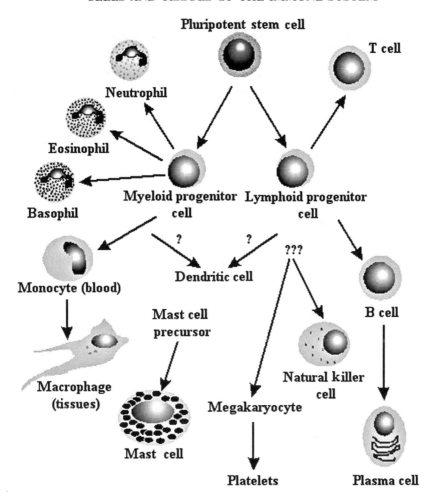

Figure 1.1 Representation of the developmental lineage of immunologically active cells

The figure shows the development of immune cells from the pluripotent stem cell in the bone marrow. Dendritic cells have been shown to derive from myeloid- or lymphoid-like cells (indicated by the question marks) but it is unclear at what precise stage this differentiation takes place. Other cells are known to derive from the bone marrow but their precise route of differentiation is unclear.

maturation) controlled by a variety of soluble secreted factors (known as **cytokines** or **lymphokines**) and hormones. The developmental lineage of those cells described in this chapter is shown in Figure 1.1.

Cytokines are "cellular hormones". They are peptides, which are produced by cells and act locally.

1.1.2 CELLS PRINCIPALLY INVOLVED IN THE INNATE IMMUNE RESPONSE

POLYMORPHONUCLEAR LEUKOCYTES

The polymorphonuclear leukocytes (PMNs) are a group of cells that have two major features in common; their nuclei demonstrate a wide range (**poly**) of different shapes (**morpho**) and they all have distinct granules in their cytoplasm. The presence of these granules has led to their being known as **granulocytes**, although this is slightly confusing since some other cells also have granules in their cytoplasm. To be a granulocyte, a cell must have both granules and the typical lobulate nucleus.

The polymorphs derive from the **myeloid progenitor cell**, which is found in the bone marrow. This cell goes through a series of replication and differentiation processes giving rise to differentiated daughter cells with distinct characteristics. This process is regulated by cytokines, particular cytokines favouring the production of neutrophils, eosinophils, basophils or mast cells. A summary of the characteristics of these cells is shown in Table 1.2.

NEUTROPHILS

Normally, 60–70% of white blood cells are granulocytes and about 90% of these are neutrophils, which provide protection from a variety of micro-organisms and are arguably the most important white blood cells in eliminating **non-viral** infections. They are relatively large cells (about 10–20 μm in diameter) and despite their important function, are relatively short-lived (about 2–3 days).

Neutrophils are the most common white blood cell. The primary function of these cells is to remove microorganisms by a process known as **phagocytosis** (a phenomenon which may be compared to the uptake of particulate matter by an amoeba).

Table 1.2   Summary of the characteristics of the polymorphonuclear leukocytes

Name	Characteristics
Polymorphonuclear leukocytes (also known as granulocytes)	Irregularly shaped nuclei; granular cytoplasm
Neutrophils	Pale blue staining, granular cytoplasm; actively phagocytic
Eosinophils	Granular cytoplasm stains red with eosin; slightly phagocytic but most important role is in allergy and resistance to parasitic infections
Basophils	Large, dark blue staining granules; blood borne; important in allergy; granules contain chemicals which have dramatic effects on muscles and blood vessels
Mast cells	Similar staining to basophils only larger granules, usually not seen in blood, only tissues

.The granular appearance of polymorphs is due to their cytoplasmic inclusions. At least four types of granules have been identified in neutrophils that emerge at different stages of the cell's development. These are the primary (azurophilic) granules (**lysosomes**), which contain acid hydrolases, myeloperoxidase and lysozyme; secondary (specific) granules, which contain lactoferrin and lysozyme but lack myeloperoxidase; tertiary granules that contain gelatinase; and secretory vesicles, which act as intracellular stores of molecules usually found anchored in the cell membrane where they act as receptors for other molecules.

Neutrophils are produced in the bone marrow whence mature cells pass into the circulation. In the major vessels these cells are in constant flow. However, in the capillary beds these cells become temporarily stationary (owing to their lack of deformability), without being attached to the **endothelial cells** that line the blood vessels. When there is local tissue damage as a result of trauma or infection, neutrophils become activated and emigrate from the capillaries and post-capillary venules into the tissues in response to gradients of particular chemicals known as **chemotaxins** and **chemokines** (chemotactic cytokines). This **directed migration** is known as **chemotaxis**. During this process, the cells may discharge the contents of their granules (**degranulation**). This may affect nearby cells or extracellular bacteria and may increase cell membrane-associated events (such as chemotaxis and the **respiratory burst**) by increased expression of particular membrane proteins. This whole process is described in detail in the section on innate immunity.

> *The respiratory burst is an ATP-dependent chemical reaction, which consumes oxygen and results in the production of highly reactive chemicals (e.g. reactive oxygen and nitrogen species) that are capable of destroying microorganisms.*

EOSINOPHILS

Eosinophils, like neutrophils, are produced in the bone marrow, which retains a reserve of mature cells. The majority of eosinophils are found in the tissues of the body and comprise only 4% of the white cells in the blood. Their life span is about 13 days and they are about 8 μm in diameter. Differentiation of precursors in the bone marrow is influenced by the cytokines **interleukin 3** (IL-3) and **granulocyte–monocyte colony-stimulating factor (GM-CSF)**. In addition, **interleukin 5** (IL-5) specifically promotes the expansion of eosinophil (and basophil) numbers. The release of mature eosinophils from the bone marrow reserves is promoted by both IL-5 and the chemokine known as **eotaxin**.

In early development, their nuclei are bilobed but with maturation, they can become multilobed like other polymorphs. Like neutrophils, they contain intracellular granules, although those in eosinophils are quite distinct. The primary granules contain Charcot–Leiden crystal protein and the characteristic secondary granules contain a crystalline core of **major basic protein** (**MBP**) and a matrix of **eosinophil cationic protein** (**ECP**), **eosinophil-derived neurotoxin** (**EDN**) and **eosinophil peroxidase** (**EPO**). The cells also contain lipid bodies that are the site of lipid mediator synthesis. The major basic protein is highly toxic to multicellular parasites. Although eosinophils are able to phagocytose, it is not their main function and these organisms are too large. Thus, the membranes surrounding the eosinophil granules fuse with the cell membrane and the contents are released outside the eosinophil. The toxic granule proteins help to destroy and eliminate the parasites. This process is dependent upon adhesion of the eosinophil to the parasite. This attachment is mediated via molecules on the surface of the eosinophil called *β*-integrins.

> *β-Integrins are adhesion molecules that are found on the surface of many cells and whose expression can be increased or decreased by local chemical influences such as cytokines.*

In addition to their anti-parasitic activity, eosinophils participate in a number of other immunological reactions, including allergy. They are able to produce a range of cytokines (e.g. IL-2, interferon gamma (IFNγ), IL-4, IL-5 and IL-10) that may enhance or decrease their own function (**autocrine action**) or that of a range of other cells (**paracrine action**). Additionally, eosinophils synthesise **prostaglandins** and **leukotrienes** from lipids found in the cell membrane. These molecules stimulate a process known as **inflammation**. Activation of eosinophils is dependent upon adhesion but also on electrical charge. Negatively charged molecules such as heparin, mucins and sialic acid may decrease activation, whilst it may be increased by positively charged molecules such as the basic granule protein.

> *Inflammation is a complex series of cellular and biochemical reactions that occur in response to tissue damage.*

BASOPHILS AND MAST CELLS

Both mast cells and basophils originate from haematopoietic stem cells in the bone marrow. Their progenitor cells are expanded in number through the influence of IL-3. Although these cells share many characteristics, their differentiation pathways are quite distinct (Figure 1.2). Basophils complete their differentiation in the bone marrow under the influence of IL-3 and the cytokine **transforming growth factor β** (TGFβ). Then they enter the circulation where they comprise <0.2% of white blood cells. Mast cell differentiation is due to the presence of **stem cell factor** (SCF; the ligand for **Kit**, a product of the c-kit proto-oncogene). They leave the bone marrow as precursors and after migrating to the tissues, proliferate and differentiate into mature mast cells.

Like other granulocytes, the nucleus of the circulating basophil is deeply lobed. However, those of mast cells in the tissues are rounded. As mentioned earlier, basophils are largely found in the circulation but enter the tissues in response to the release of chemotaxins and chemokines during inflammation.

Both cell types play a role in allergic reactions, inflammation, host responses to parasites and cancers, blood vessel generation (**angiogenesis**) and tissue remodelling. They are the only cells on whose membranes large amounts of a high-affinity receptor for a molecule known as immunoglobulin E (IgE) are expressed naturally (**constitutively**), and that store histamine in their secretory granules. These molecules play an important role in allergic and inflammatory responses respectively.

There are two main types of mast cell distinguished by the contents of their intracellular granules. Those with tryptase, chymase, carboxypeptidase and cathepsin are called MC_{TC} and are found largely in the normal skin and submucosa of the small bowel. Those with only tryptase are referred to as MC_T cells and are found in the normal airway. In addition, mast cells in different tissues may exhibit different activities in response to stimulators other than IgE. Mast cells have been shown to have different types of chemokine receptors on their surface. Since the binding of chemokines to these receptors stimulates mast cell migration into the tissues, this may explain how different types of mast cell are recruited to different tissue sites.

Activation of basophils and mast cells may be due to the cross-linking of IgE bound to the IgE receptors on their surface (IgεR; Figure 1.3). In addition, molecules produced as a result of inflammation such as C3a and C5a, eosinophil-derived major basic protein and neuropeptides may activate some mast cells and basophils.

Once activated, both basophils and mast cells release a variety of substances that can enhance inflammation and influence other cells. These can be divided into those preformed mediators stored in the secretory granules and those that are freshly generated upon activation. The former include histamine, proteoglycans and proteases; the latter include arachidonic acid metabolites, cytokines and chemokines (Table 1.3).

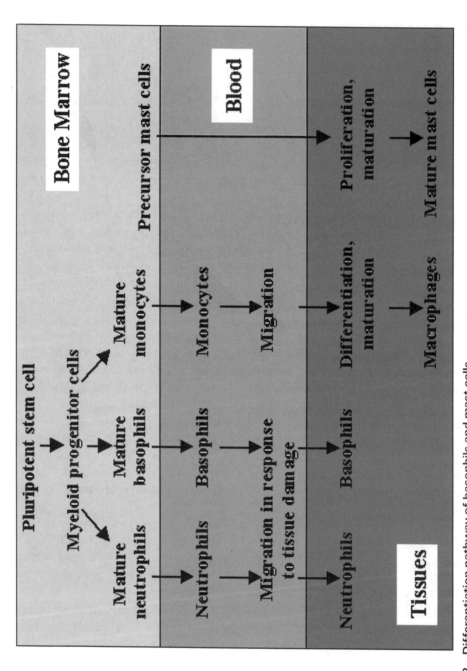

Figure 1.2   Differentiation pathway of basophils and mast cells
Basophils leave the bone marrow as mature cells whilst mast cells leave as precursors. After migrating to the tissues, precursor mast cells proliferate, and differentiate into either mucosa-associated mast cells (MMC) or connective tissue mast cells (CTMC).

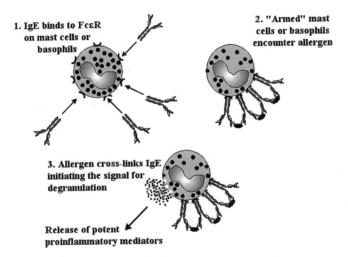

Figure 1.3 Involvement of mast cells and basophils in antibody-mediated response to allergen
Antibody (IgE) binds to specific receptors on mast cells and basophils. When cross-linked by allergen, this causes the degranulation of the cells releasing proinflammatory mediators.

Table 1.3 Secretory products of activated mast cells and basophils

Mediators	Cells
⩽5 minutes	
Histamine, tryptase	MC and basophils
Heparin, tissue plasminogen activator (tPA), fibroblast growth factor (bFGF)	MC
Chymase, carboxypeptidase, cathepsin G	MC_{TC} only
Basogranin	Basophils only
1–30 minutes	
Leukotriene C_4 (LTC_4)	MC and basophils
Prostaglandin D_2 (PGD_2)	MC
Minutes to hours	
IL-5, 6, 8, 16, TNFα, monocyte chemotactic protein-1 (MCP-1), monocyte inhibitory protein 1α (MIP-1α)	MC
IL-4, 13	MC and basophils

MEGAKARYOCYTES AND PLATELETS

Megakaryocytic progenitor cells are derived from haematopoietic stem cells. They undergo **endomitosis** (producing multiple copies of DNA within the cell) and differentiate into megakaryocytes. Thus, mature **megakaryocytes** are large, **polyploid cells** with distinct, folded membranes. A pool is maintained in the bone marrow to replenish stocks in the blood when required. This may be controlled by the lymphokine interleukin 3 (IL-3), a potent stimulator of megakaryocyte progenitor cells. Megakaryocytes give rise to platelets by a process that appears to involve cytoplasmic fragmentation of the cell. Platelet production depends on the number and size of megakaryocytes in the marrow and is stimulated by **thrombopoietin**.

Platelets have a **cytoskeleton**, a meshwork of proteinaceous fibrils, which maintains cell shape and acts as an intracellular scaffold upon which cellular reactions may take place. The cells are contractile and capable of adherence to other cells and surfaces. Upon stimulation by exposed collagen, they become activated, contract and produce finger-like projections of cytoplasm (**pseudopodia**). They express new proteins on their surface encouraging them to aggregate together (via inter-receptor fibrinogen bridges) and bind to von Willebrand factor expressed on the damaged lining (endothelium) of the blood vessels. When activated, the platelets contract releasing their granules. A major constituent of platelet alpha granules is **thrombospondin**, which plays an important role in blood coagulation. Also, **platelet-derived endothelial cell growth factor (PD-ECGF)** stimulates the growth and chemotaxis of endothelial cells *in vitro* and angiogenesis *in vivo*.

1.1.3 ANTIGEN PRESENTING CELLS AND LARGE GRANULAR LYMPHOCYTES

Antigen presenting cells and large granular lymphocytes are collections of distinct cell types, which play a role in both the non-specific and the specific immune responses. Antigen presenting cells include **monocytes** (and their tissue-based derivatives **macrophages**) and dendritic cells.

MONOCYTES AND MACROPHAGES

Monocytes derive from the myeloid progenitor cell in the bone marrow. They circulate in the blood for 1–2 days and migrate to the tissues where they differentiate into macrophages. The functional and phenotypic characteristics of the cells depend upon the tissue in which they reside, e.g. **Kupffer cells** of the liver and **microglia** of the brain are resident macrophages (Table 1.4).

This network of related cells is the **mononuclear phagocyte system** (MPS) and includes those cells in the early developmental stages (**monoblasts and promonocytes**), as well as **monocytes** and **macrophages**. Macrophages may be categorised according to their stage of development and their state of activation (Table 1.5).

Like neutrophils, monocytes and macrophages are capable of phagocytosis and have lysosomes that contain acid hydrolases and peroxidase, which are important in killing microorganisms. Although these cells have small cytoplasmic granules (lysosomes), they have regular, kidney-shaped nuclei and therefore are not granulocytes.

Table 1.4 Examples of tissue macrophages and their characteristics

Type	Source	Characteristics
Alveolar macrophage (M0)	Lung	Biochemically and functionally distinct subpopulations; life span approximately 3 months; may be self-replicating
Kupffer cells	Liver	Subpopulations based on distinct endocytic and lysosomal enzyme activity
Splenic M0	Spleen	Subpopulations based on distinct surface antigen expression distributed in defined areas of the spleen; differences may reflect different functional activity
Microglial cells	Brain	Unknown function, CD4 positive

Table 1.5 Characterisation of macrophages

Type	Description
Resident M0	Present in specific sites in normal, non-inflamed tissues
Exudate M0	Derived from monocytes with which they share many characteristics. Identifiable by peroxidase activity; thought to be precursors of resident macrophages
Elicited M0	Blood monocytes recently migrated to the tissues that are attracted to a particular tissue site by chemotactic/inflammatory stimuli. They have a range of characteristics and functions
Activated M0	Both resident and elicited M0 may become activated by appropriate signals (such as the cytokine interferon gamma). Such cells exhibit increased or new functional activities

In addition to their ability to phagocytose and kill microorganisms, MPs secrete a vast range of chemicals involved in inflammation, blood clotting and tissue remodelling. They also play an important role in stimulating immune responses to specific foreign molecules, a function known as **antigen presentation**. *In vitro*, monocytes from blood will stick to glass or plastic and can be identified by the expression of molecules known as CD14 and CD15.

DENDRITIC CELLS

Dendritic cells are irregularly shaped and actively extrude and retract thread-like "fingers" of cytoplasm and surrounding cell membrane. They are found in most tissues of the body but their stage of maturation may vary with their location. These specialised cells, like macrophages, play a critical role in initiating specific immune responses particularly to novel agents to which the body has not been previously exposed. Cells resembling dendritic cells have been found in the fluid that drains from the tissues – the **lymph**. These **veiled cells** may be derived from tissue-based dendritic cells such as **Langerhans cells** of the skin.

Dendritic cells in the tissues may be of two types, myeloid (DC1) or lymphoid (DC2). DC1 typically have high levels of receptors in their cell membrane that are involved in innate immunity and are important in binding potentially toxic products of bacteria. These immature cells are capable of taking up bacteria and their products, a process that stimulates their migration from the tissues into the blood. Maturing DCs then travel to particular areas of organised tissues known as **lymphoid tissues**. During this process, the DCs lose their ability to capture molecules but show increased ability to stimulate the specific immune response.

LARGE GRANULAR LYMPHOCYTES

Large granular lymphocytes (LGLs) are a collection of different subpopulations of cells that play a role that borders between innate and specific immunity. Generally, they are relatively large, round cells with a good deal of cytoplasm and a large, round, regular nucleus. Their cytoplasm is distinctly granular, but the granules are smaller than those found in the cells described above as granulocytes. These cells comprise approximately 4% of white blood cells and have distinct proteins exposed on their cell membranes that allow us to distinguish them from other cells and from each other.

Natural killer (NK) cells can kill certain tumour cells and some virally infected cells. They show some selectivity in their actions, being able to bind to and kill a limited range of cells (their **target cells**). This recognition is dependent on the presence of certain molecules on the target cell. These molecules are the products of a group of genes known as the **major histocompatibility complex** (MHC). There are different classes of MHC genes and NK cells "expect" to see certain products of the class I genes on the target cell surface. If this molecule is not present (or is present at too low a concentration for recognition), the NK cell will destroy the target cell through the action of molecules known as perforins and granzymes.

Killer (K) cells have molecules on their surface that act as receptors (**Fc receptors**) for a molecule known as immunoglobulin G (IgG) that can specifically recognise foreign particles in the host.

The immunoglobulin molecule consists of three major functional regions called the $F(ab)_2$ region, the hinge region and the Fc region. The $F(ab)_2$ region (Fragment antigen binding) contains the binding sites for foreign particles (or antigens), the Fc region (Fragment crystallisable) confers the biological properties of the molecule and the hinge region is where the other two meet and confers flexibility on the molecule.

Using these Fc receptors, K cells are able to bind to, and kill, cells that have immunoglobulin attached to them via their antigen-binding regions. Thus, if a

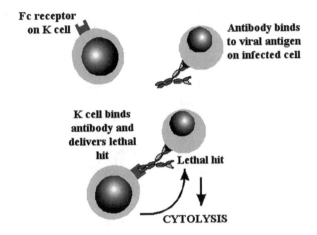

Figure 1.4 Antibody-dependent cellular cytotoxicity
In a virally infected cell, some of the viral proteins are expressed on the cell membrane allowing virus-specific antibodies to bind to them. A killer cell can attach to this antibody using its Fc receptor and is thereby activated and kills the virally infected target cell. This activity is known as antibody-dependent cellular cytotoxicity (ADCC).

cell is infected with a virus and some of the viral proteins are present in the cell membrane, antibodies formed against them will bind to the viral antigens on the surface of the cell. A killer cell can bind to this antibody, is thereby activated, and kills the virally infected (target) cell (Figure 1.4). This activity is known as **antibody-dependent cellular cytotoxicity (ADCC)** and may be performed by other cells as well.

1.1.4 CELLS INVOLVED IN THE SPECIFIC IMMUNE RESPONSE

Most of us are aware that the immune system works by recognising unusual molecules that are not usually found in the body (i.e. they are **non-self**). These chemicals may be complex (in the form of microorganisms) or simple (such as minor changes in molecules usually present in the body – **altered-self**). This ability to discriminate **between** what are sometimes very small differences in chemical structure is a property of the **specific** or **adaptive immune response** and is dependent upon the activity of a particular group of cells, the **lymphocytes**.

LYMPHOCYTES

Lymphocytes comprise about 20% of the peripheral white blood cells and derive from the common lymphoid progenitor cell in the bone marrow. They are about 6–10 μm in diameter and have a large, almost spherical nucleus surrounded by a very small, indistinct halo of cytoplasm. The prominence of this regular nucleus has led to them being referred to as **mononuclear leukocytes** (MNL). Their most important characteristic is their ability to specifically recognise foreign (**non-self**) molecules such as microorganisms, a feature not possessed by any other cell. This means the function of any lymphocyte stimulated by a foreign molecule, or **antigen**, is directed solely at that antigen and usually no other. Upon stimulation, some lymphocytes become **effector cells** performing functions designed to eliminate the antigen whilst others form long-lived **memory cells** that may persist for years and allow a more rapid response upon subsequent exposure to the antigen.

There are two major populations of lymphocytes – **T cells** and **B cells**. Although they are derived from a common progenitor in the bone marrow, they are "conditioned" or "educated" by the **Thymus** or the **Bone marrow** (respectively) before they become functionally active.

 Go to the web site to learn more about the early experiments performed to identify lymphocytes

These lymphocyte populations may be distinguished by the molecules they express on their surface membrane and by the substances they secrete. T (and other) cells produce **lymphokines**. By contrast, only B cells produce **antibodies**. These are **globular proteins – immunoglobulins (Ig)** – that are designed to recognise and bind to specific molecules or groups of molecules – **antigens**.

> *Many molecules in the immune system interact with other molecules known as receptors. This ligand–receptor interaction is often likened to the interaction between a lock and key. The key for any particular lock is shaped intricately so that it fits that one lock and no other. However, master keys may fit many different locks because they share the important common features with the different keys that allow the lock to be opened. Many cellular receptors may be considered to be like locks including the antibody molecules mentioned above. They recognise a single molecule – a particular antigen – a specific key. However, a different antigen may have the capacity to bind that antibody molecule – a cross-reacting antigen – because it acts like a master key and has the important features of the original antigen.*

T and B cell populations are distinguished by the presence or absence of particular molecules found in their cell membranes (Table 1.6).

> *All membranes are fluid lipid bilayers that have proteins inserted in them. These proteins may be distinct and have particular functions. They may act as a relay system, telling the inside of the cell about what is around outside. This may be done by the proteins reacting with particular elements in the extracellular medium, i.e. they act as receptors for these elements.*

Table 1.6   Characteristics that distinguish T from B lymphocytes

Characteristic	T cells	B cells
Cell type	Mononuclear leukocyte/lymphocyte	Mononuclear leukocyte/lymphocyte
Membrane molecules that allow binding of antigen – the antigen receptor	T cell antigen receptor (TCR)/CD3	Immunoglobulin/CD79a/b B cell antigen receptor (BCR)
Characteristic surface membrane molecules	CD3, CD4 or CD8	Membrane immunoglobulins (mIg), CD19, CD20, CD40
Chief secretory products	Lymphokines	Antibodies

Each population can be divided further into **subpopulations** based on the presence of particular receptors on the cell surface. These appear to distinguish groups of cells that are at certain stages of development or activation or those that have specific functions. These receptors or markers are classified using an internationally recognised system known as the **CD (cluster determinant) system** such that molecules are identified as CD1, CD2, etc.

T CELLS

Originally, human T cells were identified by their ability to bind to **sheep red blood cells** (SRBC); now known to be due to the presence of the **CD2** molecule on the T cell surface which acts as a receptor for certain molecules on the surface of the SRBC.

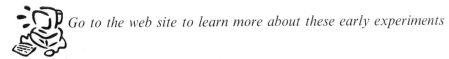 *Go to the web site to learn more about these early experiments*

Later on, another group of membrane-anchored molecules was identified that comprises the polypeptide **CD3 complex**. These molecules associate on the cell surface with the **T cell antigen receptor** (**TCR**), a group of molecules used by T cells to recognise and interact with an antigen in the form of a short string of amino acids. Since the TCR is not expressed on T cells without the CD3 complex, the latter is now used to identify T cells. Furthermore, T cells are subdivided according to the presence or absence of other surface molecules. Thus, in the blood, some T cells express the **CD4** molecule whilst a distinct set express the **CD8** molecule. Previously, these molecules were thought to define functionally distinct subsets of T cells. **CD4+** T cells were known as **helper cells** (e.g. they helped **B cells** to produce **antibody**) and **CD8+** T cells as **cytotoxic cells** (they were capable of **killing** certain cells). This division is becoming less obvious since **some CD4+ cells** may have **cytotoxic** activity.

Naïve cells which have not encountered antigen are referred to as T precursor or type 0 cells. Upon engagement of their antigen receptors, these cells secrete the cytokine IL-2. Other local cells may also be stimulated to release cytokines and these will influence the further development of the T cells. The presence of IL-18 and IL-12 will lead to the development of **type 1** effector or memory cells. The effector cells will secrete cytokines (most importantly interferon gamma – IFNγ – and tumour necrosis factor – TNF) that stimulate a range of cells leading to **cell-mediated immunity** (CMI). Conversely, the presence of IL-10 will lead to the development of **type 2** effector and memory cells. The effector cells secrete IL-4, IL-5, IL-6 and IL-13 which influence the **humoral immune response** and affect the class of antibody produced in response to the antigen (Figure 1.5). Both T helper and T cytotoxic cells develop these different cytokine secretion profiles.

B CELLS

Pre-B cells derive from the common lymphoid progenitor. They are large and have constituents of immunoglobulins in their cytoplasm. They

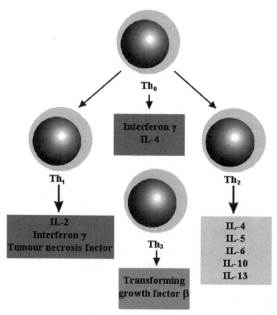

Figure 1.5   Th subpopulations and the cytokines they produce
T helper cells may be classified according to the type of lymphokines they produce. These subsets have been designated Th$_0$ (or T$_p$), Th$_1$, Th$_2$ and Th$_3$ (or T$_{reg}$) cells. The Th$_0$ cells are naïve T cells that produce cytokines typical of both Th$_1$ and Th$_2$ cells. In general, Th$_1$ cells produce lymphokines that stimulate macrophages and cytotoxic T cells whilst Th$_2$ cells produce lymphokines that stimulate B cells to proliferate and produce antibody. In contrast, Th$_3$ cells produce cytokines that are involved in the regulation or "switching off" of the immune response.

differentiate into immature and then mature B cells, which have immuno-globulin and other molecules (e.g. CD19, 20, 23, 24, 35 and 40) inserted in their membranes.

B cells comprise about 5–15% of circulating lymphocytes. A distinguishing feature of B cells is the expression of immunoglobulin on their surface (**mIg**), which acts as the **antigen receptor** for the cell. Like the TCR, the B cell antigen receptor (**BCR**) consists of more than one group of molecules. In addition to mIg, the BCR comprises a duplex of molecules known as CD79a/b (formerly Igα and Igβ) that have a single extracellular region and a cytoplasmic tail. The detailed structures of both the T and B cell antigen receptors are described in Section 2.4.

After exposure to an antigen (antigenic stimulation or challenge), B cells proliferate and differentiate either into **plasma cells** or small, resting cells, which are able to respond next time the same antigen is encountered (**memory cells**). Plasma cells secrete antibody molecules that have the same antigen specificity as the immunoglobulin found on the membrane of the parent cell. However, they lack the membrane anchoring region and cytoplasmic tail.

The genetic code for the antigen-binding region is highly variable, allowing each B cell to produce molecules that recognise only a single, distinct antigen. The **progeny** of a B cell (the new cells produced when a B cell divides) all have the same code for immunoglobulin and so recognise the same antigen as the parent cell (i.e. have the same **antigenic specificity**). However, owing to different influences during B cell division (**mitosis**), the variable sequence of the immunoglobulin produced by the daughter cells (which binds to the antigen) may be slightly different to that of the parent cell. Usually, this does not alter which antigen the antibody recognises (**antigen specificity**), but may alter the strength of attraction between the antibody and its antigen.

The fact that the progeny of a single B cell all produce antibody of the same specificity was exploited in the 1960s to produce a tool, which is widely used in many different scientific disciplines. B cells, which had been stimulated by antigen, were mixed with tumour cells derived from B cells that grow indefinitely but do not produce antibody. By using a chemical to fuse the different cells, the resulting product was a B cell that grew indefinitely and produced antibody of the same specificity as the original B cell. This meant an endless supply of highly specific, **monoclonal** (i.e. derived from a single cell and its daughters) antibody could be produced to virtually any antigen. Such **monoclonal antibodies** have allowed us to identify molecules on the surface of cells (**CD molecules**), to quantify both antibody and antigen, and are used in numerous immunological techniques.

 You can learn more about monoclonal antibodies from the web site

B cells comprise at least two main subpopulations designated B-1 and B-2. B-1 cells include B cells that express the CD5 molecule (CD5+). These cells appear to produce antibodies with poor specificity (i.e. they can recognise more than one antigen), which react with bacterial polysaccharides and lipopolysaccharides. These cells do not appear to require help from T cells in their responses to antigens but may be influenced by the cytokines produced by T cells. By contrast, B-2 cells include the majority of circulating B cells (65–89%) and are dependent upon help from T cells for their activity.

KEY POINTS FOR REVIEW

- *Polymorphonuclear leukocytes are white blood cells with granular cytoplasm and deeply lobed nuclei. They include the neutrophils, eosinophils and basophils.*
- *Neutrophils are the most numerous white blood cells in the circulation and are vital in combating non-viral infections.*
- *Eosinophils play key roles in the inflammatory allergic response and in combating parasitic infections.*
- *Basophils and mast cells are responsible for the adverse signs and symptoms of allergy. They secrete a wide range of chemical mediators, which have diverse effects on a range of cells.*
- *Antigen presenting cells play a role both in innate and specific immune responses. They include dendritic cells and monocyte-derived macrophages.*
- *Natural killer cells are part of the innate immune response but are capable of recognising certain molecules – the MHC antigens – allowing them selectivity in killing target cells. They are responsible for the elimination of certain tumour or virally infected cells.*
- *Lymphocytes are the active arm of the specific immune response. They have receptors that bind antigen (the BCR or TCR) and their activities are influenced by cytokines.*
- *B cells produce antibodies or differentiate into long-lived memory cells in response to antigen challenge.*
- *When stimulated by antigen, T cells produce cytokines, develop effector functions (cytotoxicity), or differentiate into memory cells.*
- *Both T cells and B cells comprise a number of subpopulations that are identified by their surface molecules (CD molecules) or their functional activity.*

1.2 LYMPHOID TISSUES

Although lymphocytes are found circulating in the blood, a large proportion of them are found either in discrete clusters or organised in specific tissues. This distribution increases the chance of an antigen meeting a cell that bears a receptor capable of binding it. The components of this lymphoid system may be categorised as primary, secondary or tertiary lymphoid tissue.

> *Imagine arranging to meet a friend in a busy shopping mall. If you did not state a precise meeting point the likelihood of the two of you meeting amongst the crowd would be very remote. However, arranging to meet at a particular place would ensure that you would do so, provided you waited long enough for your friend to arrive. This is the logic behind the organisation of lymphoid tissue. Antigen-specific cells are located in a tissue through which any foreign molecules will eventually drain, thus increasing the likelihood of the cells meeting their specific antigen.*

1.2.1   PRIMARY LYMPHOID TISSUES

Primary lymphoid tissues are involved in the development and differentiation of lymphocytes and include the thymus (T lymphocytes) and the "bursa equivalent" tissues, which are the foetal liver and the adult bone marrow (in man). They are responsible for the production of mature, **virgin**, lymphocytes, i.e. those that have not yet been exposed to antigen.

> *Glick, Chang and Joap (1963) performed a series of experiments using newborn chicks. In some birds they removed a small organ near the cloaca (equivalent of the mammalian anus) called the bursa. When challenged with antigen, these chicks were unable to produce specific antibody, which led the authors to conclude that in chickens, B cells develop in the bursa of Fabricius.*

THE THYMUS

During development, the thymus is the first organ to produce lymphocytes and provides an environment for T cell maturation. It has two lobes divided by **trabeculae** (or connective tissue "walls") into **lobules**, each of which has an outer **cortex** and an inner **medulla**. **Epithelial cells**, and other supporting cells (including **interdigitating reticular cells** and macrophages), surround the thymic lymphocytes. In the cortex, these cells include the **thymic nurse cells**, which are thought to influence the development of thymocytes. In the medulla, and at the junction between the cortex and medulla where most blood vessels are situated, there are interdigitating cells, which are derived from the bone marrow and are a type of dendritic cell. The characteristic **Hassal's corpuscles** found within the medulla of the thymus are concentric agglomerations of epithelial cells.

The epithelial cells of the thymus produce a number of hormones, which are required for the differentiation of thymic precursors into mature cells. **Thymocytes** (immature, pre-T cells) are attracted to the thymus from the bone marrow by these hormones. They differentiate into mature T cells as they pass from the cortex to the medulla whence they are released to populate the peripheral lymphoid tissue (Figure 1.6).

Approximately three-quarters of all the lymphocytes in the thymus are located in the deeper cortex. These cells express CD1 and both CD4 and CD8 (T cells in the blood express either CD4 or CD8). Cells, which express antigen receptors that readily recognise molecules usually present in the body (self-antigens) in association with products of the MHC, are induced to die by a process called **apoptosis** (non-necrotic cell death which prevents the release of intracellular molecules). If such self-reactive cells were released to the periphery, they might cause damage to normal body cells (**autoimmune T cells**). Indeed, the majority of cells produced in the thymus die there.

As the cells pass into the medulla, they lose either CD4 or CD8 expression reflecting genetic rearrangement. These naïve, mature T cells then pass into the peripheral circulation.

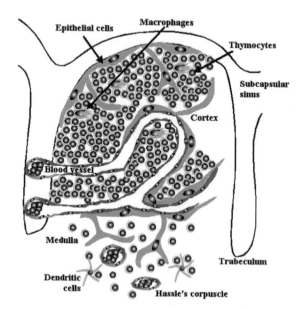

Figure 1.6 The thymus
The thymus comprises an outer cortex and inner medulla. Naïve cells enter the thymus from the bone marrow through the subcapsular sinus. They migrate through the cortex and medulla where they undergo a process of selection. Those cells that do not strongly recognise self-antigens undergo differentiation, express CD3 and either CD4 or CD8 and leave the thymus as mature T cells.

MAMMALIAN "BURSA EQUIVALENTS"

The **bursa of Fabricius** in birds is a lymphoepithelial organ located near the cloaca. Birds which have this organ removed are not able to mount a normal antibody response when stimulated with an antigen. Thus, the bursa is a primary lymphoid tissue concerned with the development and differentiation of B cells. In mammals, those tissues that most closely resemble the bursa include the **gut-associated lymphoid tissues** (GALT; including the **appendix** and **Peyer's patches**), the **foetal liver** and, following birth, the **bone marrow**.

B CELL DEVELOPMENT IN THE BONE MARROW

All lymphocytes develop initially from haemopoietic stem cells in the bone marrow. Unlike precursor T cells, which migrate to the thymus for further development, immature B cells remain in the bone marrow and develop into mature cells under local influences.

The immature B cells interact with the bone marrow stromal cells that provide signals for the precursor cells to undergo a number of defined developmental steps. These processes are influenced by a series of cell surface ligands and cytokines (particularly IL-7).

1.2.2 SECONDARY LYMPHOID TISSUES

Secondary lymphoid tissues are designed to allow the accumulation and presentation of antigen to both virgin and memory lymphocyte populations.

The lymphoid tissues are further subdivided into discrete microenvironments, each characterised by a distinct complement of lymphocyte subsets and **stromal cells** (non-specialised cells which form the "skeleton" of the tissue or organ). This distribution arises as a result of **lymphocyte homing**; a phenomenon whereby lymphocytes seek out and localise to specific microenvironments in response to a number of molecular signals. These homing mechanisms play a vital role in the distribution of naïve and memory lymphocytes that are required for effective **immune surveillance**.

THE LYMPHATIC SYSTEM

Within the body, there are two circulatory systems, the blood and the lymph. Blood flows around the body through a complex of arteries, veins and capillaries. Components of the blood that leave the vessels and enter the tissues comprise the extracellular fluid. This fluid returns to the blood by draining into a network of vessels called **lymphatics**. At the junction between major lymphatic vessels are small, bean-shaped, discrete aggregates of tissue called **lymph nodes**. Several vessels may bring the lymph to a particular node (afferent lymphatics) and usually a single vessel (the efferent lymphatic) carries it away. The lymph carries antigen from the tissues to the lymph nodes where immune responses are initiated.

Lymphocytes can enter the lymphatic circulation directly from the blood to which they return via the **thoracic duct** – a lymphatic vessel draining into the circulation close to the heart. This traffic of lymphocytes is known as **recirculation** (Figure 1.7) and occurs at specialised sites called **high endothelial venules** (HEV) found particularly in lymph nodes and the Peyer's patches (collections of lymphoid tissue in the gut). HEV are blood vessels in which the endothelial cells that line them have a high columnar structure, which is distinct to that in other areas. However, the presence of HEV and even lymph nodes is not essential for lymphocyte recirculation.

Leukocytes have special membrane molecules called homing receptors, which allow them to bind to particular HEV and other endothelia. As a result, lymphocytes adhere to the walls of vessels in a process called **margination** and then pass between the cells of the blood vessels in a process called **diapedesis** into the surrounding tissues, from whence they return via the lymph back to the blood.

The movement or **traffic** of cells through the body to certain areas in response to specific stimuli is called **migration**. However, when splenic T cells are reinjected into the blood, a large number of the cells return to this organ rather

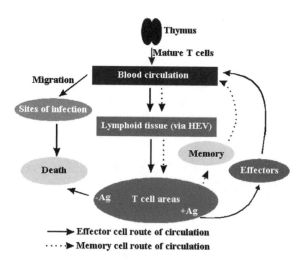

Figure 1.7   Lymphocyte recirculation
Lymphocytes can enter the lymphatic circulation directly from the blood to which they return via the thoracic duct. This traffic of lymphocytes is known as recirculation and occurs at specialised sites called high endothelial venules. Leukocytes have molecules on their membranes called homing receptors which allow them to bind to the walls of blood vessels at certain sites and pass into the tissues whence they return, via the lymph, back to the blood.

than to other sites. This non-stimulated, directed migration of cells to particular tissue sites is called **homing**.

LYMPH NODES

The lymph nodes are bean-shaped structures usually found at the junction between major lymphatic vessels. They range between 1 and 25 mm in diameter but become much larger during an infection. A normal, resting lymph node has three main areas, the **cortex**, the **paracortical areas** and the **medulla**. It is surrounded by a **capsule** and the cells within it are supported by a fine meshwork known as a **reticulum**. Lymph (in the afferent lymphatic vessels) comes into the lymph node at the **subcapsular sinus**. In addition, lymph nodes have a blood supply and lymphocytes may enter the node directly from the blood through **high endothelial venules** in the **paracortex**. The flow of cells is towards the medulla at the centre (**centripetal**) where they drain into the major efferent lymphatic duct in the hilus of the node to be conducted away.

Once in the lymph node, lymphocytes locate according to type such that T lymphocytes tend to collect in the paracortical areas and B cells go to the outer edge of the cortex. This pattern of distribution may be affected by other cells in these areas, e.g. interdigitating cells in the T cell areas and follicular dendritic cells in the B-dependent areas. The paracortical region contains large lymphocytes and blast-like cells and is easily distinguished from the cortex. Also, the medulla contains numerous plasma cells which actively secrete antibody.

Typical T and B lymphocytes in the secondary lymphoid organs are long-lived cells that are selected from a large pool of short-lived precursor cells in the primary lymphoid organs. The bulk of mature T and B cells are immunologically naïve and remain inactive for long periods of time. Contact with specific antigen causes these cells to proliferate rapidly and differentiate into a mixture of **short-lived effector cells** and **long-lived memory cells**. Survival of memory cells appears to require persistent contact with antigen.

The B cells form dense aggregates, which are known as **follicles**. **Primary follicles** are very dense and uniform, the centre of which may contain some larger cells often associated with macrophages. When follicles are not involved in antigen responses, the principle cellular components are naïve, recirculating B cells passing through a network of follicular dendritic cells. This zone is known as the **germinal centre**. Following exposure to antigen, the lymph node shows an increased turnover of lymphocytes. The follicles of the cortex become much larger, with prominent germinal centres composed of metabolically active and mitotic cells. They are known as **secondary follicles**.

Germinal centres last for about 3 weeks following immunisation. After subsequent exposure to the same antigen, they reappear but their size decreases with successive immunisations. In the next few months, follicular memory B **blast** cells continue to proliferate. These cells probably provide the source of plasma and memory cells needed to maintain antibody production and memory.

SPLEEN

The spleen is a secondary lymphoid organ but also performs several other non-immunological functions. Like the lymph nodes, it has a **capsule** with fibrous partitions (**septae**) that penetrate the body of the spleen. There are two main types of tissue, the **white and red pulp**. The erythroid **red pulp** serves as a filter for damaged or aged red cells. Unlike lymph nodes, lymphocytes enter and leave the spleen predominantly via the blood stream.

The **white pulp** consists of cells and tissues surrounding the major arterial branches – **the periarteriolar sheath (PALS)** – and associated clusters of lymphocytes – **the lymphatic follicles or nodules**. These follicles have a similar cellular arrangement to those described in lymph nodes. Thus, the B cell-dependent area of the spleen consists of the lymphoid follicles and the T cell-dependent area consists of the PALS.

The histological changes seen in the spleen after antigenic stimulation are similar to those described in the lymph node, with the development of distinct germinal centres in secondary follicles.

1.2.3 TERTIARY LYMPHOID TISSUES

The majority of other tissues in the body possess poorly organised collections of lymphoid cells. The latter may be very few in number but may undergo a rapid and substantial increase during an immune response. Such collections include the intraepithelial lymphocytes (IEL) and the mucosa-associated lymphoid tissue and are collectively known as the tertiary lymphoid tissues.

MUCOSA-ASSOCIATED LYMPHOID TISSUE

This term is used to describe the diffusely distributed lymphoid tissues in the linings (**mucosa**) of the gastrointestinal, respiratory and urogenital tracts. However, the gut-associated lymphoid tissue (**GALT**) and the bronchus-associated lymphoid tissue (**BALT**) are the best characterised.

GALT is made up of **Peyer's patches** and isolated follicles in the tissue beneath the mucosa of the colon (**colonic submucosa**). Lymphocytes are also found in the lamina propria, the intestinal epithelium and in the lumen of the intestine. Peyer's patches are aggregates of lymphocytes where the B cells form a central follicle and are surrounded by T cells and macrophages which help T cells recognise antigen (i.e. they act as antigen presenting cells). These patches have efferent lymphatics that drain into mesenteric lymph nodes, but no afferent lymphatics. They are covered by a specialised lymphoepithelium consisting of a microfold of cells known as **M cells**. Antigens in the gut can enter the Peyer's patches via the M cells and pass to the lymphoid follicles.

BALT is structurally similar to GALT. It consists of large collections of lymphocytes (the majority of which are B cells), organised into aggregates and follicles with few germinal centres. These are found primarily along the main bronchi in the lungs. The epithelium covering BALT follicles lacks goblet cells and cilia. M cells, which cover the follicles of the BALT, are structurally similar to intestinal M cells. BALT contains an elaborate network of capillaries, arterioles and venules, and efferent lymphatics. This suggests that it may play a role in sampling antigen not only from the lungs but also from the systemic circulation.

INTRAEPITHELIAL LYMPHOCYTES

Large numbers of lymphocytes are intrinsically associated with the epithelial surfaces of the body. Particularly in the reproductive tract, the lung and the skin. These collections of lymphoid cells play a key role in the development of both local and systemic specific immune responses to antigens present at the body surface. These and other aspects of mucosal immunity are described further in Section 4.5.

KEY POINTS FOR REVIEW

- *The majority of responses to specific antigen are precipitated in the lymphoid tissues.*
- *Lymphoid tissues may be classified as primary, secondary, or tertiary.*
- *Primary lymphoid tissues include the thymus and the bone marrow.*
- *T cells are "educated" in the thymus and self-reactive T cells are eliminated by apoptosis.*
- *B cells are "educated" in the bone marrow.*
- *Secondary lymphoid tissues include the spleen and the lymph nodes. These facilitate the interaction between antigen-specific lymphocytes and antigen presenting cells, particularly dendritic cells.*
- *Tertiary lymphoid tissues include the mucosa-associated lymphoid tissues, which are largely unstructured agglomerations of lymphoid cells, which can expand upon antigenic stimulation.*

BIBLIOGRAPHY

Askin DF, Young, S. (2001) The thymus gland. Neonatal Netw, 20; 7–13.
Burrows PD, Cooper MD. (1997) B cell development and differentiation. Curr Opin Immunol, 9; 239–244.
Hartgers FC, Figdor CG, Adema GJ. (2000) Towards a molecular understanding of dendritic cell immunobiology. Immunol Today, 21; 542–545.
Hayday A, Viney JL. (2000) The ins and outs of body surface immunology. Science, 290; 97–100.
Karre K. (2002) NK cells, MHC Class I molecules and the missing self. Scand J Immunol, 55; 221–228.
Moretta L, Biassoni R, Bottino C, Mingari MC, Moretta A. (2002) Natural killer cells: a mystery no more. Scand J Immunol, 55; 229–232.
Neutra MR, Mantis NJ, Kraehenbuhl JP. (2001) Collaboration of epithelial cells with organized mucosal lymphoid tissues. Nat Immunol, 2; 1004–1009.
Robinson DS, Kay AB, Wardlaw AJ. (2002) Eosinophils. Clin Allergy Immunol, 16; 43–75.
Schwartz LB. (2002) Mast cells and basophils. Clin Allergy Immunol, 16; 3–42.
Wiedle G, Dunon D, Imhof BA. (2001) Current concepts in lymphocyte homing and recirculation. Crit Rev Clin Lab Sci, 38; 1–31.
Youinou P, Jamin C, Lydyard PM. (1999) CD5 expression in human B-cell populations. Immunol Today, 20; 312–316.

http://www.keratin.com/am/am025.shtml
This web site lists the CD antigens, their cellular expression, functions and other names.

NOW TEST YOURSELF!

Pick the single, best answer, further questions are available on the web site.

1.   Which of the following statements concerning lymphoid tissues is CORRECT?
(a)   Lymphoid tissues are subdivided into discrete microenvironments which all contain the same lymphocyte subsets and stromal cells.
(b)   Stromal cells are specialised cells which form the skeleton of the tissue or organ.
(c)   Tertiary lymphoid tissues contain large numbers of lymphocytes which are activated in an inflammatory reaction.
(d)   The distribution of lymphocyte subsets in lymphoid tissues arises as a result of lymphocyte trafficking.
(e)   Lymphocyte homing regulates the distribution of naïve and memory cells in lymphoid tissues.

2.   The bursa of Fabricius in birds is a lymphoepithelial organ located near the cloaca. Which of the following is NOT considered to be part of the equivalent organ in humans?

(a) The appendix.
(b) Peyer's patches.
(c) The foetal liver.
(d) Post-natal and adult bone marrow.
(e) The spleen.

3.   Which of the following statements concerning the lymphatic system and lymphatic fluid is INCORRECT?

(a) Components of the blood which leave the vessels and enter the tissues comprise the extracellular fluid.
(b) At the junction between the major lymphatic vessels are small bean-shaped structures called lymph nodes.
(c) Several vessels may bring the lymph to a particular node – the efferent lymphatics – and a single vessel – the afferent lymphatic – carries it away.
(d) Lymph carries antigens from the tissues to the lymph node, where immune responses are initiated.
(e) Lymphocytes can enter the lymphatic circulation directly from the blood, to which they return directly via the thoracic duct.

4.   Which of the following is characteristic of lymph nodes?

(a) Lymph nodes are bean-shaped structures usually found at the junction of major blood vessels.
(b) Lymph nodes range in size between 1 and 2.5 cm in diameter, although they may be much larger during an infection.
(c) A normal resting lymph node has only two main areas, the cortex and the medulla.
(d) The lymph node is covered by a capsule and the cells within it are supported by the trabeculae.
(e) The flow of cells through the node is centripetal, the cells draining into the major efferent lymphatic duct in the hilus of the node.

5.   The spleen is a secondary lymphoid organ but also performs several other functions. Which of the following is NOT typically part of the structure of the spleen?

(a) The T cell-dependent area of the spleen consists of the lymphoid follicles and the B cell-dependent area consists of the periarteriolar lymphoid sheath.
(b) The red pulp filters damaged or aged red cells.
(c) The white pulp comprises the periarteriolar sheath and the lymphatic follicles or nodules.
(d) The splenic lymphatic follicles have a similar cellular arrangement to those in lymph nodes.
(e) A capsule with fibrous partitions or septae that penetrate the body of the spleen.

6. The common myeloid progenitor cell gives rise to:
(a) Neutrophils alone.
(b) Neutrophils, basophils, eosinophils and mast cells.
(c) Polymorphonuclear leukocytes and mononuclear leukocytes.
(d) Polymorphonuclear leukocytes and monocytes.
(e) Neutrophils, eosinophils, basophils, monocytes and macrophages.

7. Phagocytic cells include:
(a) Monocytes and macrophages alone.
(b) Monocytes, macrophages and lymphocytes.
(c) Neutrophils, monocytes and macrophages alone.
(d) Neutrophils, basophils, monocytes and macrophages.
(e) Neutrophils, eosinophils, monocytes and macrophages.

8. Which of the following characteristics distinguishes B lymphocytes from other mononuclear cells?
(a) Phagocytosis.
(b) Secretion of antibody.
(c) Expression of the surface antigen CD3.
(d) Large cytoplasmic granules.
(e) Production of cytokines.

9. Neutrophils provide protection from a variety of microorganisms and are arguably the most important white blood cells in eliminating:
(a) Non-viral infections.
(b) All fungal infections.
(c) Viral infections.
(d) All bacterial infections.
(e) Parasitic infections.

10. Which one of the following statements is CORRECT?
(a) T lymphocytes are conditioned by the bone marrow.
(b) B lymphocytes are conditioned by the thymus.
(c) T cells produce antibodies.
(d) B cells produce antibodies.
(e) T cells do not produce cytokines.

2

ANTIGENS AND THEIR RECEPTORS

An important characteristic of the immune system is that the cells are able to distinguish between those molecules that are normally present in the body, i.e. **self** and those that are not, i.e. **non-self**. This is a vital distinction. The term "non-self" may mean a foreign invader such as a microorganism or a protein expressed on a cell in an abnormal way.

This chapter is designed to introduce you to the terms used to describe those substances which stimulate an immune response – **immunogens**. It will discuss those characteristics which make a molecule a good immunogen and will distinguish between an immunogen and an **antigen** – a molecule or group of molecules which bind specific receptors but may not alone induce an immune response. We will look at an important group of self-antigens, which are coded for by genes of the **major histocompatibility complex**. In addition, we will examine the structure and function of those molecules on cells that are capable of recognising antigens.

2.1 CHARACTERISTICS OF ANTIGENS AND IMMUNOGENS

An **immunogen** is any molecule (or group of molecules) that can induce an immune response, whilst an **antigen** is any substance that can react with antigen-specific receptors found on the surface of certain white blood cells. Thus, an antigen differs from an immunogen in that although an antigen can interact in a specific way with the immune system, it cannot by itself stimulate an immune response; other stimuli are required. Thus, all immunogens are antigens but not all antigens are immunogens. Although these terms are interchangeable, it is common to refer to molecules as antigens even if they are immunogens. We shall follow this practice.

Immunology for Life Scientists, Second Edition. Lesley-Jane Eales.
© 2003 John Wiley & Sons, Ltd: ISBN 0 470 84523 6 (HB); 0 470 84524 4 (PB)

When an antigen is recognised by the immune system, it interacts with specific receptors on the surface of a group of white blood cells called lymphocytes. That part of an antigen which binds to these receptors is known as the **antigenic determinant** or **epitope**.

An antigen may be protein, lipid, carbohydrate or any combination of these. It may be soluble or particulate, simple or complex with many different antigenic determinants (e.g. a bacterium may have antigenic determinants on the cell wall, the flagellum or on pili). Although an antigen may have many different antigenic determinants each of which comprises a small number of amino acids (4–6) or sugar residues, the resulting immune response may comprise antibodies which recognise only a few of these. If the same antigen is introduced in two different people, the epitopes recognised may be quite different suggesting that the range of epitopes recognised is under genetic control.

Since antigens can be of almost any chemical composition, the proteins and carbohydrates present in the membranes of our cells may be antigenic if the cells are introduced into another person or an animal. It was just this principle that was exploited in the production of monoclonal antibodies. Injecting human cells into mice (where they are recognised as foreign) meant that mice produced antibodies to the different molecules on the surfaces of the cells. By fusing a single antibody producing B cell with a replicating, transformed, cell the product was an immortalised clone of cells constantly producing antibody of a single specificity. That allowed us to identify individual molecules (antigens) on the surface of cells and to use them to identify and classify different cell types. Thus, a molecule on the surface of a cell (i.e. inserted through the membrane of the cell) may also be referred to as a **surface antigen**.

2.1.1 FACTORS AFFECTING IMMUNOGENICITY

Various physical and biochemical characteristics affect a substance's immunogenicity. It is important to understand how an antigen's immunogenicity may be modified since this may for example affect the ability of a candidate vaccine to stimulate a protective response.

FOREIGNNESS

The immune system is designed to eliminate anything that does not belong in the normal healthy body, i.e. it is capable of distinguishing between "self" and "non-self"; it can recognise things that are foreign to it. The more foreign a molecule is, the more likely it is that the immune system will react to it and the more **immunogenic** it will be.

It is important to remember that although a molecule may not be immunogenic in the normal host, if it is introduced into a different host, it may become so. For example, rabbit serum albumin injected into a rabbit will not be immunogenic. The same molecule injected into a dog will stimulate an immune response.

SIZE

The size of a molecule appears to affect its immunogenicity. Generally, substances with molecular weights greater than 100 kDa are potent immunogens, whilst those of less than 10 kDa may not stimulate an immune response at all.

Although some small molecules may contain antigenic determinants and can bind antigen-specific receptors on cells, they are not large enough to stimulate an effective immune response. However, these molecules may be made immunogenic by attaching them to a larger molecule known as a **carrier**. Under these circumstances, the small antigenic molecule is known as a **hapten**.

CHEMICAL COMPLEXITY

The chemical complexity of a molecule may affect its ability to stimulate an immune response. Large polymers of amino acids might be expected to be good immunogens (because of their size) but only prove to be so when they consist of a mixture of amino acids.

The type of amino acids present in a peptide also affects its immunogenicity. Aromatic amino acids make a molecule more immunogenic than non-aromatic molecules because non-covalent, hydrophobic, forces govern the interaction between an antigen and its specific receptor on a cell.

ROUTE OF ADMINISTRATION

The type of immune response elicited by an immunogen may be very different at one particular site in the body compared to another. Thus, the route by which an antigen gains access to the immune system may affect its immunogenicity. For example an organism that normally causes infection when introduced in the lungs (a respiratory pathogen) may be destroyed by the acid in the gut if swallowed.

DOSE

The dose of an antigen may also affect its ability to be immunogenic. Given at too high or too low a dose, the immune system may fail to respond to an antigen, which at the correct dose is immunogenic. This failure to respond is known as **immunological tolerance**.

HOST GENETIC MAKE-UP

Since the immunogenicity of a molecule is determined by the size of the subsequent immune response, and an individual's ability to mount an immune response is genetically controlled, then the genetic make-up of the host must play a role in determining the relative immunogenicity of a molecule. This is demonstrated by the fact that some antigens, which stimulate an immune response in man are non-immunogenic in other animals.

All the factors affecting the immunogenicity of a molecule are summarised in Table 2.1.

APPROACHES USED TO INCREASE IMMUNOGENICITY

One of the aims of an immune response is to eliminate whatever has stimulated it, e.g. a microorganism. Obviously, in the case of infection, elimination must be quick and effective to prevent extensive damage to the host (**pathology**). However, where an immunogen is introduced specifically to stimulate a long-lasting immunity (e.g. in the case of immunisation), the longer it is present, the stronger and more long-lasting the resulting immune response will be. This persistence can be achieved by mixing the immunogen with an **adjuvant**.

There are a number of adjuvants which are commonly used, and whilst their precise method of action is not known exactly, they all increase the strength and longevity of an immune response to a particular immunogen. It is thought that this effect may be achieved in one or more of the following ways: increasing the effective size of the immunogen; enhancing the persistence of the immunogen; activating cells such as macrophages and lymphocytes.

Table 2.1   Factors affecting the immunogenicity of a molecule

Size	Large molecules are better than small (>100 kDa)
Foreignness	The more foreign a molecule the better the immunogen
Complexity	Heterogeneous amino acid composition improves immunogenicity
Amino acids	Aromatic amino acids make a molecule more immunogenic
Route of administration	Immunogenicity may be affected by route of administration, e.g. respiratory tract pathogens may be destroyed in the gut
Dose of antigen	Too high or too low a dose fails to stimulate a response and may prevent response on subsequent exposure
Genetic make-up of host	The generation of an immune response is under genetic control

- *Antigens bind to specific receptors on immune cells.*
- *Immunogens bind to specific receptors on immune cells and provide the signals required to stimulate an immune response.*
- *A number of factors can influence whether or not a molecule is a good antigen including size, foreignness, molecular make-up, route of administration, dose and host genetic make-up.*
- *The effectiveness of an immunogen to stimulate an immune response may be enhanced by the use of an adjuvant.*

2.2 THE MAJOR HISTOCOMPATIBILITY COMPLEX

As explained previously, the membrane of a cell is composed of a lipid bilayer, which has proteins, glycoproteins and other compound molecules inserted in it. Such molecules may act as antigens when introduced to a foreign host (cell surface antigens). Probably the best example of this is the blood group antigens A, B and O. An individual of blood group A will have erythrocytes which express this antigen (A+). If this individual is given group B blood (which expresses the B antigen B+), their immune system will recognise the B antigen as foreign and will destroy the transfused blood. This is why it is vital to cross-match blood.

All other cells of the body have a variety of surface antigens, the nature of which are determined by the genetic make-up of the host. These tissue antigens are quite distinct in each individual and when an organ is transplanted, the donor must be matched to the recipient. If the tissues are not matched, the recipient's immune system will recognise the donor tissue antigens as foreign and will destroy the transplant.

These **human leukocyte antigens (HLA)** are the molecules that are identified when an individual is 'tissue-typed'. They are the products of a group of genes known as the **major histocompatibility complex (MHC)**.

The MHC comprises a large number of separate genes and in man they occupy about 1/3000th of the total genome (Figure 2.1). The genes are divided into three classes. Class I includes the A, B and C region genes, Class II includes the D region genes and Class III includes those genes which produce some of the enzymes and control elements involved in antigen processing and presentation and genes coding for members of a group of serum proteins known as **complement** (see Section 3.1).

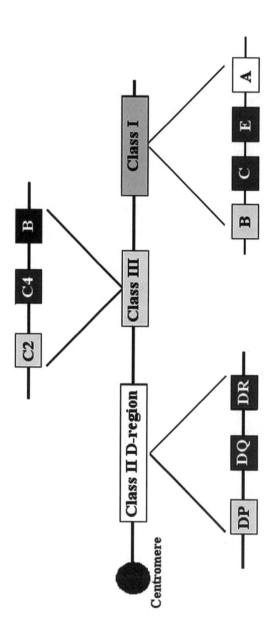

Figure 2.1   The major histocompatibility complex

The MHC comprises a large number of separate genes which, in man, occupy about 1/3000th of the total genome. The genes are divided into three classes: Class I includes the A, B and C region genes; Class II includes the D region genes; Class III includes those which produce some of the enzymes and control elements which form part of a group of serum proteins known as complement.

Antigens coded for by MHC Class I genes are found on the surface of **all nucleated cells and platelets**. The antigenically distinct molecules are coded for by different regions within the Class I genome (on chromosome 6). These regions are known as A, B and C and the molecules coded for by these regions are classed as A1, A2, B1, B2, etc. More than 100 alleles have been identified in the HLA-A and B loci so far.

Class I molecules have one glycosylated polypeptide chain encoded for by the MHC (Figure 2.2). This chain has a relative molecular weight of 45 kDa and is anchored through the cell membrane. It is non-covalently linked with another molecule – β_2 **microglobulin** (12 kDa) – which is not coded for by the MHC and is not membrane bound. The heavy or α- **chain** has five distinct regions or **domains**, three of which are extracellular and hydrophilic (the $\alpha1$, $\alpha2$ and $\alpha3$ globular domains), one of which is transmembraneous and hydrophobic, and one of which is cytoplasmic and hydrophilic.

The majority of the differences which distinguish the Class I antigens from each other (i.e. the antigenic determinants) result from amino acid differences in the $\alpha1$ and $\alpha2$ domains. The existence of a number of antigenically distinct versions of the same molecule is known as **polymorphism**.

β_2 microglobulin is a polypeptide chain with a single domain, which is structurally similar to MHC domains. This molecule plays a vital role in transporting newly synthesised MHC proteins to the cell surface.

Class I molecules are involved in stimulating an immune response by presenting processed antigen to those cells of the immune system capable of recognising them. This ability to present antigen is related to the structure of the molecule. Each of the $\alpha1$ and $\alpha2$ domains consists of four β strands and an α helix. Together these β strands form a β-pleated sheet, which acts as a platform that supports the α helices. This creates a groove or cleft, which forms the antigen-binding site of the molecule (Figure 2.3). The β_2 microglobulin is key to the stability of the structure formed by the $\alpha1$ and $\alpha2$ domains.

Most of the polymorphism of Class I molecules is found within the antigen-binding cleft. These differences affect the ability of a particular MHC Class I molecule to bind a specific processed antigen and restrict the range of antigens presented. HLA-A alleles differ from each other by 20 to 30 amino acids. This affects the shape of the antigen-binding cleft allowing the alleles to bind a distinct range of peptides.

The peptide binding groove of Class I molecules is restricted at both ends, a feature that presumably dictates the binding of peptides of restricted size (8–10 amino acids). Also, the ends of the bound peptide are fixed in the binding groove allowing the peptide to arch away from it in the centre. Peptides, which share a particular sequence of amino acids with similar spacing and charge, will bind to the same Class I molecule.

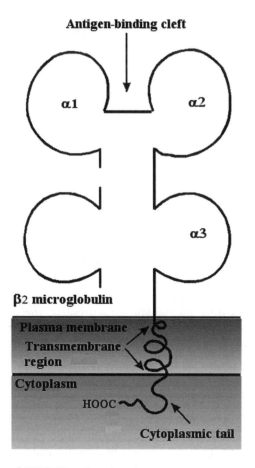

Figure 2.2   Structure of MHC Class I molecules
Class I molecules have one glycosylated polypeptide chain encoded for by the MHC which is anchored through the cell membrane. It is non-covalently linked with another molecule – β_2 microglobulin (12 kDa) – which is not coded for by the MHC and is not membrane bound. The heavy or α- chain has five distinct regions or domains, three of which are extracellular and hydrophilic (the α1, α2 and α3 globular domains), one of which is transmembraneous and hydrophobic and one of which is cytoplasmic and hydrophilic.

The groove is lined by pockets, which vary in size. Peptides produced by antigen processing have short extensions like side-chains that may fit into these pockets (named A–F) and mediate binding of the peptide via hydrogen bonds and van der Waals forces. Studies have shown that specific pockets bind particular amino acids (**anchor residues**).

Many Class I molecules do not have precisely defined functions. However, their presence on the surface of all nucleated cells and their ability to present antigen means that they are important in promoting the immune response to viruses since these organisms may infect any cell in the body. Antigen receptors on white blood cells will recognise a particular viral peptide only in the context of a particular Class I molecule. This phenomenon is termed **HLA-restriction**.

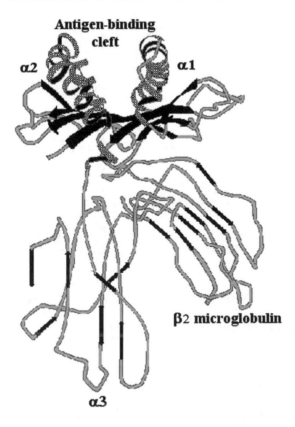

Figure 2.3 Representation of the molecular structure of an MHC Class I molecule showing the antigen-binding cleft
Class I molecules present antigen to T cells. Each of the α1 and α2 domains consists of four β strands and an α helix. Together these β strands form a β-pleated sheet which acts as a platform and supports the two α helices. Thus, a groove or cleft, which is closed at both ends, is created that forms the antigen-binding site of the molecule.

When foreign antigens are not occupying the cleft, self-antigens associate with the Class I molecules. During the development of antigen-specific white blood cells, those recognising self-antigens are eliminated or inactivated preventing the development of a response, which would damage host tissues – **an autoimmune response**.

2.2.2 CLASS II MHC MOLECULES

The MHC Class II molecules **HLA-DR, -DP and -DQ** are expressed on antigen presenting cells (e.g. dendritic cells, macrophages and B cells), which stimulate an immune response. However, under appropriate conditions, cells that do not normally express them can be induced to do so (e.g. activated T cells).

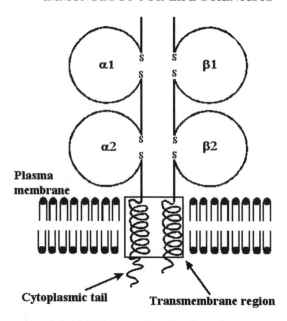

Figure 2.4   Structure of the MHC Class II molecules
Class II molecules consist of two, linked, glycoproteins (α and β) both of which are coded for by the
genes of the MHC. Each consists of four regions: two extracellular, hydrophilic regions (α1, α2 or β1,
β2 domains), a transmembraneous, hydrophobic region and an intracellular hydrophilic region
which anchors the molecule in the cell membrane.

These molecules consist of two, linked, glycoproteins (α and β), composed of
229 and 237 amino acids, respectively (Figure 2.4). Each is coded for by genes of
the MHC and consists of four regions; two extracellular, hydrophilic regions (α1
and α2, or β1 and β2 domains), a transmembraneous, hydrophobic region; and
an intracellular, hydrophilic, region that anchors the molecule in the cell
membrane.

Study of the structure of the HLA-DR1 allele has shown that the α1 and β1
domains combine to form a single peptide-binding site composed of two α
helical loops supported by a platform of eight anti-parallel β strands – similar
to that seen in the Class I molecules. The polymorphism in different MHC Class
II alleles is usually concentrated in these domains. In the HLA-DR molecule,
polymorphism is confined to the β chain, the α chain being conserved.

Peptides that bind Class II molecules are different to those that bind Class I.
The latter are limited in size and both ends are anchored within the antigen-
binding groove. Those peptides that bind Class II molecules may be of variable
length owing to the fact that the antigen-binding groove is open at both ends
and does not enclose the C- and N-termini of the peptide. This means that the
bound peptide is a twisted structure that extends beyond the antigen-binding
groove at both ends.

Three asparagine residues are conserved in all Class II molecules, which
enable the formation of **hydrogen bonds** with the main chain of amino acids

in the bound peptide. In addition, other conserved residues are found in key positions to stabilise the peptide–Class II association through hydrogen bonds. These strong bonds result in the peptide being maintained in an extended helix causing the peptide backbone to twist in the binding groove of the molecule.

As with Class I molecules, the peptide also associates with the Class II molecule through interactions with the pockets formed by the polymorphic amino acids within the molecule. This increases the specificity of the binding and hides a considerable part of the peptide surface.

Peptide binding may be dependent upon a few key molecules for a particular allele. These molecules are known as **allele-specific peptide binding motifs**. However, these motifs may not be essential since poor interactions with one pocket may be compensated for by enhanced interactions further along the peptide. Peptides lacking the key motifs may still bind and activate T cells but they have high dissociation rates, making the process less efficient.

2.2.3 NON-CLASSICAL HLA MOLECULES

The non-classical Class I molecules include HLA-E, F and G. These molecules are expressed at much lower levels on tissues than the classical Class I molecules. In contrast to this, during the development of the placenta and the foetus, classical Class I molecule expression is downregulated whilst that of HLA-G is increased. The latter is not recognised by natural killer cells, thus protecting these specialised tissues from destruction.

Non-classical Class II molecules (HLA-DM and DO) are not directly involved in antigen binding. However, they do have a role to play in the processing of antigen and the association of peptides with the classical Class II molecules (see Section 4.1).

KEY POINTS FOR REVIEW

- *The major histocompatibility complex comprises three groups of genes – MHC Class I, Class II and Class III.*
- *Class I gene products are expressed on the surface of all nucleated cells and platelets.*
- *Class II gene products are expressed on the surface of antigen presenting cells (dendritic cells, macrophages and B lymphocytes).*
- *The level of expression of these molecules may be regulated by cytokines and infectious agents such as some viruses.*

- *Class I molecules comprise an alpha chain which associates with β_2 microglobulin. The $\alpha1$ and $\alpha2$ domains form a structure comprising alpha helices bordering a β-pleated sheet. This forms the antigen-binding groove.*
- *Class II molecules have an alpha and a beta chain, the $\alpha1$ and $\beta1$ domains form the structure enclosing the antigen-binding groove.*
- *Class I molecules bind shorter peptides than Class II molecules since in the latter, the antigen-binding groove is open at each end.*
- *MHC gene products may be classical or non-classical, the latter having a different distribution, expression or function to the classical antigens.*

2.3 ANTIGEN RECEPTORS ON CELLS

The major structures responsible for the recognition of antigens leading to an immune response and the removal of the specific antigen are the **B cell antigen receptor (BCR)** and the **T cell antigen receptor (TCR)**. The BCR comprises membrane-bound immunoglobulin and the CD79a/b molecules whilst the TCR comprises the CD3 complex and the α/β or γ/δ TCR chains.

2.3.1 THE B CELL ANTIGEN RECEPTOR

B cells bind antigen via membrane-bound immunoglobulin molecules (mIg). Normal B cells in the peripheral blood have 10^4–10^5 molecules of antibody in their membrane, which differ from the secreted form due to the presence of spacer, transmembrane and cytoplasmic sequences at the Fc (carboxyl) end of the heavy chains. When antigen binds to mIg, the cell must be made aware of this event. This is achieved through a series of biochemical events collectively known as **signal transduction**. This is usually achieved by the interaction of particular cellular proteins (e.g. G proteins or tyrosine kinases) with specific regions in the cytoplasmic tail of mIg. However, the most prevalent mIgs, IgM and IgD, do not possess such regions in their tails, suggesting that the required signals are transmitted in some other way. Other similar receptor systems have associated proteins which perform the task of signal transduction. On B cells, mIg is non-covalently associated with a dimeric protein consisting of two, disulphide-linked glycoproteins. These molecules (known as **Igα and Igβ** or **CD79a and b**) have molecular masses of about 32/33 kDa and 37 kDa (Figure 2.5). The amino acid sequences of the chains indicate that both have a single, extracellular domain, which shows similarity in both sequence and structure to those in immunoglobulin molecules. Thus, the genes coding for all these molecules (CD79a/b or **mb-1** and **B29**) are considered to belong to the

Membrane Immunoglobulin (mIg)

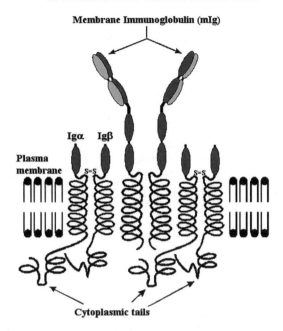

Igα Igβ

Plasma
membrane

Cytoplasmic tails

Figure 2.5 Representation of the structure of the B cell antigen receptor
mIg on the surface of B cells is non-covalently associated with a dimeric protein consisting of two, disulphide-linked glycoproteins. These molecules are known as CD79a (Igα) and CD79b (Igβ).

same family, which has become known as the **immunoglobulin supergene family**. We will come across more members of this family shortly.

The CD79 molecules have intracellular tails, which contain a particular sequence of molecules known as **immunoreceptor tyrosine-based activation motifs (ITAMs)**. It is thought that when clustering of the BCRs occurs as a result of binding to antigen, tyrosine kinases pre-bound to the receptors are brought into association with the ITAMs leading to further signal transduction and cellular activation.

IMMUNOGLOBULINS

Immunoglobulins are a group of globular glycoproteins found in the serum and body fluids and play a vital role in the immune response. Since they are capable of specifically recognising and binding to antigens, they are also known as **antibodies**.

> *Tiselius and Kabat (1939) showed that antibodies were gamma globulins by incubating serum from an immune animal with specific antigen. The immune complexes formed between the antigen and antibodies precipitated out of solution and the remaining serum was analysed. The gamma globulin portion of the serum was severely diminished.*

Immunoglobulins are also found on the surface of **B cells** where they are inserted through the cell membrane (**mIg**). When B cells are activated by antigen, they proliferate and may differentiate into **plasma cells**, which manufacture and secrete large amounts of antibody. This antibody binds the same antigen as the mIg on the B cell from which the plasma cell was derived (i.e. they have the same **binding specificity**).

There are five major **classes** of immunoglobulin (**IgG, IgA, IgM, IgE** and **IgD**), which differ from each other in size, charge, amino acid sequences and carbohydrate content. Within the classes, there are distinct differences (heterogeneity) and **subclasses** can be distinguished, e.g. IgG1, IgG2, IgG3 and IgG4. The number of subclasses varies depending on the host species and each differs in biological function.

ANTIBODY STRUCTURE

The basic structure of all immunoglobulins consists of two pairs of chains (heavy and light) linked together by covalent, **disulphide bonds** and non-covalent forces (Figure 2.6). The **heavy chains** dictate the **class** of immunoglobulin, i.e. μ chains are present in IgM, γ chains in IgG, etc. The light chains may be either κ or λ type. These chains are antigenically distinct and only one type of light chain is present in any single antibody molecule. This four-chain structure is seen in IgG, IgD and IgE. By contrast, IgA occurs in both monomeric and polymeric forms (comprising more than one basic four-chain unit structure) whilst IgM occurs as a **pentamer** with five basic units.

> *Edelman received the Nobel prize for his work on determining the structure of the immunoglobulin molecule. For this purpose, he used myeloma proteins. Multiple myeloma results from the uncontrolled growth of a cell which normally produces antibodies. The cell replicates unchecked and the daughter cells all produce antibody of the same type and specificity as the original cell. This leads to a high serum concentration of homologous antibody. Using this myeloma protein, Edelman identified the heavy and light chain structure of antibody molecules. After unfolding the proteins in 6 M urea, the disulphide bonds were disrupted by mercaptoethanol and prevented from reforming by alkylation. After this treatment, he found two types of molecule with molecular weights of 20 kDa (light chain) and 50 kDa (heavy chain). Their relative concentrations suggested that the basic antibody unit consisted of two heavy chains and two light chains.*

Each of the chains comprises a number of **globular** regions (called **domains**) formed by intra-chain disulphide bonds. At the amino terminal of both the heavy and light chains is a single **variable region** or domain (**VL** or **VH**) consisting of 110 amino acids. The variable regions of one light chain and one heavy chain form one of the antigen-binding sites of the antibody.

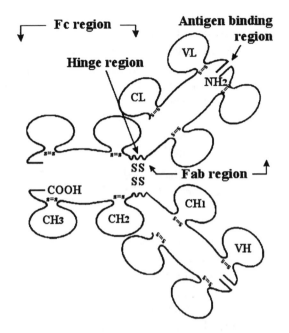

Figure 2.6   Representation of the basic structure of immunoglobulins
The basic structure of all immunoglobulins consists of two pairs of chains (heavy and light) linked together by covalent, disulphide bonds and non-covalent forces. Each chain comprises a number of globular regions (called domains) formed by intra-chain disulphide bonds. At the amino terminal of both the heavy and light chains is a single variable region or domain (VL or VH). The number of heavy chain constant regions (CH) in an antibody molecule varies depending on the class.

The number of heavy chain constant regions (CH) in an antibody molecule varies; being three in IgG, A and D and four in IgM and E. Light chains have only one constant region (CL). These regions are called constant because there is very little difference in the secondary and tertiary structure of the proteins in these areas.

There are several genes that code for immunoglobulins and unusually each chain of an antibody molecule is the product of more than one of these. The variable region is coded for largely by a V gene and the constant region by a Cγ, Cμ, Cα, Cε or Cδ gene.

Individual CH genes are organised such that different exons code for the structural domains of the protein. Thus, the **Cμ** genes contain **four exons** to code for the **four constant domains** of the mu chain. The Cγ genes each have an additional small exon between the first and second CH domain exons that encodes the **hinge region**. The Cδ gene is organised somewhat differently from the other H chain genes in that it contains an extended hinge and lacks a CH2 domain.

Each class of antibody may exist in either a secreted or membrane-bound form. With the exception of IgD, the carboxy-terminal sequences of the secreted forms are contiguous with the terminal C region domain. By contrast, the unique sequence of the membrane-bound forms is encoded by an exon (or exons) downstream of the terminal CH exon. This sequence comprises a series of 26 hydrophobic amino acids, which spans the plasma membrane and a hydrophilic, cytoplasmic tail varying in size from 3 to 28 amino acids. For IgD, the exons for both the secreted and membrane-bound forms of the molecule are separate. The production of membrane-bound or secreted immunoglobulin is probably regulated at the level of RNA processing.

V region genes code for the variable regions of the antibody. Specific V region genes associate with a constant region product of either a heavy chain or a light chain, i.e. VH with CH and VL with CL gene products. However, any of the products of the CH genes may associate with any of those of the VH genes.

Kappa chains have V region subgroups differing in the number and position of amino acid substitutions and deletions. These molecules share a degree of structural similarity, which distinguishes them from lambda V or VH region products. Similar subgroups also exist for lambda and heavy chain V regions.

All V gene products have regions which are relatively conserved, and it is these that define the type of the V gene product (VH or VL) and the subgroup to which it belongs. In addition, they have extremely variable zones or "hot spots". These are the **hypervariable regions**, which are involved in the formation of the antigen-binding site. Light chains have three hypervariable regions whilst heavy chains have four.

All immunoglobulins are covalently bonded to carbohydrates in the form of simple or complex side-chains. This carbohydrate may assist in secretion of the antibody by plasma cells and may affect the biological functions of the molecule, which are associated with the constant regions of the heavy chains.

Immunoglobulins consist of two functional domains: the Fab fragment (Fragment antigen binding) consists of the two VH–CH1 domains and the two VL–CL domains; the Fc fragment (Fragment crystallisable) consists of the CH2 and CH3 domains (and CH4 in IgM and IgE) of both heavy chains. The antigen specificity of the molecule resides in the Fab fragment but the majority of the biological function resides in the Fc region. The **hinge region** binds these two fragments. As its name suggests, this area allows slight relative motion between the two fragments. This mobility is important in antigen binding. The hinge region contains a high number of proline and cysteine residues; the latter form inter-chain disulphide bonds, which maintain the integrity of the molecule. These bonds also prevent folding in this area making it especially vulnerable to enzymatic cleavage. The number of these disulphide bonds varies between classes and subclasses of antibody.

ISOTYPES

As we mentioned earlier, when antibodies are injected into another person or a different species, they can act as antigens and antibodies will be raised against any part of the molecule that is foreign to the host. Thus, if human immunoglobulins are injected into mice, antibodies will form that will react with a range of epitopes on the human immunoglobulins.

> *Isotypic antibodies react with those parts of a heavy or light chain which distinguishes it from all other classes of heavy or light chains.*

Although all the immunoglobulin heavy chains have a similar structure, they have different molecular weights and therefore must have differences in their amino acid sequences and carbohydrate substitution. Thus, they must have distinguishing antigenic epitopes, which are known as **isotypes**. Antibodies may be raised to these isotypes and thus may be used to distinguish between immunoglobulin classes and subclasses.

ALLOTYPES

In the same way that isotypic antibodies identify antigenic differences between the classes of immunoglobulins, allotypic antibodies identify differences **within** a class (or subclass) of immunoglobulin. For example, the amino acid sequence for IgG1 in one person (A) may vary slightly from that in another (B) due to the inheritance of different alleles of IgG1 or to mutation. Thus, when the antibody from A is introduced into B, the differences are recognised as foreign and antibodies are formed to that part which is different – the **allotype**.

IDIOTYPES

In contrast to allotypic differences, idiotypic differences are associated with the antigen-binding region of an antibody. If a mouse is exposed to an antigen for the first time, it forms antibodies that have antigen-binding sites that specifically recognise the inducing antigen. If that antibody is isolated and injected into a genetically identical mouse, which has not been exposed to the antigen, the only part of the antibody that would appear foreign to the recipient is the antigen-binding site. Since B cells recognise conformational (3-D) antigenic determinants, the antigen-binding site may contain novel conformations, which the recipient may recognise as foreign and to which it may form antibodies (**anti-idiotypes**). Such antibodies define the **idiotype** of the eliciting antibody. Each antigenic determinant is known as an **idiotope**.

2.3.2 ANTIBODY CLASSES

Antibodies may be classified into different classes according to the type of heavy chain present. These different molecular structures confer distinct biological properties on the molecules.

IMMUNOGLOBULIN G

IgG comprises 70–75% of the circulating immunoglobulins. It has a molecular weight of 146 kDa and a sedimentation coefficient of 7S. It is the major immunoglobulin produced during a secondary immune response and is the only antibody with antitoxin activity. It has four subclasses IgG1, 2, 3 and 4. These molecules vary in molecular weight, the number and position of inter-chain disulphide bonds and in their functional properties (Table 2.2).

IgG is the only antibody to be transported across the placenta. However, not all the subclasses have the same properties; IgG2 being transported more slowly than the other subclasses. One serum protein – namely C1q – binds to the CH2 domain on IgG. C1q is involved in the activation of a group of serum proteins, which comprise the **complement pathway** and are involved in innate immunity. Different subclasses of IgG fix C1q with decreasing efficiency in the order IgG3, IgG1, IgG2. Indeed, IgG4 cannot fix C1q but may be active in the alternative complement pathway (see Section 3.1).

Many cells (including polymorphs, monocytes/macrophages, B cells, NK cells and some T cells) bear molecules on their surface, which bind IgG through the Fc region. These are known as **Fc receptors**. Fc receptors on macrophages, some T cells and killer cells allow these cells to bind antibodies attached to specific antigens on cells (**target cells**) and can lyse these target cells through a mechanism known as **antibody-dependent cellular cytotoxicity (ADCC)**.

Table 2.2 General biological properties of the IgG subclasses

	IgG1	IgG2	IgG3	IgG4
% IgG in serum	60–71	19–31	5–8	0.7–4
Average serum concentration (g/l)	8	4	0.8	0.4
Range in normal serum (g/l)	5–12	2–6	0.5–1	0.2–1
% Circulating B cells	40	48	8	1
Placental transfer	++	+	++	++
Rate of catabolism (days)	21–23	20–23	7–8	21–23
Complement fixation	++	+	++	–

IgG is also found in mucous membrane secretions and therefore has a role to play in immunity to infection at mucosal surfaces. This activity is considered in more detail in the section on specific immunity.

IMMUNOGLOBULIN M

IgM comprises about 10% of circulating immunoglobulins. It has a molecular weight of 970 kDa and comprises five, four-chain units, which are linked at the CH3 domains by inter-heavy chain disulphide bonds (Figure 2.7). The heavy chains have four constant regions and the whole unit is stabilised by a **J (joining) chain**. This immunoglobulin is largely confined to the peripheral circulation and is the principal antibody produced in a primary response. It is produced early in a secondary response, and with certain antigens is the sole antibody produced, e.g. natural blood group antibodies. IgM, with IgD, is found on the surface of the majority of mature B cells. It binds C1q more efficiently than any other class of antibody.

IMMUNOGLOBULIN A

IgA comprises about 15–20% of the circulating immunoglobulin pool. In man, the majority of serum IgA (80%) occurs as a basic four-chain monomeric unit.

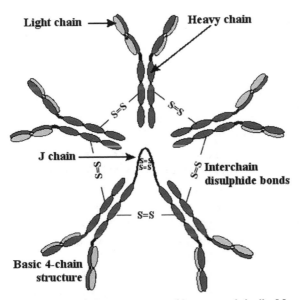

Figure 2.7 Representation of the structure of immunoglobulin M
IgM comprises five, four-chain units which are linked at the CH3 domains by inter-heavy chain disulphide bonds. The heavy chains have four constant regions and the whole unit is stabilised by a J (joining) chain.

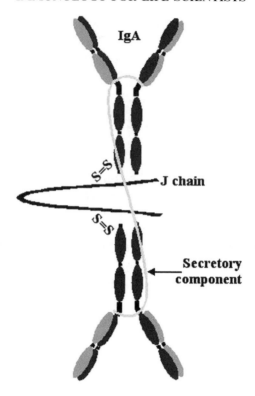

Figure 2.8   Representation of the structure of secretory immunoglobulin A
In man, the majority of IgA occurs as a basic four-chain monomeric unit. However, when it is
secreted at mucous membranes, it exists predominantly as a dimer which is held together by a
J chain. On passing through the epithelial cell layers it acquires the secretory component. This is
bound by strong covalent bonds and aids release of the dimer at mucosal surfaces.

However, in other mammals it occurs chiefly as a dimer, which is held together
by a J chain synthesised by plasma cells.

IgA is the chief antibody secreted at mucous membranes where it exists
predominantly as a dimer of molecular weight 385 kDa (Figure 2.8). Dimeric
IgA, with its associated J chain, passes through the epithelial cell layers where it
acquires the **secretory component**. This is bound by strong covalent bonds, aids
release of the dimer at mucosal surfaces, and protects it from proteolytic attack.
Mucosal IgA probably exerts its protective effect by blocking access to the
immune system rather than by destroying the antigen.

There are at least two different subclasses of IgA, IgA1 and IgA2. IgA1
predominates in serum but IgA2 predominates in mucous secretions. This
difference may have evolved as a protective response owing to the fact that
many microorganisms at the mucosal surface release proteases capable of
destroying IgA1 (e.g. meningococci).

Neither of the subclasses activates complement via C1q, but both may activate it via an alternative pathway.

IMMUNOGLOBULIN D

Although IgD comprises only less than 1% of serum Ig, it is expressed (with IgM) on the surface membrane of many B cells. This expression appears to indicate the differentiation of a pre-B cell into a mature B cell. The biological role of IgD is largely unknown but the molecule is thought to be involved in antigen-triggered lymphocyte differentiation. IgD has a tendency to undergo spontaneous proteolysis and is more sensitive to proteolytic cleavage than IgG1, 2, IgA or IgM. It is also easily destroyed by heat.

IgD may be able to enhance a protective humoral response, interfere with viral replication, and participate in the generation and maintenance of B cell memory. It may be important in the change from non-responsiveness to responsiveness to a particular antigen. In addition, the presence of IgD appears to be related to the ability of monocytes to produce the cytokines tumour necrosis factor (TNF), interleukin 1β (IL-1β), and IL-1 receptor antagonist.

IMMUNOGLOBULIN E

Only trace amounts of IgE are present in the serum, the majority of this antibody is found bound to the surface of mast cells and basophils. It is functionally associated with those reactions that occur in individuals who are undergoing an allergic reaction. It can activate complement via an alternative pathway to C1q. IgE also has a role to play in immunity to helminthic infections.

Along with IgM, IgE has an extra heavy-chain constant domain.

2.3.3 ANTIBODY FUNCTION

Functionally, antibodies show a spectrum of activities ranging from those that are beneficial (such as the neutralisation of viruses) to those which cause damage to the host (such as the prevention of nervous impulse conduction in *Myaesthenia gravis*). These functions are covered in more detail in the appropriate chapters and a summary is given in Table 2.3.

Table 2.3   Summary of the biological functions of immunoglobulin

Function	Description
Neutralisation	Antibodies may block cellular receptors for toxins, bacteria or viruses preventing toxicity/infection
Complement fixation	Activation of the classic pathway occurs as a result of complement components binding to the CH2 region Ig
Opsonisation	Phagocytosis of an object is greatly enhanced when it is coated by antibodies – a process known as opsonisation
Allergy and anaphylaxis	Antigen-specific IgE may bind to receptors on mast cells and promote their degranulation leading to the signs and symptoms of allergy
Antibody-dependent cellular cytotoxicity	Antibodies stimulated by virus infection bind to viral antigens expressed on the surface of infected cells. The Fc portion binds to FcR-bearing cells which are able to lyse the virally infected cells
Agglutination	Each antibody molecule has at least two sites to which antigen can bind. Thus they may "stick together" or agglutinate a number of organisms
Effect on microbial physiology	Some antibodies inhibit the movement organisms by attaching to flagella. Also, some antibodies inhibit the metabolism or growth of microorganisms

2.3.4 Fc RECEPTORS

As mentioned earlier, certain cells express surface membrane receptors, which bind the Fc region of immunoglobulins. These **Fc receptors (FcR)** may be classified according to the class of antibody they bind, e.g. FcεR (IgE receptor), FcαR (IgA receptor), FcγR (IgG receptor), etc. The FcγR may be divided further into three groups: FcγRI, FcγRII, FcγRIII, which differ in their affinity for IgG and immune complexes. The properties and cellular distribution of these receptors are summarised in Table 2.4.

2.3.5 THE T CELL ANTIGEN RECEPTOR

The identity of the molecule on the surface of T cells which binds antigen took many years to determine. T cells had been shown experimentally to exhibit antigen specificity and so it seemed logical that they must express antigen-specific receptors. Finally, the **T cell antigen receptor (TCR)** was identified (by using antibodies with unique specificity for a particular clone of T cells) as an 80–90 kDa, cell surface, dimeric, glycoprotein (Figure 3.5). The disulphide-

Table 2.4 Summary of the function and distribution of Fc receptors for IgG

Receptor	MW (kDa)	Function	Cellular distribution
FcγRI (CD 64)	72	Binds monomeric IgG; high affinity receptor; binds IgG in CH2 region; important in clearance of immune complexes and ADCC	Monocytes, macrophages. Expression is increased on monocytes treated with the cytokine interferon gamma
FcγRII (CDw32)	40	Low affinity receptor for aggregated IgG; occupation triggers IgG mediated phagocytosis and triggers an oxidative burst in monocytes and neutrophils; simultaneous binding to mIg and occupation of FcγRII on B cells provides a negative signal	FcγRII comprises a group of proteins coded by a number of closely related genes. All types are expressed on monocytes, FcγRII B is present on B cells and FcγRIIB and C are expressed by neutrophils
FcγRIII (CD 16)	50–80	Low affinity receptor for aggregated IgG; mediates phagocytosis and ADCC	There are two distinct forms of FcγRIII, a transmembrane form and a glycosylphosphatidylinositol linked form (GPI-linked form). The transmembrane form is expressed on macrophages and NK cells; the GPI-linked form on neutrophils

linked α and β chains each consist of two extracellular domains, one constant and one variable, with a joining segment in between. A short cytoplasmic tail connects the extracellular domains via a transmembraneous region, which is next to a group of about 20 amino acids (containing cysteines) which comprise the connecting peptide where the inter-chain disulphide bridges are formed.

The development of antigen-specific T cell clones (T cells derived from a single antigen reactive cell which therefore recognise the same antigenic determinant) allowed the structure of the T cell antigen receptor to be determined. Basically, cloned, antigen-specific T cells were injected into a mouse and monoclonal antibodies were produced. Antibodies which recognised determinants expressed only by the cells used to immunise the mice were identified. Since the only difference between these and other T cells should be the molecules which recognise antigen, the monoclonal antibodies were assumed to recognise the T cell antigen receptor (TCR). Partial confirmation of this was obtained by incubating the T cell clone with the monoclonal antibody and stimulating with antigen. The antibody blocked antigen recognition and the cells failed to proliferate. The antibody was used to isolate the receptor by labelling cells, lysing them, and incubating them with the monoclonal. The immune complexes were then removed by reacting them with a substance that binds the Fc region of Ig (protein A) and analysed by sodium dodecyl sulphate polyacrylamide gel electrophoresis (SDS-PAGE). The proteins from the cells were labelled with a radioactive substance. Thus, when the SDS-PAGE gels were exposed to film, bands containing cell-derived proteins could be visualised.

The variable regions of the α and β chains together form the antigen-binding site of the receptor. Amino acid sequence analysis suggests that the variable regions show a β-pleated sheet structure similar to that seen in the variable regions of MHC molecules. Within the variable domain, at least three **hypervariable regions** have been identified which are directly involved in antigen binding. The structural similarity between antibody molecules and the TCR chains has led to the inclusion of the genes coding for the TCR in the "Ig supergene family".

Following the identification of the $\alpha\beta$TCR, cells were isolated which expressed a different chain – the γ **chain** (55 kDa). Although similar to the $\alpha\beta$ molecules, the γ chain lacks glycosylation. It was found to be non-covalently associated with a protein of molecular weight 40 kDa – the δ **chain**. The $\gamma\delta$TCR is expressed on a proportion of mature T cells and thymocytes; its presence precluding the expression of the $\alpha\beta$TCR.

$\gamma\delta$T CELLS

$\gamma\delta$T cells are typically found within epithelia, in the peripheral blood, and in lymphoid tissue parenchyma. They are not found concentrated in the areas typically associated with sampling of diverse antigens. This led to the suggestion that $\gamma\delta$T cells might react with non-classical MHC molecules (Class Ib antigens). Subsequent studies demonstrated that $\gamma\delta$T cells could respond to the MHC Class Ib molecules **MICA** and **MICB** expressed on stressed cells or those undergoing malignant transformation. Blocking of the TCR with specific antibodies could eliminate this activation and the subsequent lysis of the MICA/B expressing cells. Importantly, there was no evidence of a peptide associated with the antigen-binding groove of the MHC Class Ib molecules suggesting that these molecules may be indicators of cell stress or malignancy.

$\gamma\delta$T cells have been shown to express the **natural killer cell activating receptor – NKG2D**. Some evidence suggests that the $\gamma\delta$TCR and NKG2D both recognise MICA in a similar manner to the $\alpha\beta$TCR/CD8 recognition of the antigen-MHC Class I complex (see Section 4.3.2).

THE CD3 COMPLEX

As mentioned earlier, the TCR was identified by precipitation of labelled cell membrane-associated proteins using monoclonal antibodies. When different detergents were used and the precipitated proteins separated by two-dimensional electrophoresis, sequentially under non-reducing and reducing conditions, further molecules (γ, δ, ε) were identified which associated with the TCR (Figure 2.9). Originally, these were known as the **T3 complex** and

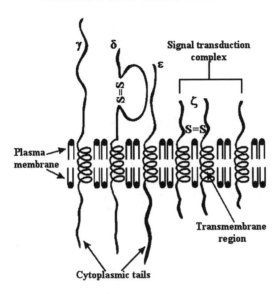

Figure 2.9   The molecular make-up of the CD3 complex
CD3 molecules are expressed on a proportion of thymocytes and on all peripheral T cells in association with the TCR chains. The presence of CD3 is vital for the expression of the TCR chains and thus for the presence of a functional receptor on the cell membrane.

subsequently as the **CD3 complex**. Later work identified a further molecule associated with the TCR, the ζ chain.

CD3 molecules are expressed on a proportion of thymocytes and on all peripheral T cells in association with the TCR chains. Its presence is vital for the expression of the TCR chains and thus for the presence of a functional receptor on the cell membrane.

> *Ohashi et al. (1985) showed that mutant cells which have lost the ability to express one or other of the TCR genes have neither the TCRα chain nor the CD3 complex on their membranes. If the cells are transfected with a competent β chain gene, the cells are able to express a functional αβTCR and the CD3 complex.*

When cells are incubated with antibodies that bind CD3 (anti-CD3 antibodies), antigen-specific T cell proliferation may be inhibited due to the **capping** (movement of a molecule within the plane of the membrane to the pole of the cell) and **recycling** of CD3. It has been shown that the TCR co-caps with CD3. This treatment reduces the expression of the antigen receptor thereby inhibiting antigen-induced activation. Conversely, when anti-CD3 is anchored to a solid support it can cross-link TCR–CD3 complexes and provides a similar signal to that which is delivered when an antigen binds the TCR.

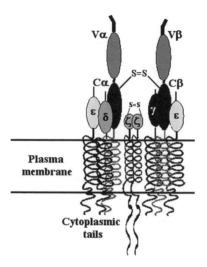

Figure 2.10   Representation of the spatial association of molecules of the TCR and CD3 complex
The γ, δ and ε chains of CD3 are non-covalently linked, transmembraneous polypeptides and are thought to associate with the $\alpha\beta$ chains of the TCR so that an ε molecule associates with each chain of the TCR.

The γ, δ and ε chains of CD3 are non-covalently linked, transmembraneous polypeptides. The molecules of CD3 associate with the $\alpha\beta$ chains of the TCR so that an ε molecule associates with each chain of the TCR (Figure 2.10). The transmembrane regions of both the δ and ε chains of CD3 have aspartate molecules forming salt bridges with lysine molecules in the equivalent part of the TCR chains.

FUNCTION OF THE TCR-CD3 COMPLEX

As its title suggests, the $\alpha\beta$ chains of the TCR are responsible for recognising specific antigen whilst the CD3 γ, δ, ε and TCR ζ chains provide the appropriate information to the cell concerning this interaction. These signal transduction molecules form an immunoreceptor signal transduction subunit and possess immunoreceptor tyrosine-based activation motifs critical to successful signalling. Each of the γ, δ and ε chains contains one ITAM whilst the ζ chain contains three. These motifs are phosphorylated by tyrosine kinases of the **Src family**. Activation of tyrosine kinases following engagement of the $\alpha\beta$TCR leads to the recruitment and phosphorylation of a group of enzymes and adapter proteins resulting in the reorganisation of the cytoskeleton and transcription of multiple genes leading to T cell proliferation, differentiation, and/or effector function (Figure 2.11).

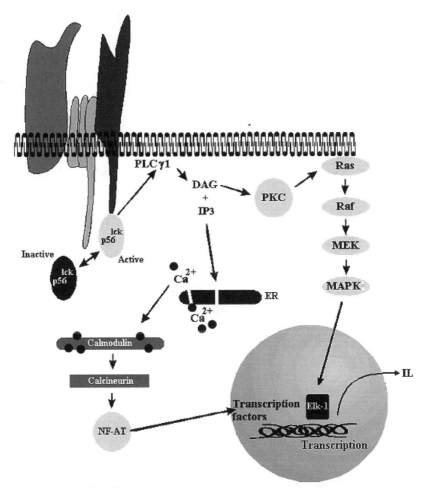

Figure 2.11 T cell receptor signalling
The T cell receptor (TCR) is activated upon binding antigen causing the activation of p56^{lck}, one of the Src family of tyrosine kinases. p56^{lck} phosphorylates (and therefore activates phospholipase C$\gamma 1_1$ (PLC$\gamma 1_1$)) which hydrolyses phosphatidylinositol 4,5-bisphosphate (PIP$_2$), resulting in the production of diacylglycerol (DAG) and inositol trisphosphate (IP$_3$). DAG activates protein kinase C (PKC) to phosphorylate the GTPase Ras, which in turn activates Raf leading to the mitogen-activated protein (MAP) kinase (MEK, MAPK) cascade and activation of the Elk transcription factor. Stored calcium released by IP$_3$ binds to calmodulin causing the activation of calcineurin (a Ca^{2+}/calmodulin-dependent protein phosphatase). The latter dephosphorylates the transcriptional regulator of interleukin 2 gene expression – NFAT – which can then migrate to the nucleus and induce the transcription of the IL-2 gene.

2.3.6 THE NATURAL KILLER CELL RECEPTOR

Natural killer (NK) cells are a group of large granular lymphocytes capable of killing a limited range of tumour and virally infected cells. Work in recent years has demonstrated that NK cell activity is dependent upon a form of antigen recognition. It does not display the exquisite specificity associated with T and B cell antigen recognition but does involve presentation of antigens in association with MHC Class I gene products.

Three distinct gene families have been identified which code for receptors on NK cells capable of recognising MHC Class I gene products. The **killer cell Ig-like receptors (KIR)** are transmembraneous molecules belonging to the immunoglobulin supergene family. Another group belonging to this family are the **immunoglobulin-like transcripts (ILT)**. These are expressed mainly on lymphocytes and myeloid cells but may be found on NK cells. The third family of receptors comprise heterodimers of **CD94** covalently bound to a molecule from the **NKG2** family. These receptors are known as **C-type lectins** and mostly bind the non-classical HLA-E molecule. Ligands for the KIR and some of the ILT receptors include the classical MHC Class I products and the non-classical HLA-G molecule. Within each of these families are receptors that despite binding similar if not identical ligands, have opposing outcomes, i.e. stimulation or inhibition of cellular activities. The outcome of this interaction is either to activate or prevent NK-mediated lysis. The outcome of the interaction appears to depend on the presence of certain conserved epitopes on the ligand. Evidence suggests that the type of peptide present in the cleft of the Class I molecule may also play a role in the outcome of NK cell recognition.

KEY POINTS FOR REVIEW

- *Major structures involved in recognising antigens are the BCR and TCR.*
- *The BCR comprises mIg and the CD79a/b molecules.*
- *The TCR comprises the CD3 complex in association with either the α/β or γ/δ chains.*
- *Immunoglobulins are globular proteins found on the surface of B cells and in the serum.*
- *There are five major classes of Ig – IgG, A, M, E and D.*
- *The basic structure of Igs comprises two heavy chains (γ, α, μ, ε or δ) and two light chains (κ or λ).*
- *The chains have constant, variable and hinge regions which affect their function and classification.*
- *Antibodies may be classified according to their type, isotype, allotype or idiotype.*
- *Different classes of antibody have different functions with regard to their ability to fix complement, traverse the placenta, act as opsonins, etc.*
- *The TCR belongs to the immunoglobulin superfamily of molecules.*
- *The CD3 complex acts as the signal transduction complex of the TCR.*

- *γδT cells recognise antigens in association with non-classical MHC Class I molecules and may express the NK cell activating receptor – NKG2D.*
- *Natural killer cells also express receptors capable of recognising antigen.*
- *NK cells have receptors that either stimulate or inhibit the activation of NK cells.*

2.4 GENERATION OF ANTIGEN RECEPTOR DIVERSITY

The effectiveness of the specific immune response is dependent in part on its ability to develop memory, allowing a rapid response upon subsequent exposure to antigen. However, the real key is the ability of the specific immune response to distinguish between different antigenic epitopes. The immune system is exposed to an enormous variety of antigens in the form of infectious agents or chemicals and must be able to respond to such a challenge. However, the number of genes required to code for every possible antigenic determinant would be enormous. Thus, logically, a balance is required. Since it is important that the immune system does not react to self-antigens, the range of possible antibody specificities (**the antibody repertoire**) must be great enough to prevent extensive cross-reactivity between self-antigens and those on infectious agents but small enough that there is space for the genetic material required. This logic must also be extended to the T cell antigen receptor where the specificity is not as exquisite as that found in antibodies but must be great enough to allow some distinction between antigens.

2.4.1 THEORIES CONCERNING ANTIBODY DIVERSITY

Over the years, many theories have been proposed to explain the range of antigenic determinants recognised by antibodies. Two particular theories received the most attention and have been given greatest credence. The **germ line theory** proposes that there must be a gene in the germ line (i.e. the original chromosome complement present at conception) to code for every antibody variable region and that these genes arose by **duplication** during evolution. By contrast, the **somatic mutation theory** proposes that only a small number of variable region genes are present in the germ line and that the products of these genes may vary greatly due to **point mutation** or **recombination** during lymphocyte differentiation, thus giving rise to a unique antibody repertoire in each person. If diversity were dependent on this theory alone, would have to exist [special mechanisms] for selecting variants due to the normally low rate of

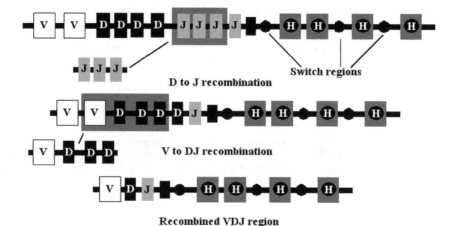

Figure 2.12 Recombination of genes comprising the antigen-binding region of an antibody
The antigen-binding site of an antibody is made up of the V(ariability), D(iversity) and J(oining) regions of the heavy chain and the VJ regions of the light chain. The number of VH, VL, DH, JH and JL genes influences the diversity of the antibody response due to recombination between the different genes.

mutation. Studies using DNA cloning techniques suggest that both of the theories contribute to antibody diversity but the relative contribution of each in generating antibody diversity remains unknown.

2.4.2 THE GENETIC BASIS OF ANTIBODY DIVERSITY

During B cell development, rearrangement of Ig genes results in the surface membrane expression of antibody with a single antigenic specificity. Although there may be more than one type of antibody expressed on the surface of a single B cell (commonly IgM and IgD are co-expressed), all the molecules use the same VH and VL genes. The antigen-binding site of an antibody is made up of the V(ariability), D(iversity) and J(oining) regions of the heavy chain and the VJ regions of the light chain (Figure 2.12). Immunoglobulin diversity is affected by a variety of genetic mechanisms but the number of VH, VL, DH, JH and JL genes is highly influential.

V, D AND J REGION HEAVY CHAIN GENES

DNA sequence and Southern blotting analyses have resulted in the VH region being divided into seven or eight subfamilies each having between four and more than 100 members. However, recent work has suggested that this severely underestimates the number of VH genes present in the germ line.

Currently in man, there is thought to be between 10 and 20 D region genes and nine J region genes (including three pseudogenes).

THE LIGHT CHAIN V AND J GENES

Unlike their counterparts in heavy chains, light chains do not contain D regions. The V region is divided into a leader exon and one further exon, which codes for the bulk of the V region. In mice, the V region comprises two alleles, each of which is associated with two J region alleles. In contrast to this, the number of genes in the human Vλ region is much greater than in mice, which may reflect the greater usage of this L chain in humans.

The Vκ locus in both man and mouse comprises a number of Vκ genes (estimated to be between 50 and 300 in man) and five Jκ genes. Analysis using Southern blotting has allowed the subdivision of Vκ genes into families similar to those of the VH genes.

2.4.3   GENERATION OF ANTIBODY DIVERSITY

The primary antibody repertoire of an individual includes the specificity of all those antibodies which normally circulate in the blood stream. They do not result from exposure to specific antigen and arise through the random combination of immunoglobulin heavy and light chain V, D and J segments; a process resulting in combinatorial diversity. However, the repertoire is increased further as a result of the imprecision in joining the different gene segments, i.e. **junctional diversity**. Since each amino acid is coded for by a group of three bases, errors in joining gene segments together may result in a frame shift or the replacement of one amino acid by another. This may lead to a conformational change, which will affect the binding specificity of the antibody.

Studies in mice have shown that the bone marrow produces enough primary B cells every few days to completely renew the peripheral blood pool. These cells, if they do not encounter antigen, have a short life of between 4 and 7 days. Thus, the B cell antigen-recognition repertoire is constantly changing through the production of cells, which are using different VDJ gene combinations. Thus, in an infection, if none of the primary B cells expresses an antibody which recognises the antigen, it is likely that one with effective affinity will be produced within a few days through combinatorial and junctional diversity.

Following exposure to an antigen, reactive B cells undergo a process of hypermutation within the Ig gene loci. This results in the maturation of the immune response with the production of antibodies of increased affinity.

Table 2.5   Estimate of the number of antibody specificities possible through combinatorial diversity

	IgH	Igk
V region genes	1000	200
D region genes	15	–
J region genes	4	4
Combinatorial joining	6×10^4	8×10^2
Combinatorial association	$\sim 5 \times 10^7$	

However, only a minor proportion of the point mutations which occur actually contribute to the observed increase in antibody affinity.

COMBINATORIAL AND JUNCTIONAL DIVERSITY

Before the genetic code for an antibody is transcribed, segments of the Ig gene loci are rearranged in a two-step process to give rise to the code for the functional protein. Firstly, a particular **D region** gene associates with a **J region** gene. The second step results in a **V region** gene being associated with the **rearranged DJ genes**. The multiplicity of genes in each region gives rise to a wide range of different combinations (Table 2.5), i.e. **combinatorial diversity**. In pre-B cells those VH genes closest to the JH genes are preferentially recombined. However, this preference does not persist in mature B cells suggesting that **antigenic pressure** may affect the VH repertoire.

Further diversity is introduced into the antibody repertoire through the imprecision of the joining process. The point at which V, D and J gene segments join may differ by as much as 10 bases which may result in removal of nucleotides from the ends of the regions leading to codon changes and amino acid differences in the processed protein (**junctional diversity**). The result of this imprecision is that the majority of the gene rearrangements are non-productive because the joining has resulted in non-translatable base sequences. However, if the joining process is productive (i.e. the joins are 'in frame') each cell undergoes further gene rearrangement involving the L chain, V and J region genes. Once the L chain genes have been productively rearranged and a functional antibody has been assembled, further H and L chain rearrangement is prevented, thus ensuring that the cell produces mIg of a single specificity.

Since the antigen-binding region of an antibody is formed by the VH and VL regions, further diversity can be introduced through the association of different rearranged heavy and light chain regions, i.e. **combinatorial association**. However, some VH and VL combinations prevent the association of functional H and L chains. Such failure to produce functional antibodies could be very wasteful and thus during maturation, L chain gene rearrangement only ceases once a fully assembled, functional protein is produced.

Further diversity may be introduced in the variable regions of **heavy** (but not light) chains through the addition of nucleotides, which are not coded for by either of the gene segments to be joined. The insertion of these **N-regions** correlates with the level of activity of an enzyme called **terminal deoxynucleotidyl transferase (TdT)** and their compositions reflect the preference of this enzyme for guanosine nucleotides.

CONTROL OF VDJ GENE REARRANGEMENT

It has been shown that the V, D and J gene segments are flanked by either a conserved series of **seven bases** or a less conserved **nine-base sequence**. These regions are separated by a spacer whose length is either **12 or 23 bases**, which approximates to one or two turns of the double helix. It is the length, rather than the sequence, of the spacer which directs recombination since a segment with a **12 base spacer** can only recombine with a segment containing a **23 base spacer** (the '12–23' rule). This means that **VH–D** and **D–JH** joins may occur whilst **VH–JH** association may not. However, rearrangement of VH region genes to non-rearranged D region genes is not normally seen, suggesting that there must be other mechanisms controlling the VDJ rearrangement.

The **recombinase enzyme complex**, which includes the recombination-activating genes **RAG-1** and **RAG-2**, regulates the joining of the gene segments.

MECHANISMS OF V(D)J REARRANGEMENT

As we mentioned earlier, the gene sequences to be joined are flanked on either side by either a heptamer or nonamer and are separated by a spacer region. These flanking sequences with the intervening spacer are together known as the **recombination signal sequence (RSS)**, which is removed in the joining process. Commonly, gene segments are joined by a **deletional method** where the intervening DNA is **looped out** and lost from the genome (Figure 2.13a). However, not all recombination can be accounted for in this way and some may result from **inversion** or **unequal sister chromatid exchange** (Figure 2.13b,c).

DIVERSITY DUE TO SOMATIC MUTATION

During the later stages of B cell maturation, antibody diversity is increased further through **somatic mutation**. This results in single base changes throughout the VH and VL regions. However, certain areas within these regions are particularly susceptible to somatic mutation. Such mutation is

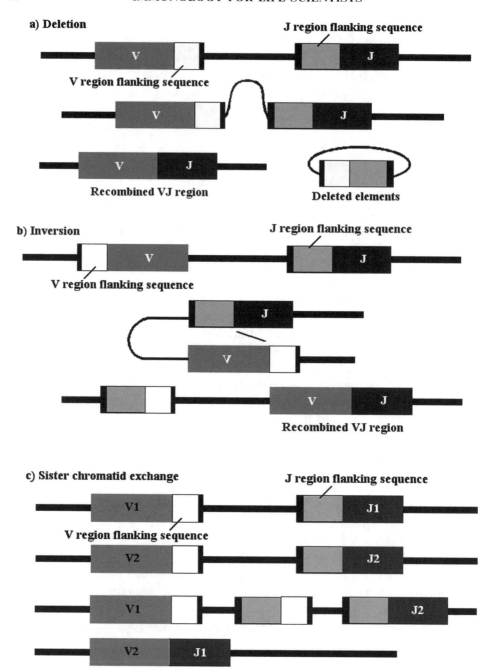

Figure 2.13 Methods of gene recombination which give diversity to the antibody response

Commonly, gene segments are joined by a deletional method where the intervening DNA is looped out and lost from the genome (a). However, not all recombination can be accounted for in this way and some may result from inversion (b) or unequal sister chromatid exchange (c).

thought to **increase the affinity** of the antibody for its antigen and thus to contribute to **maturation** of the antibody response. For example, it is probable that those B cells that proliferate, particularly in limiting antigen concentration, have undergone somatic mutation and as a result have membrane immunoglobulin with higher affinity for antigen.

2.4.4 ANTIBODY MATURATION

Antibody maturation is restricted to T-dependent antigens and is brought about in one of two ways: (i) the germ line genes used in the primary response are different to those used in a memory response; (ii) diversification of the primary repertoire is enhanced through repeated mutation leading to random changes in both heavy and light chain genes which occasionally result in increased affinity of the antibody for its antigen. Cells producing these higher affinity antibodies preferentially differentiate into memory cells.

2.4.5 GENETIC BASIS OF T CELL ANTIGEN RECEPTOR DIVERSITY

T cell antigen receptor diversity is generated in a manner similar to that observed with membrane immunoglobulin. A large number of genes have been identified in the germ line, which contribute to TCR diversity. However, in contrast to the generation of antibody diversity, TCR diversity is rarely, if ever, affected by somatic mutation.

As with immunoglobulins, the T cell antigen receptor is coded for by **variability** (V) and **joining** (J) region genes but lacks **diversity** (D) region genes in all but one of the identified components (the β chain). Whilst the TCR repertoire used in response to a particular antigen may be quite diverse, studies have shown that such responses may also be extremely restricted. Such restriction reflects not only limited V and J gene usage (for both α and β chains) but also relatively conserved amino acid usage in the junctional regions. In contrast to this, it has been shown that diverse responses reflect unrestricted usage of V and J region genes (apart from the preferential use of certain $V\beta$ genes), and heterogeneous amino acid composition in the junctional regions of both α and β chains. These extremes may be explained by the **similarity to self** rule.

'SIMILARITY TO SELF RULE' – LIMITED DIVERSITY

When an antigen is similar to one or more normally present in the body, the T cell repertoire is limited. This is to reduce the possibility of the foreign antigen

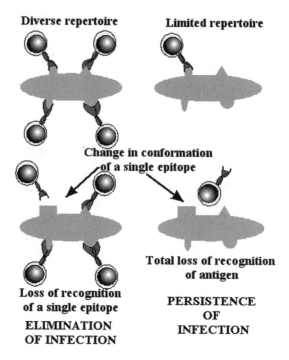

Figure 2.14   Dependence on TCR diversity for the elimination of infection
Microorganisms are constantly underoing mutation. If the TCR showed a limited repertoire, mutation in a dominant antigen on the microorganism would prevent its recognition by T cells and lead to persistent infection. Such a mutation will not prevent elimination if the T cell repertoire is diverse enough to recognise alternate epitopes on the microorganism.

stimulating cross-reactive T cells which recognise self-proteins and thus minimise the risk of developing an autoimmune response (i.e. one which recognises and destroys antigens present in the normal healthy body thus leading to tissue damage, disease and possibly death).

DIVERSE TCR REPERTOIRE

An infectious agent may have a wide range of antigenic determinants. The development of a diverse TCR repertoire in response to microbial infection is advantageous to the host since this would increase the rate of patient survival and decrease the likelihood of the pathogens escaping recognition. Rapidly replicating microorganisms undergo mutations relatively frequently; if such a mutation were to affect the only antigenic determinant recognised by a limited TCR repertoire, the microorganism would be able to grow unchecked. However, if the TCR repertoire were diverse enough to recognise several determinants on a single organism, such mutation would not prevent elimination of the infection (Figure 2.14).

GENOMIC ORGANISATION – THE TCRα CHAIN

The TCRα gene locus comprises a single constant region gene associated with a group of Jα and Vα genes. The extracellular part of the constant region, which includes a short connecting peptide, is coded for by two exons; a third exon coding for the transmembrane region and intracellular cytoplasmic tail. The large number of Jα region genes (estimated to be about 50) are spread out along the genome, the entire locus extending over about 100 000 bases. Despite difficulties in estimating the size of the Vα germ line repertoire, in both mouse and man it has been calculated to comprise 50–100 gene segments, divided into at least 10 different subfamilies, which range in size from one to 10 members.

GENOMIC ORGANISATION – THE TCRβ CHAIN

The genome which codes for the TCRβ chain contains a duplicated set of one Cβ and D region gene and several J region genes. The two Cβ genes are highly conserved, with only four amino acid differences in the mouse and six in humans. They have identical organisation, being encoded by four exons. The first exon encodes the extracellular constant region domain and part of the connecting peptide, the remainder of which is encoded by the second exon and part of the third exon. The transmembrane region is encoded by the remainder of the third exon and the cytoplasmic tail by the fourth exon.

Each D region gene (Dβ1 and Dβ2) is located about 600 bases from its J region gene segment (Jβ1 and Jβ2 comprising six and seven genes respectively). The Vβ region comprises about 20 genes in the mouse and 50–100 genes in the human. Part of the translated V region (about 15–17 amino acids) is coded for by genes of the J region.

GENOMIC ORGANISATION – THE TCRγ CHAIN

The organisation of the genome for the TCRγ chain is complex. Humans have two Cγ genes about 16 000 bases apart. Each of these genes consists of three exons; one codes for the extracellular domain and the second codes for the majority of the connecting peptide. The third exon also encodes the extracellular domain as well as the remainder of the connecting peptide, the transmembrane region, and the cytoplasmic tail. In mice, there are four Cγ genes.

In humans, three Jγ gene segments have been identified associated with one of the Cγ gene segments and two with the other. All of these genes have been shown to be used by T cell clones. By contrast, in mice, each C gene is associated with a single J gene. No Dγ gene segments have been demonstrated in either the human or murine genomes.

Eight Vγ genes have been identified in humans. These are located upstream of the two Cγ genes. In mice, there are seven Vγ genes, one associated with each of the first three Cγ genes and four with the last.

GENOMIC ORGANISATION – THE TCRδ CHAIN

The delta chain is coded for by a **constant gene** segment and at least **one J** and **one D gene** segment. These genes are located between the variable and joining region genes of the alpha chain and have been shown to use some of the latter during recombination.

2.4.6   GENERATION OF T CELL ANTIGEN RECEPTOR DIVERSITY

As stated earlier, the mechanisms involved in the generation of diversity in the T cell antigen receptor are similar to those found in B cells, i.e. gene duplication in the germ line coupled with combinatorial diversity and joining diversity. As with antibody, gene rearrangement during TCR transcription is controlled by the **12–23 rule** which allows Vβ–Dβ–Jβ, Vβ–Jβ and even Dβ–Dβ joining.

As with antibodies, TCR gene rearrangement results in substantial **junctional diversity** due to the lack of precision in the joining process. This is particularly important for generating diversity in the TCRγ chains, which have a comparatively small number of genes in the germ line. Also, **N-region diversity** of the variable regions has also been shown in α, β and γ chains of the TCR. As with antibodies, **terminal deoxynucleotidyl transferase** (TdT) has been associated with this process in T cells and is found to be highly active in the **thymus** where the TCR repertoire is generated.

SIZE OF THE T CELL REPERTOIRE

As with antibody, the size of the TCR repertoire may be estimated by considering the number of V(D) and J region genes and their possible combinations. However, due to the elimination of autoreactive T cells in the thymus and the requirement for MHC restriction, the repertoire expressed in the periphery is less than that estimated using these values.

- *The repertoire of antigens recognised must be great enough to prevent cross-reactivity between foreign antigens and self-antigens but small enough to accommodate the genetic material required.*
- *Current concepts propose both the germ line theory and the somatic mutation theory are instrumental in the generation of diversity of antigen receptors.*
- *Antibody diversity depends upon recombination events affecting the V, D and J region genes.*
- *Further diversity is introduced through imprecision in the joining mechanisms.*
- *V, D, J gene segment joining is governed by the '12–23' rule.*
- *Similar rules govern the generation of diversity in the TCR.*
- *Fewer germ line genes means that there is less diversity in the TCR but this probably relates to the limited size/complexity of the peptides presented to T cells.*

BIBLIOGRAPHY

Allan DSJ, Lepin EJM, Braud VM, O'Callaghan CA, McMichael AJ. (2002) Tetrameric complexes of HLA-E, HLA-F and HLA-G. J Immunol Meth, 268; 43–50.
Bengten E, Wilson M, Miller N, Clem LW, Pilstrom L, Warr GW. (2000) Immunoglobulin isotypes: structure, function, and genetics. Curr Top Microbiol Immunol, 248; 189–219.
Bjorkman PJ, Burmeister WP. (1994) Structures of two classes of MHC molecules elucidated: crucial differences and similarities. Curr Opin Struct Biol, 4; 852–856.
Borrego F, Kabat J, Kim D-K, Lieto L, Maasho K, Pena J, Solana R, Coligan JE. (2001) Structure and function of major histocompatibility complex (MHC) class I specific receptors expressed on human natural killer cells. Mol Immunol, 38; 637–660.
Borst H, Brouns GS, de Vries E, Verschuren MCM, Mason DY, van Dongen JJM. (1993) Antigen receptors on T and B lymphocytes: parallels in organisation and functions. Immunol Rev, 132; 49–84.
Jefferis R. (1993) What is an idiotype? Immunol Today, 14; 119–121.
Moss PA, Rosenberg WM, Bell JI. (1992) The human T cell receptor in health and disease. Ann Rev Immunol, 10; 71–96.
Natarajan K, Li H, Mariuzza RA, Margulies DH. (1999) MHC class I molecules, structure and function. Rev Immunogenet, 1; 32–46.
Nelson CA, Fremont DH. (1999) Structural principles of MHC class II antigen presentation. Rev Immunogenet, 1; 47–59.
O'Callaghan CA, Bell JI. (1998) Structure and function of the human MHC class Ib molecules HLA-E, HLA-F and HLA-G. Immunol Rev, 163; 129–138.
Ramsden DA, van Gent DC, Gellert M. (1997) Specificity in V(D)J recombination: new lessons from biochemistry and genetics. Curr Opin Immunol, 9; 114–120.
Steel CR, Oppenheim DE, Hayday AC. (2000) $\gamma\delta$T cells: non-classical ligands for non-classical cells. Curr Biol, 10; R282–R285.

Van Leeuwen JEM, Samelson LE. (1999) T cell antigen-receptor signal transduction. Curr Opin Immunol, 11; 242–248.

Vladutiu AO. (2000) Immunoglobulin D: properties, measurement and clinical relevance. Clin Diag Lab Immunol, 7; 131–140.

http://depts.washington.edu/rhwlab/dq/3structure.html
Excellent models of Class I and II molecules with and without bound peptide.

http://www.library.uq.edu.au/bio/lectures/vets3001_2002/i2_intro_immunology.ppt
An interesting Powerpoint presentation giving basic information about antigens, epitopes and immunogens.

http://www.researchd.com/rdikits/rdisubbk.htm
Useful resource on IgG.

http://people.ku.edu/%7Ejbrown/antibody.html
What the heck is an antibody?!

NOW TEST YOURSELF!

1.   Which of the following statements is TRUE?

(a) *An antigen can interact specifically with the immune system but requires other stimuli in order to initiate an immune response.*

(b) *An antigen is any molecule or group of molecules, which can induce an immune response.*

(c) *All antigens are immunogens but not all immunogens are antigens.*

(d) *An immunogen can interact specifically with the immune system but cannot itself stimulate an immune response.*

(e) *An immunogen is any molecule or group of molecules, which can react only with antigen-specific receptors on T cells and B cells.*

2.   Antigens bind to specific receptors on lymphocytes. One of the following statements is CORRECT:

(a) *That part of the antigen that binds to lymphocyte antigen receptors is called the antigenic determinant or epitope.*

(b) *The antigen-specific receptor on T cells is membrane-bound immunoglobulin.*

(c) *The antigen-specific receptor on B cells is made up of two groups of molecules, one being a duplex of molecules, the other being CD3.*

(d) *Each antigen-specific receptor on a single B cell binds a distinct epitope on the same antigen.*

(e) *T cell antigen receptors bind the same epitope as those on B cells.*

3.   Which of the following is NOT typically characteristic of an antigen?

(a) *An antigen may be protein, lipid, carbohydrate or any combination of these.*

(b) *An antigen may be simple or complex, with many different antigenic determinants.*

(c) *A complex antigen will elicit antibodies to all the different antigenic determinants it expresses. Thus the same antigen introduced into two different individuals will elicit an identical range of antibodies.*
(d) *Antigenic determinants comprise a small number of amino acids or sugar residues.*
(e) *An antigen may be soluble or particulate.*

4. Which of the following does NOT affect the immunogenicity of a substance?
(a) *Making the molecule more foreign (less like a self-antigen).*
(b) *Making a molecule larger.*
(c) *Adding identical subunits to a large molecule with identical repeating subunits.*
(d) *Altering the dose of a molecule.*
(e) *Increasing the chemical complexity of a molecule by adding particular amino acids.*

5. Which of the following statements concerning the foreignness and size of an antigen is INCORRECT?
(a) *The immune system is designed to eliminate anything which is foreign, i.e. non-self.*
(b) *Substances with molecular masses greater than 50 kDa are potent immunogens.*
(c) *The more foreign a molecule is, the more likely it is that the immune system will react to it.*
(d) *Substances with molecular masses less than 100 kDa tend to be poor immunogens.*
(e) *Smaller molecules may be made immunogenic by attaching them to a carrier molecule.*

6. The human leukocyte antigens are a group of molecules expressed on the surface of cells. Which of the following statements concerning these molecules and the genes which code for them is INCORRECT?
(a) *When cells are introduced into a genetically distinct individual, the human leukocyte antigens act as immunogens and stimulate an immune response.*
(b) *The human leukocyte antigens are identified when an individual is tissue typed.*
(c) *The human leukocyte antigens are the products of a group of genes known as the major histocompatibility complex.*
(d) *The MHC genes are divided into three classes, Class I, II and III.*
(e) *Class I MHC genes include the A, B and C region genes. Class II include the D region genes. Class III include the E region genes and some enzymes and control elements.*

7. **Which of the following statements is INCORRECT?**
(a) *MHC Class I gene products are found on the surface of all nucleated cells and platelets.*
(b) *MHC Class I gene products are only found on the surface of antigen presenting cells.*
(c) *MHC Class I gene products are the antigens which are typed when an individual needs an organ transplant.*
(d) *MHC Class I gene products are antigenically distinct and are coded for by different regions within the Class I genome.*
(e) *The regions of the Class I genome are known as A, B and C.*

8. **Which of the following CORRECTLY describes the structure of Class I gene products?**
(a) *A bimolecular structure comprising two glycosylated polypeptide chains encoded by the MHC.*
(b) *The molecule has a polypeptide chain of molecular mass 45 kDa which is anchored through the cell membrane and is covalently bound to beta-2 microglobulin.*
(c) *The polypeptide chain has three extracellular (and hydrophilic) domains, one transmembraneous (and hydrophobic) domain and one cytoplasmic (and hydrophilic) domain.*
(d) *The polypeptide chain has four distinct domains.*
(e) *Beta-2 microglobulin is encoded by the MHC and is membrane bound.*

9. **Which of the following statements concerning MHC Class II genes and their products is CORRECT?**
(a) *The MHC Class II molecules are expressed normally (in humans) on antigen presenting cells such as activated B lymphocytes, macrophages, dendritic cells, resting T cells.*
(b) *Products of MHC Class II molecules are HLA-DR, HLA-DS, HLA-DQ alone.*
(c) *The molecules consist of two glycoprotein chains (alpha and beta), the alpha chain alone being coded for by genes of the MHC.*
(d) *Other cells such as endothelial cells and thyroid cells can be induced to express MHC Class II molecules.*
(e) *Each glycoprotein chain consists of five regions, three extracellular, one transmembraneous and one intracellular which anchors the molecule in the cell membrane.*

10. **Which of the following is INCORRECT?**
(a) *The antigen-binding cleft of Class II molecules is created by the alpha-1 and beta-1 domains of the glycoprotein chains.*
(b) *The cleft is composed of eight beta strands and two alpha helices such that the resulting structure is similar to that of MHC Class I molecules.*

(c) *Polymorphism of Class II molecules is located in the cleft, thus restricting the range of peptides bound by a single molecule.*
(d) *Like Class I molecules, the antigen-binding site of a Class II molecule is able to bind a range of different antigens.*
(e) *The Class II peptide-binding groove is closed at both ends, restricting the size of peptides to 8–10 amino acids. That in Class I molecules is open at one end, allowing slightly larger peptides (14 amino acids) to bind.*

11. Which of the following statements concerning the basic structure of immunoglobulins is INCORRECT?
(a) *The basic structure of all immunoglobulins comprises two pairs of chains – the heavy and light chains.*
(b) *The light chain dictates the class of the antibody molecule.*
(c) *Heavy chains may be either mu, gamma, alpha, epsilon or delta.*
(d) *Light chains are either kappa or lambda and are antigenically distinct.*
(e) *In any single antibody molecule only one type of light chain is present.*

12. Which of the following associations may NOT occur?
(a) *VH with CH.*
(b) *VL with CL.*
(c) *V kappa with C kappa.*
(d) *V lambda with C lambda.*
(e) *VL with CH.*

13. Which of the following statements concerning antibody regions and their genes is INCORRECT?
(a) *V region gene products have relatively conserved regions which define the type of V gene product.*
(b) *C region gene products have extremely variable zones or hot spots known as hypervariable regions.*
(c) *Hypervariable regions are involved in the formation of the antigen-binding site.*
(d) *Light chains have three hypervariable regions whilst heavy chains have four.*
(e) *V kappa region products share a degree of structural similarity which distinguishes them from lambda or VH regions.*

14. Which of the following statements concerning IgD is CORRECT?
(a) *IgD comprises 1% of serum immunoglobulin.*
(b) *Expression of IgD in association with IgM appears to indicate the differentiation of a pre-B cell into a mature B cell.*
(c) *The biological role of IgD is clearly understood. IgD stimulates differentiation of T cells in response to antigen stimulation.*
(d) *Unlike other classes of antibody, IgD does not undergo spontaneous proteolysis.*

(e) IgD is more sensitive to proteolytic cleavage than IgG1, IgG2, IgA or IgM but is not easily destroyed by heat.

15. One of the following is INCORRECT. Gamma/delta T cells:
(a) Are found in various locations including the epithelium and peripheral blood.
(b) Are functionally more like natural killer cells than cytotoxic T cells.
(c) May recognise antigens associated with non-classical MHC molecules.
(d) Comprise a variable proportion of mature T cells.
(e) Are the most common cells found in the germinal centres of lymph nodes.

16. The T cell antigen receptor (TCR) alpha chain gene locus:
(a) Comprises two constant region genes.
(b) Comprises about 50 J α region genes which are spread out along the genome.
(c) Comprises two exons which code for an extracellular region which includes the transmembrane region.
(d) Comprises a third exon which codes for a short connecting peptide.
(e) Comprises a group of J α, V α and D α genes.

17. With regard to the genome which codes for the TCR beta chain:
(a) The genome contains a duplicated set of one C β, two D region genes and one J region gene.
(b) The genome contains an exon which encodes the extracellular constant region domain and part of the connecting peptide.
(c) The genome contains a second exon which encodes the transmembrane region.
(d) The genome contains a third exon which encodes the cytoplasmic tail.
(e) The V β region comprises about 20 genes in humans.

18. Antibody diversity due to somatic mutation occurs in B cells. Which of the following statements is FALSE?
(a) During the early states of B cell maturation, antibody diversity is increased through somatic mutation.
(b) Somatic mutation results in single base changes throughout the VH and VL regions.
(c) Mutation is thought to increase the affinity of the antibody for its antigen.
(d) Increased antibody affinity for its antigen is thought to contribute to the maturation of the antibody response.
(e) B cells which proliferate in limiting antigen concentration have probably undergone somatic mutation.

19. VDJ rearrangements are closely controlled. Which of the following statements concerning this control is INCORRECT?
(a) V, D and J gene segments are flanked by either a conserved series of seven bases or a less conserved nine-base sequence.

(b) *The flanking regions are separated by a spacer whose length is either 12 or 23 bases.*

(c) *According to the "12/12; 23/23" rule, a segment with a 12 base spacer can only recombine with a segment containing a 12 base spacer, whilst a 23 base spacer can only recombine with a segment containing a 23 base spacer.*

(d) *According to the rule, VH–D and D–JH joins may occur, whilst VH–JH association may not.*

(e) *Two recombination-activating genes have been identified and the products of these genes are thought to participate in the events leading to recombination by forming an essential part of the recombinase enzyme complex.*

20. Other processes result in the generation of antibody diversity. Which of the following statements is TRUE?

(a) *Since the antigen-binding region of an antibody is formed by both the VH and CH regions, further diversity can be introduced through the association of different rearranged heavy chain regions, i.e. junctional association.*

(b) *All VH and CH combinations prevent the association of functional H chains.*

(c) *During maturation, H chain gene rearrangement only ceases once a fully assembled, functional protein is produced.*

(d) *Further diversity may be introduced in the variable regions of heavy (but not light) chains through the addition of nucleotides which are not coded for by either of the gene segments to be joined.*

(e) *The insertion of additional nucleotides correlates with the level of activity of an enzyme called terminal deoxynucleoside transferase (TdT) and the type of nucleotide inserted reflects the preference of this enzyme for adenine nucleotides.*

3

THE INNATE IMMUNE RESPONSE

When tissue damage occurs as a result of trauma or infection, a complex series of cellular and biochemical events occur, which are designed to limit the spread of infection/degree of tissue damage, eliminate any microorganisms and repair the damaged tissue. Initially, these activities are limited to the innate immune response, i.e. they do not require specific identification of the precipitating organism but often a successful outcome requires the combined activity of both the innate and specific immune responses. In this chapter, we are going to look at the cellular and molecular events that occur early in a response to tissue damage – the innate immune response.

As a result of trauma and/or infection, cells in your tissues are damaged and release their contents into the lymph, which bathes the tissues. One of the earliest consequences of tissue damage or infection is the release of cytokines from activated tissue macrophages and mast cells, in particular the **colony-stimulating factors (CSF)** G(ranulocyte)-CSF and G(ranulocyte)M(onocyte)-CSF. This causes the release of granulocytes and monocytes from the bone marrow providing a ready reserve of these front-line cells. Other cytokines released include those responsible for the increased expression of **adhesion molecules** on the endothelial cells lining the blood vessels and on leukocytes in the vicinity. The interaction of these adhesion molecules allows cells to attach to the endothelium. Other factors released at the site of damage/infection affect the vascular tone and the integrity of the endothelial layer, giving attached cells the opportunity to escape into the underlying tissues. This they do in response to certain cytokines known as **chemokines**. Once at the site of infection/damage, the cells may actively **phagocytose** material recognised either through a group of molecules known as **pattern recognition receptors** or as a result of binding antibody or proteins of the **complement** pathways which encourage phagocytosis (i.e. they act as **opsonins**). As a result of phagocytosis, the organism may be destroyed by the action of **defensins** or antimicrobial enzymes found in the cellular granules. Alternatively, stimulation of the **oxidative (respiratory) burst**

Immunology for Life Scientists, Second Edition. Lesley-Jane Eales.
© 2003 John Wiley & Sons, Ltd: ISBN 0 470 84523 6 (HB); 0 470 84524 4 (PB)

may lead to the production of reactive oxygen radicals, which can destroy the microorganism. This chemical and cellular response involves a number of other cells and molecules, which collectively are known as the **inflammatory** response. It is intimately associated with the **kinin system** (responsible for the recognition of pain), the **clotting cascade** and the **fibrinolytic pathway**. The following sections describe some of these key mediators/functions in detail.

3.1 THE COMPLEMENT CASCADES

Complement is a term used to describe a group of serum and cell surface proteins, which have a number of important functions including lysis of cells and microorganisms, opsonisation of microorganisms (a mechanism which increases phagocytosis) and regulation of inflammatory and immune responses. Owing to these wide-ranging and often dramatic effects, the complement components are present as **inactive precursors** in the blood. There are three major pathways by which complement may be activated. These are the **classical**, **alternative** and **lectin pathways**.

The components of the complement system interact with each other in a sequential manner such that the product of one reaction forms the enzyme for the next. This leads to the formation of an enzyme complex, which binds and cleaves **C3** – the third component of the complement cascade. This component is central to the complement activation pathways and forms the point at which they converge. Subsequent components and complexes act to form the membrane attack complex (MAC), which ultimately causes lysis of the cell/ microorganism on which it forms.

Cleavage fragments of complement molecules are identified by an adjunct. Classically, the **small** fragments have been denoted by **a** (e.g. C3a, C5a) and the **large** fragments by **b** (e.g. C3b, C5b). Unfortunately, the fragments of **C2** do not follow this notation and the larger fragment is designated "a" and the smaller fragment is "b".

3.1.1 THE CLASSICAL COMPLEMENT PATHWAY

The classical complement pathway is normally activated by **immune complexes** (antibody bound to specific antigen), containing **IgG** or **IgM**, which bind to the first component, C1. In addition, the acute phase protein – C reactive protein – endotoxin (a component of some bacterial cell walls) and certain viruses may directly activate the classical pathway.

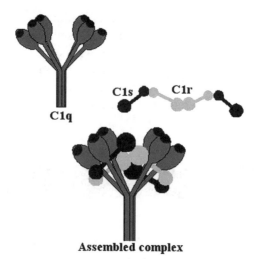

Assembled complex

Figure 3.1   Representation of the structure of the first component of the complement cascade
C1q comprises six subunits with globular heads and associates with two molecules each of C1s and C1r.

Table 3.1 Effectiveness of different classes of antibody in classical pathway activation		
Class	Subclass	Classical pathway
IgM		++++
IgG		
	IgG1	++++
	IgG2	+
	IgG3	+++
	IgG4	–
IgA		–
IgE		–
IgD		–

C1

C1 comprises three different types of molecule – **C1q**, **C1r** and **C1s** – which, in the presence of calcium, are held together (Figure 3.1). The Fc portion of an antibody in an immune complex binds to the globular heads of the **six subunits**, which comprise C1q. The affinity of C1q for immunoglobulin alone is very weak but when several antibodies are closely associated (as in an immune complex), the affinity of the binding is greatly increased. Not all forms of immunoglobulin bind to C1 with the same affinity; some classes are better than others at activating the classical complement pathway (Table 3.1).

The **enzymatic activity** of C1 resides in the **C1r** and **C1s** chains. Each molecule of C1 comprises one molecule of C1q and two molecules each of C1r and C1s. Binding of antibody to C1q leads to the cleavage of the two chains of C1r, which in turn cleaves the C1s chains into long and short fragments. This results in the appearance of an enzymatic site on C1s which acts on the next component in the pathway, **C4**.

C4

C4 has three chains, the largest of which – the alpha chain – is cleaved by C1s causing the release of a small fragment, C4a. The larger fragment – C4b – binds to the target antigen (an infected cell or a microorganism) via the formation of covalent amide or ester bonds. In the presence of magnesium ions, C4b bound to the target antigen is capable of interacting with, and binding, the next component of complement, C2.

C2

C2 is a single chain molecule, which binds to **C4b** and, in the presence of C1s, is cleaved. The larger fragment – **C2a** – contains the enzymatic site of the C2 molecule and remains in the complex whilst the smaller fragment is released. This new complex – **C4b2a** – acquires the ability to activate the next component in the classical pathway, C3. This complex is also known as the **classical pathway C3 convertase**[1] (Figure 3.2).

Both C4b and C2a have labile active sites and most of the molecules formed lose their binding sites before achieving association with membranes or with one another, diffusing away as inactive reaction products. In addition, C4b2a is unstable and quickly loses the C2 peptide, which becomes inactive upon dissociation. C4b bound to an activator can accept another molecule of C2 and, in the presence of active C1, will form an active enzyme capable of continuing the complement cascade.

C3

C3 has two disulphide-linked chains (α and β) and like C4 has an internal thiolester bond in the α chain. When this bond is cleaved, the molecule undergoes a conformational change, which leads to an alteration in its biochemical properties.

---

[1] You may see this referred to as C4b2b in some texts that do not use the classical notation.

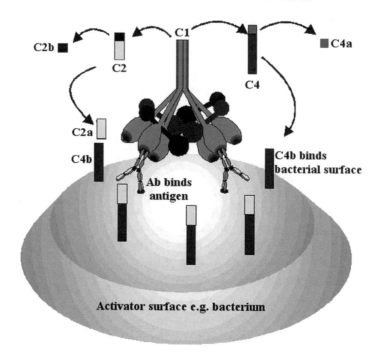

Figure 3.2   Formation of the classical pathway C3 convertase
C1 is activated by immune complexes and splits C4 and C2. C4b binds the activator surface and C2a to form the C3 convertase. The C4a and C2b are soluble fragments with other biological properties.

When C4b2a acts on C3, a small peptide is cleaved from the α chain, **C3a**. This exposes a thioester bond in the remaining fragment – **C3b** – which will interact with any suitable acceptor in the environment (e.g. molecules with exposed reactive hydroxyl or amino groups). If this thiolester bond does not form a covalent bond with an appropriate acceptor, it is hydrolysed through interaction with water in the tissues. The majority of cleaved C3 molecules fail to bind to an activator.

The attachment of C3b to membranes leads to the formation of **C4b2a3b**, which is covalently bound to the antigen (via the C3 thiolester linkage) and forms the **classical pathway C5 convertase** (Figure 3.3). This cleaves C5 into two fragments – C5a and C5b – the larger of which, C5b, associates with the convertase and can interact with subsequent components of the complement cascade leading to lysis of membranes and microorganisms.

The smaller fragments released by the actions of the enzymes of the classical complement pathway – i.e. **C3a**, **C4a** and **C5a** – have a number of potent biological effects which are important in inflammation and will be discussed later.

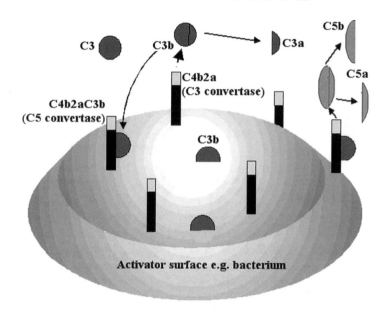

Figure 3.3 Formation of the classical pathway C5 convertase
The C3 convertase attached to the activator splits C3, the larger fragment of which (C3b) attaches to the activator leading to the formation of C4b2a3b which is covalently bound to the antigen and forms the classical pathway C5 convertase.

3.1.2 THE ALTERNATIVE COMPLEMENT PATHWAY

In the alternative complement pathway, C3 exists in two molecular forms: the native form, which circulates in the serum, and a conformationally altered form in which the thiolester bond has been hydrolysed. This altered C3 can bind another factor in the presence of magnesium ions – Factor B of the alternative pathway. In the presence of Factor D (a serine protease), Factor B may be cleaved giving rise to the fragment Bb. These proteins are analogous to the C4b, C2 and C1 of the classical pathway respectively. Together they form the alternative pathway C3 convertase – C3bBb (Figure 3.4). Like the convertase of the classical pathway, it catalyses the breakdown of C3 to C3a and C3b. The C3b so formed may either continue the alternative pathway activation by binding Factor B or it may bind the C3 convertase to form the alternative pathway C5 convertase – $(C3b)_n Bb$. This compound is extremely unstable under normal physiological conditions and is stabilised by another serum protein – properdin ($C3b_n PBb$).

Activation of the alternative pathway may be achieved through the presence of surfaces to which the conformationally altered C3 may attach, e.g. rabbit erythrocytes, Gram-negative bacteria, aggregates of IgA and certain

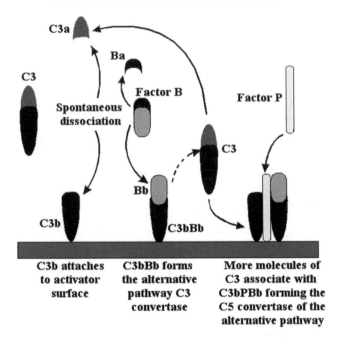

Figure 3.4 Formation of the alternative pathway C3 convertase
C3 can naturally exist in an altered form which can bind Factor B of the alternative pathway. In the presence of Factor D (a serine protease), Factor B may be cleaved – Bb. These proteins are analogous to the C4b, C2 and C1 of the classical pathway respectively. Together they form the alternative pathway C3 convertase – C3bBb.

B-lymphocytes. Once attached, the alternative pathway C3 convertase becomes highly active and is able to act on large numbers of C3 molecules to produce C3a and C3b. Like the classical pathway, the alternative pathway may be activated by immune complexes, IgA-containing complexes being the most efficient (Table 3.2).

Table 3.2 Effectiveness of different classes of antibody in alternative pathway activation

Class	Subclass	Classical pathway
IgM		++
IgG		
	IgG1	++
	IgG2	++
	IgG3	++
	IgG4	++
IgA		+++
IgE		++
IgD		++

3.1.3 THE LECTIN PATHWAY

The third complement activation pathway is the lectin pathway (Figure 3.5). Lectins are carbohydrate-binding proteins, which are able to bind to a wide range of microorganisms. There are two major types found in serum: the **ficollins** (consisting of a fibrinogen- and a collagen-like domain) and the mannose-binding lectin (MBL). Both of these lectins can activate complement. Like the classical pathway, which involves the activation of the serine proteases C1r and C1s, the lectin pathway is activated by the binding of carbohydrates on pathogens followed by the activation of two novel serine proteases (MBL-associated serine proteases – MASPs), which are responsible for the subsequent activation of the lectin pathway. The structural similarities between the initial activating complexes of the classical and lectin pathways suggest that the former may have evolved from the latter to take advantage of the evolution of the specific immune response and the presence of immune complexes.

MBL is a member of a family of proteins containing a collagen-like domain and a carbohydrate recognition domain (CRD) as is seen in C1q. These proteins are called **collectins**. Structurally, MBL consists of three identical chains but these structures can cross-link giving a final structure similar to that of C1q. MBL binds certain carbohydrates such as mannose and N-acetyl glucosamine (GlcNAc) on bacterial surfaces. It associates with MASPs, the whole structure

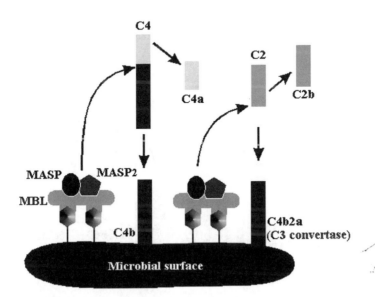

Figure 3.5 Lectin pathway of complement activation
Carbohydrates on pathogens bind to mannose-binding lectin (MBL) or ficollins found in the serum. This causes the activation of MASPs (MBL-associated serine proteases – MASPs), which activate the lectin pathway in a manner analogous to C1q.

forming the first active enzyme in the complement cascade. MASP 1 cleaves C3 and C2 while MASP 2 cleaves C4 and C2.

MASPs also associate with ficollins. Ficollins possess a fibrinogen-like domain responsible for binding to carbohydrates. They do not bind mannose but bind GlcNAc in proximity to galactose and elastin. Thus, these lectins bind a distinct range of carbohydrates compared to MBL. In addition, ficollins are found expressed on cell membranes such as monocytes and aid in the phagocytosis of organisms such as *E. coli*.

3.1.4   THE MEMBRANE ATTACK COMPLEX

The **membrane attack complex (MAC)** is formed by complement components C5 to C9. Upon attachment to its convertase (derived from either the classical or alternative pathways), C5 is cleaved into C5a and C5b. The latter binds to its ligand, C6. Failure to do so results in its swift inactivation. The C5b6 complex so formed binds C7. The resulting complex, being relatively hydrophobic, interacts with lipids present in the membranes surrounding the immunogen (Figure 3.6).

The C7 molecule, when bound to the C5b6 complex, can insert in the membrane and may bind a single molecule of C8. The resulting small, highly charged channel is stabilised by the incorporation of several molecules of C9 giving rise to a cylindrical, pore-like structure which spans the membrane (Figure 3.7). The stability of this membrane attack complex – $C5b678(9)_n$ –

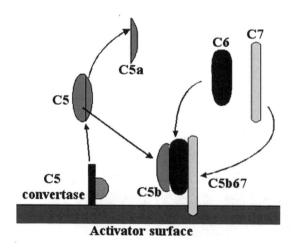

Figure 3.6   Formation of the C5b67 complex
The C5 convertase splits C5, allowing the fragment C5b to attach to the antigen. This binds to C6 and the C5b6 complex so formed binds C7. This complex is relatively hydrophobic and interacts with lipids present in the membranes surrounding the antigen.

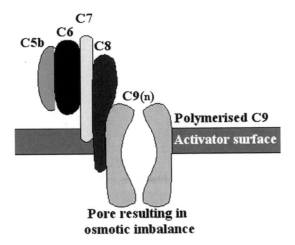

Figure 3.7 Formation of the membrane attack complex
The C7 molecule, when bound to the C5b6 complex, can insert in the membrane and may bind a single molecule of C8. The resulting small, highly charged channel is stabilised by the incorporation of several molecules of C9 giving rise to a cylindrical, pore-like structure which causes lysis of the cell.

arises from the association between the hydrophobic exterior of the MAC with membrane lipids. The hydrophilic interior of the channel allows the loss of water and small ions from the target cell, thus eliminating its osmotic and chemical balance and resulting in lysis.

3.1.5 REGULATION OF COMPLEMENT ACTIVATION

Since the formation of the MAC is antigen-independent and may attach to cell surfaces in the vicinity and cause lysis of nearby host cells, it is vital to maintain strict control of the complement system. It has powerful lytic and inflammatory activities and if uncontrolled may lead to serious tissue damage.

Neither the classical, nor the alternative pathway can be activated by antibody alone; it must be bound to antigen to be effective. In addition, a single antibody molecule bound to antigen is ineffectual; more than one must coat the antigen before complement can be activated. This limitation is probably an important method of regulation since relatively large amounts of specific antibody must be formed before complement activation can occur. Infections, which are controlled quickly and effectively by other mechanisms, may only stimulate a small antibody response. If the organism has already been eliminated, activation of complement would probably lead to pathology (tissue damage). By contrast, a poorly controlled infection with increasing microorganismal load will stimulate a strong antibody response leading to complement activation, which may help to eliminate the infecting agent.

However, complement may be activated in the absence of specific antibody and so regulation at different stages of activation is achieved through the involvement of other proteins.

C1 INHIBITOR (C1INH)

This prevents the function of activated C1s and C1r by binding to their active sites. It also inhibits activated **Hageman factor** (one of the components of the **clotting cascade**) and all the systems activated by Hageman factor fragments. Thus, C1INH regulates enzymes of the **kinin-generating system** (chemicals which stimulate the sensation of pain), the **clotting system** and the **fibrinolytic system** (molecules involved in the regulation of blood clotting and wound repair). The importance of this regulatory protein in prevention of pathological damage is evidenced by the immunodeficiency disease **hereditary angioedema** (**HAE**) where sufferers are unable to produce normal levels of functional C1INH. This is discussed further in Section 5.3.

REGULATORS OF COMPLEMENT ACTIVATION (RCA) FAMILY

These proteins downregulate the activity of C3 convertases in the classical and alternative pathways, either by causing their decay and/or by acting as cofactors for the serine protease Factor I in the breakdown of C3b and C4b.

One member of the RCA family is the **C4-binding protein** (C4BP). As its name suggests, it binds C4b which may be cleaved (and therefore inactivated) by the protease Factor I. The latter, in the presence of another member of the RCA family, Factor H, may cleave the α chain of hydrolysed C3 or C3b to form a partially degraded molecule, iC3b. This molecule does not play a part in the complement cascade but is capable of promoting phagocytosis. In addition, under appropriate conditions, Factor I can degrade iC3b further to C3dg. Regulation by Factors I and H is dependent upon the surface to which C3b is bound. If the surface is that of a microorganism, the C3b is protected from Factors H and I, which are unable to bind, and the complement cascade proceeds to its termination with the formation of the MAC. By contrast, when C3b is bound to host cell membranes, Factors H and I are able to interact with it causing its degradation and preventing the continuation of the pathway. This difference in ability to bind to certain surfaces appears to be related to the presence of charged carbohydrates such as sialic acid on mammalian cells, which promote the binding of Factor H. Other members of the RCA family are shown in Table 3.3.

Table 3.3   Some members of the RCA family and their activities

RCA component	Activity
CR1 (CD35)	Unknown
CR2 (CD21)	Expressed on B cells and is a receptor for breakdown products of C3 including C3dg
CD46 (membrane cofactor protein)	Found on a wide variety of human cells and binds C3/C4
CD55 (decay-accelerating factor)	Promotes breakdown of the two C3 convertases and is expressed on many human cells

REGULATORS OF THE MEMBRANE ATTACK COMPLEX

Regulation of the formation of the membrane attack complex also occurs. Vitronectin (S protein) binds to C5b67 complexes and prevents their binding to cell membranes. Although C8 and C9 can still bind to the complex in the fluid phase it cannot insert into membranes and cause lysis.

KEY POINTS FOR REVIEW

- *Complement is a group of serum proteins that are in an inactive state but when appropriately stimulated, form an enzyme cascade designed to stimulate inflammation and kill infectious agents.*
- *There are three main complement activation pathways: the classical, alternative and lectin pathways.*
- *The classical pathway of complement is activated through C1q binding to immune complexes.*
- *The classical pathway involves the activity of C1–C5.*
- *The alternative pathway is activated by a shift in the normal metabolic 'tick-over' of C3 by partially hydrolysed C3 binding to the surface of micro-organisms.*
- *The alternative pathway involves the activity of components designated as factors.*
- *The lectin pathway is activated by microorganisms.*
- *The membrane attack complex can directly lyse microorganisms.*
- *Byproducts of the activation of complement such as C3a and C5a are anaphylatoxins which cause inflammation.*
- *Byproducts also act as chemoattractant for immunologically active cells.*

• *The complement pathways are highly damaging and therefore are tightly regulated to prevent unnecessary host cell damage.*

3.2 PHAGOCYTOSIS

The process of phagocytosis may be divided into a number of sequential stages: recognition, ingestion and digestion; we shall discuss each of these in turn. Although tissue macrophages are often the first cells to encounter and ingest an invading microorganism, they are not very efficient at killing. This is best achieved by neutrophils, which may be attracted to the site of infection as a result of mediators released by macrophages (chemokines). Neutrophils are by far the most efficient of the professional phagocytes. However, newly recruited macrophages (derived from blood monocytes attracted to the site of infection) also show the ability to kill phagocytosed organisms. Eosinophils, which are also efficient killers, are geared to killing extracellular pathogens that are too large to phagocytose such as parasites like *Schistosoma* spp.

3.2.1 PATTERN RECOGNITION RECEPTORS

Once at the site of inflammation, phagocytes have to recognise the causative agent. They have a number of cell surface receptors, which help to identify the agent as foreign and attach to them. These receptors are known as **pattern recognition receptors** and bind to groups of molecules known as **pathogen-associated molecular patterns** (PAMPs). These PAMPs have three chief characteristics: (i) they are found on microorganisms and not on host cells; (ii) their structure is relatively constant within a given group of organisms; (iii) they are essential for microbial survival. PAMPs are the ligands for pattern recognition receptors (PRR) on host cells, which allow the innate system to discriminate between "self" and "non-self" in a general manner. These pattern recognition receptors may be secreted (e.g. lipopolysaccharide-binding protein, mannose-binding protein), membrane bound (e.g. CR3, CD14, Toll-like receptors (TLRs), macrophage scavenger receptor, mannose receptor, surfactant protein A receptor) or intracellular. PRRs are found on the surface of those cells recruited early in an immune response, i.e. neutrophils, mononuclear phagocytes and NK cells. These cells rapidly respond to microbial invaders owing to recognition of non-self via pattern recognition receptors. Some of these will be described below.

COMPLEMENT RECEPTOR 3 (CR3)

CR3 (CD11b/CD18) is a member of a group of molecules known as the alpha$_2$ integrins. The members of this family share a common molecule – CD18 – and are expressed only on white blood cells. Other major members of the family include leukocyte function antigen-1 (LFA-1 or CD11a/CD18) and CR4 (CD11c/CD18). LFA-1 promotes migration of neutrophils and T cells across the endothelium and acts in concert with CR3 to promote migration of monocytes. CR3 provides a critical link between cells and the extracellular matrix. It exists in both inactive and active states. When activated, it promotes phagocytosis by binding complement opsonised microorganisms. In addition to its ability to bind to the extracellular matrix, C3bi and its cellular counter-receptors (intercellular adhesion molecules 1 and 2), CR3 is also able to bind to a range of molecules found on the surface of microbes including lipopolysaccharide (LPS), polysaccharides from *Mycobacterium tuberculosis* and zymosan from yeast.

CD14

CD14 is expressed on monocytes, macrophages and on neutrophils. It binds to lipopolysaccharide (either alone or in conjunction with the soluble LPS-binding protein). It is also known to bind to the exotoxin *Staphylococcus aureus* protein A and the lipoarabinomannan from mycobacteria. Recent studies suggest that CD14 acts in cooperation with members of the Toll family to discriminate between ligands, CD14 acting as the signalling unit directing the cellular response to the ligand.

TOLL-LIKE RECEPTORS

Toll receptors were first identified in the fruitfly *Drosophila*. Structurally similar molecules were subsequently identified in mammals and the group of molecules have been defined both structurally and functionally. These TLRs are able to discriminate between different PAMPs leading to the stimulation of an appropriate immune response. The binding affinities of the Toll receptors are shown in Table 3.4.

TLR4 has been demonstrated on the surface of macrophages and dendritic cells, its activation causing upregulation of co-stimulatory molecules, increased antigen presentation, secretion of proinflammatory cytokines and microbicidal activity.

Most TLRs show limitations in the range of PAMPs that they recognise. TLR2 does not appear to do so. However, it has been suggested that perhaps TLRs are able to associate with each other to form heterodimers with distinct ligands, thus explaining the apparent promiscuity of TLR2.

Table 3.4   Binding specificities of human Toll-like receptors

TLR	Function
TLR2	Lipotechoic acid, peptidoglycan, lipoarabinomannan, lipopeptide, atypical LPS
TLR3	Viral double-stranded RNA
TLR4	Lipopolysaccharide (LPS)
TLR5	Bacterial flagellin
TLR9	CpG DNA

The binding of a ligand to a Toll receptor results in the production of cytokines such as interleukin 1 and tumour necrosis factor. This is achieved through the interaction of a series of cytoplasmic molecules that transduce the signal from the receptor to the nucleus resulting in the transcription of specific genes (see Figure 3.8).

MACROPHAGE SCAVENGER RECEPTORS

There are two classes of scavenger receptors, SR-A and SR-B. The class A macrophage scavenger receptor (SR-A) was identified as one of the main receptors mediating the endocytosis of lipids by macrophages. However, as more functions have been attributed to these receptors (including macrophage growth and maintenance, adhesion to the substratum, cell–cell interactions, phagocytosis and host defence), it is thought that their earliest evolutionary roles involved their scavenger function related to innate immunity but that they have evolved to play a vital role in cellular transport of fatty acid and the regulation of angiogenesis.

SR-A: The class A macrophage scavenger receptors bind to modified low-density lipoproteins (LDLs) such as oxidised LDL and acetylated LDL. Three class A scavenger receptors have been identified. SR-AI and SR-AII are encoded by the same gene and the third receptor – MARCO (macrophage receptor with collagenous structure) – has a structure related to SR-AI. MARCO is expressed on a subgroup of macrophages. These cells are found in distinct tissue locations and are thought to be important in scavenging foreign material and debris. By contrast, SR-A is found on all macrophages and on some endothelial cells.

SR-B: The class B scavenger receptor family includes the molecule CD36, which is expressed on the endothelium of the microvasculature, dendritic cells, platelets, monocytes and macrophages. Initially, the chief role of CD36 was thought to be facilitation of cell–cell (platelets and monocytes) and tumour cell–extracellular matrix interactions but recent work has demonstrated its role in cellular lipid transport.

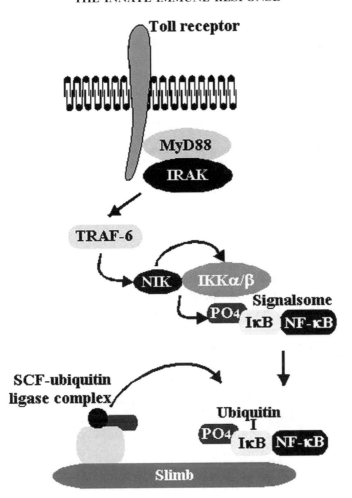

Figure 3.8   Toll receptor signalling
Upon activation the Toll receptor binds the adapter molecule MyD88 which has a modular structure:
the C-terminal domain binds the TollR whilst the N-terminal portion is a "death-domain" module,
which recruits the IL-1R-associated kinase (IRAK) to the signalling complex. Downstream, IRAK
interacts with the adapter molecule tumour necrosis factor receptor-associated factor 6 (TRAF6)
that binds them to the protein kinase NF-kB-inducing kinase (NIK). Activated IKK phosphorylates
IκBα in the NFκB signalsome leading to recognition by the specific ubiquitin–protein ligase
complex (SCF–ubiquitin–Slimb) resulting in the association of ubiquitin with the signalsome. This
leads to the rapid degradation of IκB, exposing the active NFκB which translocates to the nucleus
and initiates transcription of the target genes.

*CD36 is the receptor for thrombospondin-1 (TSP-1) which is found in the extracellular
matrix and platelet α granules. TSP-1 is involved in cell–cell interactions, cellular
proliferation, TGFβ activation and angiogenesis.*

3.2.2 OPSONISATION

Once recognition has occurred, the attachment between cell and microbe may be enhanced by the presence of **opsonins**.

> *An opsonin is something that coats a particle and makes it easier to phagocytose. For example, complement activation at the site of inflammation causes C3b to be deposited on the causative agent (which may be a microorganism or an inert particle). Both neutrophils and macrophages have receptors for C3b, which allows them to bind the complement-coated particles.*

There are three main types of opsonin: IgG antibodies, fragments of the complement protein C3 and the lectins described earlier. Each may act as a bridge between the particle and the phagocytic cell. Acute phase proteins (such as C reactive protein (**CRP**)) can bind to the surface of microorganisms and, having a structure similar to C1, activate the classical complement pathway leading to opsonisation by complement.

Molecules that bind IgG (Fc gamma receptors or **FcγR**) and those binding carbohydrates (lectins) are always in an active state and stimulate ingestion immediately following ligand–receptor interaction. By contrast, the C3-fragment receptors (Table 3.5) are inactive and require a further signal in the form of fibronectin or an **acute phase protein** before activation may occur.

However, it has been shown that C3bi on the surface of bacteria or fungi may bind to CR3 and trigger phagocytosis due to the interaction between polysaccharides on the microbial surface and a lectin-like site on CR3.

3.2.3 INGESTION

The process of taking extracellular material inside a cell is known as **endocytosis**. The active uptake of particulate material through the formation

Table 3.5	Complement receptors involved in opsonisation
Receptor	Ligands
CR1	C3b
CR2	C3dg > C3d > iC3b > C3b
CR3	C3bi

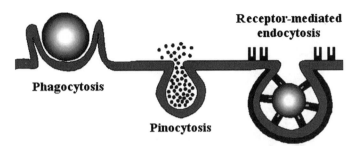

Figure 3.9 Illustration of the different methods for uptake of extracellular material
The process of taking extracellular material inside a cell is known as endocytosis. The active uptake of particulate material through the formation of pseudopodia is known as phagocytosis. Pinocytosis is the process by which cells take up soluble material.

of finger-like projections of cell membrane and cytoplasm (pseudopodia) is known as **phagocytosis**. **Pinocytosis** is the process by which cells take up soluble material (Figure 3.9).

The process of phagocytosis involves alterations in the cell membrane caused by changes in the structure of the cytoskeleton, the latter also affecting cell motility. When a particle attaches to a phagocyte (either non-specifically through chemical attraction or specifically via receptor–ligand interaction), phagocytosis is only initiated if the cell surface signals are sufficient to activate the process. Additional required signals include receptor clustering, receptor activation through co-stimulation by cytokines, chemoattractants or other microbial products, or cooperation with another type of receptor. Once the cell has been activated, the cell membrane forms pseudopodia that surround the particle. They ultimately fuse together, engulfing the particle in a membrane-bound vesicle known as a **phagosome**. Once formed, the phagosome moves to the interior of the cell where degradation of its contents occurs (Figure 3.10).

The process of phagocytosis is achieved by the transformation of the fluid cytoplasm (**cytosol**) into a gel by interaction with actin-binding proteins located on the inner surface of the cell membrane. This gelation results from the polymerisation of **actin** in the cytoplasm to form filaments which connect with each other and with **myosin**, giving a more rigid gel-like consistency, and is stimulated by the activation signal received as a result of the occupancy of an opsonin receptor. The activated actin transmits a signal to the myosin, which contracts leading to the streaming of the cytosol pushing the plasma membrane in one direction and thus forming the pseudopod (Figure 3.11). This reorganisation of the cytoskeleton is regulated by a family of small GTPases known as Rho (Rho, Rac and Cdc42). Members of this family have clearly defined roles in the process. CR3-mediated phagocytosis requires the activity of Rho and through sequential **ligand–receptor binding** (the zipper effect) results in a tight-fitting phagosome. In contrast to this, FcR-mediated phagocytosis depends on the activity of Rac and Cdc42 resulting in a more spacious phagosome. These differences between CR3- and FcR-mediated phagocytosis

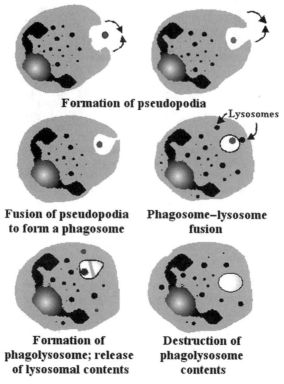

Figure 3.10   Phagocytosis

may also explain the lack of an oxidative burst and other proinflammatory signals in the former but not the latter, since Rho is not involved in the activation of NADPH oxidase.

3.2.4   DIGESTION

Digestion of the phagosomal contents is achieved by a variety of enzymes, which are introduced into the phagosome when cytoplasmic granules (polymorphs) and lysosomes (polymorphs and mononuclear phagocytes) empty their contents into the phagosome. These membrane-bound organelles fuse with the phagosomal membrane forming a larger **phagolysosome**. This fusion may start before the phagosome is closed and thus, destructive enzymes may be released outside the cell, resulting in the tissue damage associated with some immunological reactions.

One of the first events to occur immediately after ingestion is the acidification of the phagosome. This starts before the granule contents are released and is caused

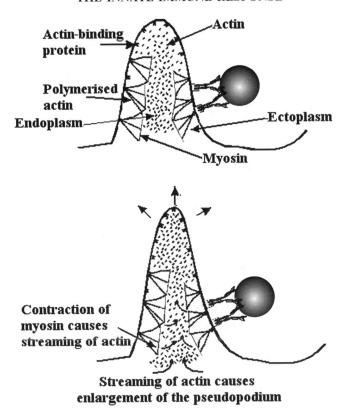

Figure 3.11 Intracellular processes leading to pseudopodia formation
Pseudopodium formation is thought to occur due to the transformation of the fluid cytoplasm (cytosol) into a gel by interaction with actin-binding proteins located on the inner surface of the cell membrane. This gelation results from the polymerisation of actin in the cytoplasm to form filaments which connect with each other and myosin, giving a more rigid gel-like consistency. The activated actin transmits a signal to the myosin which contracts leading to the streaming of the cytosol which pushes the plasma membrane in one direction thus forming the pseudopod.

by the accumulation of lactic acid and hydrogen ions produced by the **respiratory burst**. The hydrogen ions are actively moved into the lysosomes by special pumps, which derive their energy from **adenosine triphosphate (ATP)**. The pH rapidly reduces to about 4, assisted by the release of the acidic granule contents. Few microorganisms can survive or multiply in an acid environment and the lysosomal enzymes that bring about their destruction are most efficient at a low pH.

Once the contents of the phagolysosome have been destroyed, the debris must be eliminated. Some products of degradation may be re-used, such as amino acids, nucleotides, sugars and lipids. Other, more indigestible parts, may be **exocytosed** (although this is undesirable since tissue-damaging enzymes are released at the same time), or may be stored within the cell until it dies and is eliminated from the body, e.g. in the faeces or sputum.

3.2.5 THE RESPIRATORY BURST

Upon activation, the phagocyte undergoes a respiratory burst (also known as the **oxidative** or **metabolic burst**), which is characterised by a rapid, marked increase in the consumption of oxygen by the cell and results in the production of toxic oxygen metabolites. Mitochondrial enzymes normally mediate respiration. However, the respiratory burst involves the action of a group of enzymes found in the cytoplasm and associated with the membrane of the phagosome known as the **nicotinamide adenine diphosphate oxidase (NADP-oxidase)**. The principal effect of this group of enzymes is to convert molecular oxygen to the **superoxide anion** – a highly reactive molecule, which has two unpaired electrons each available for association with another electron. Addition of one electron leads to the formation of **superoxide**; a second electron converts it to **peroxide** (Figure 3.12). This conversion is mediated by the

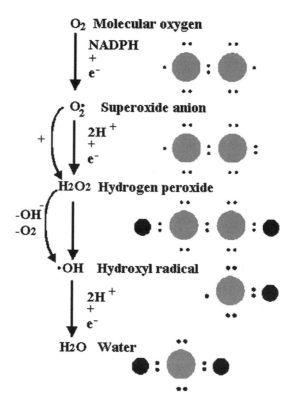

Figure 3.12   Conversion of molecular oxygen to reactive intermediates
The respiratory burst involves the action of a group of enzymes known as the nicotinamide adenine diphosphate oxidase (NADPH-oxidase). These enzymes convert molecular oxygen to the superoxide anion − a highly reactive molecule which has two unpaired electrons each available for association with another electron. Addition of one electron leads to the formation of superoxide; a second electron converts it to peroxide.

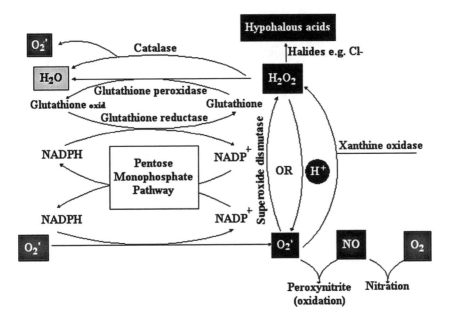

Figure 3.13 The production of toxic oxygen metabolites and other microbicidal compounds during the oxidative burst

reduced form of **NADP (NADPH)**. Interaction between superoxide and hydrogen peroxide leads to the formation of the hydroxyl anion or radical. All molecules with unpaired electrons are called **free radicals**. They are highly unstable and are capable of damaging proteins, lipids, DNA and cell membranes. Thus, they may be responsible for the destruction of phagocytosed microorganisms. Normally, endogenous, scavenger, enzymes (e.g. superoxide dismutase, catalase, glutathione peroxidase) destroy free radicals and hydrogen peroxide. However, in activated phagocytes they are produced in greater quantities than can be destroyed allowing them to accumulate and indeed to be secreted by the cells. Although the oxygen radicals are extremely short lived, **superoxide** and H_2O_2 are released in the tissues; their persistence (and hence the degree of resulting tissue damage) depends on the ability of the cells in the locality to destroy them. In addition to these toxic oxygen metabolites, other microbicidal compounds are generated during the oxidative burst including hypohalous acids (Figure 3.13).

3.2.6 OTHER ANTIMICROBIAL ACTIVITIES OF LYSOSOMES

As we have discovered in the previous section, lysosomes contain a wide variety of enzymes and chemicals involved in the destruction of microorganisms. One of the major granule constituents in neutrophils is a group of proteins that have broad-spectrum antimicrobial activity against bacteria, fungi, mycobacteria and enveloped viruses. These proteins, which are found in a wide range of other cells, are highly conserved between species and are known as **defensins**.

DEFENSINS

There are two main types of defensin, the α defensins found in neutrophils and the Paneth cells of the small intestine and the β defensins found in a range of other tissues including the skin, salivary glands and airway epithelial cells.

Defensins are usually linear polypeptides that are folded, their conformation being maintained by intra-chain disulphide bonds. These molecules are positively charged and therefore interact with negatively charged PAMPs from microbial membranes such as lipopolysaccharide from Gram-negative bacteria and lipotechoic acid from Gram-positive bacteria. Thus, defensins are electrostatically specific for microbial cells. The production of defensins is positively regulated by the interaction between PRRs and PAMPs.

It has been suggested that defensins aggregate to form pores in the cytoplasmic membranes of Gram-positive bacteria. In Gram-negative bacteria, the defensins, which have a high affinity for LPS, are thought to displace the stabilising Ca^{2+} and Mg^{2+} ions from the outer membrane, leading to disruption.

Defensins can also activate the classical complement pathway and, through their ability to regulate cytokine production and adhesion molecule expression, may influence the inflammatory response.

α-Defensins: These are preformed as pre-propetides that are processed enzymatically and stored as the functional peptide in the granules of neutrophils. They stimulate chemotaxis in monocytes, dendritic and T cells at concentrations as low as 10^{-10} M. In addition, α-defensins inhibit fibrinolysis by modulating tissue-type plasminogen activator and plasminogen binding to fibrin and endothelial cells. Thus, in pathological conditions, defensins released in the circulation may adhere to the endothelium and contribute to the inflammatory process.

β-Defensins: These are constitutively expressed in epithelial cells, their expression being increased as a result of infection or inflammation. They may influence the immune response by binding to the chemokine receptor CCR6 on dendritic and memory T cells.

KEY POINTS FOR REVIEW

- *Phagocytosis may be considered to have a number of phases, recognition and attachment, ingestion and digestion.*

- *Pattern recognition receptors on phagocytes bind to pathogen-associated molecular patterns, which are not found on host cells.*
- *CR3 is an alpha$_2$ integrin providing a critical link between cells and the extracellular matrix.*
- *CD14 is found on monocytes, macrophages and neutrophils and binds lipopolysaccharide, Staphylococcus aureus enterotoxin A and lipoarabino-mannan.*
- *Toll-like receptors discriminate between pathogen-associated molecular patterns, binding of which produces lymphokines that influence the immune response.*
- *Macrophage scavenger receptors play an important role in the transport of fatty acids and regulation of angiogenesis.*
- *Opsonins such as antibody, complement fragments and acute phase proteins enhance phagocytosis.*
- *Material taken up by phagocytes is broken down in acidified endosomes, which fuse with lysosomes.*
- *The respiratory burst that may occur as a result of phagocytosis produces reactive oxygen intermediates that are toxic to microorganisms.*
- *Other antimicrobial products of phagocytes include the defensins, which can destroy bacteria and activate complement.*

3.3 INFLAMMATION

Inflammation is the body's reaction to an injury such as invasion by a microorganism or mechanical or chemical damage and is characterised by five cardinal signs: heat (calor), pain (dolor), redness (rubor), swelling (tumour) and (in extreme cases) loss of function. The response may be initiated by the release of chemicals from damaged tissue cells either as a direct response to trauma or as a result of factors released from microorganisms such as toxins. However, it is difficult to define precisely what triggers the inflammatory response since it involves a large number of different cells and mediators. All the events occurring during inflammation are geared towards increasing the local blood flow (caused by dilation of the blood vessels) and the permeability of the vasculature (blood vessels). This allows cells and serum components increased access to the area of tissue damage in order to limit the spread of infection and tissue damage and to promote healing.

The inflammatory process involves the concerted action of the **immune, kinin, fibrinolytic** and **clotting systems** which interact to maintain the integrity of the vascular system and to limit the spread of infection/damage. Figure 3.14 illustrates the complexity of the interaction between the components of the

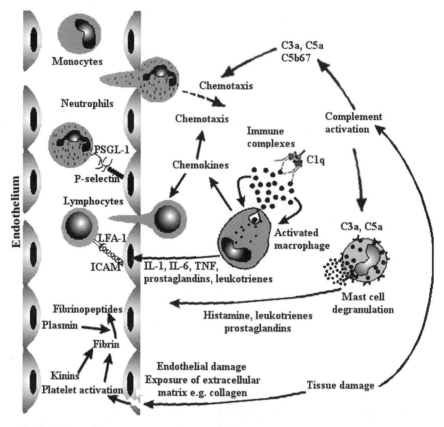

Figure 3.14   The cells and chemicals involved in inflammation
As a result of infection or tissue damage, complement is activated leading to the release of complement fragments that can activate local mast cells leading to the release of vasoactive chemicals such as leukotrienes, prostaglandins and histamine. These agents and a range of cytokines are also released by activated tissue macrophages. They have an effect on the local endothelium increasing the expression of a range of adhesion molecules (ICAM, P-selectin), encouraging the tethering, rolling and immobilisation of leukocytes. Chemokines and chemotaxins (such as C3a, C5a) released in the tissues encourage local extravasation of leukocytes where they are able to remove damaged tissue and any causative agents and initiate repair. Endothelial damage leads to platelet activation and the formation of fibrin, breakdown of which by plasmin results in the formation of chemotactic fibrinopeptides. This ensures a constant supply of leukocytes at the site of damage, ensuring repair of any tissue damage.

inflammatory response. The following sections will describe some of the chemicals and cellular functions involved in inflammation.

3.3.1   INFLAMMATORY MEDIATORS

Toxins from microorganisms and enzymes from the lysosomes of polymorphs cause or enhance tissue damage through the release of chemicals from a variety of cells. Amongst these are the **prostaglandins (PGs)** and **leukotrienes (LTs)**, which belong to a family of unsaturated fatty acids derived from **arachidonic acid** (a component of most cell membranes) by the phospholipase A2/ cyclooxygenase and 5-lipoxygenase pathways. Prostaglandins cause blood vessel dilatation and enhance the effects of histamine and bradykinin on vascular permeability. Leukotrienes stimulate the migration of leukocytes into the tissues. Interestingly, metabolites of prostaglandins help resolve inflammation through the inhibition of key intracellular molecules involved in gene transcription. Thus, the different molecules produced during inflammation have different effects but overall are responsible for the induction of pain, fever, vascular permeability and chemotaxis of polymorphonuclear leukocytes (Table 3.6).

Although mast cells and basophils are the principle producers of these inflammatory mediators, other cells such as eosinophils, neutrophils and platelets are also capable of doing so. Substances released as a result of tissue damage may activate mast cells. Their degranulation results in the release of **vasoactive amines** such as **histamine**. In addition, basophils and platelets release both **histamine** and **serotonin (5-hydroxytryptamine)**. These mediators cause increased **capillary permeability**. They are also important in the repair of tissue damage as demonstrated in patients treated with large doses of anti-histamines. Such individuals showed considerable impairment in the healing of surgical wounds. Indeed, evidence suggests that histamine (and perhaps other inflammatory mediators) may play a role in normal growth – especially foetal growth.

When tissue injury occurs, enzymes are released and surfaces are exposed which cause the activation of **Hageman factor** (Factor XII) of the **clotting cascade**. This in turn activates, and is activated by, Factor XI of the clotting cascade and **kallikrein** of the **kinin system**. The kinin system (a series of serum peptides which are sequentially activated) produces **bradykinin**, which causes pain, vasodilation and increased capillary permeability. This allows cells and serum proteins such as components of the complement cascade to pass into the tissues at the site of injury. If microorganisms are present at the site, the complement cascade may be activated and fragments of complement, particularly C3a and C5a, are released. These have dramatic, proinflammatory effects, which are summarised in Table 3.7. Indeed, studies in complement-deficient animal models have suggested that complement activation is vital for the development of acute inflammation.

3.3.2 CELLULAR RESPONSES IN INFLAMMATION

As a result of the action of inflammatory mediators, the flow of cells within the blood vessels slows, the cells becoming located along the walls of the vessel. The

Table 3.6 Biochemical mediators of inflammation

Substance	Chemistry	Produced by/from	Characteristics/functions
Heparin	Proteo-glycan	Degranulation of mast cells	It is an anti-coagulant, i.e. it prevents blood clotting. It temporarily suspends blood clotting allowing inflammatory cells to enter the area of tissue injury
Histamine	Vasoactive amine	Mast cells and basophils. Stored in cytoplasmic granules	Released on degranulation caused by cross-linking of FcR. Acts on endothelial cells of blood vessels causing them to become less tightly associated. This makes the blood vessels "leaky", allowing inflammatory cells and serum proteins, such as Ab and complement to enter the area of tissue damage. Also causes the contraction of bronchiolar and vascular smooth muscle and increased secretion by nasal and bronchial mucous glands. Effects are maximal after 1–2 minutes and last for $\sim$10 minutes
Serotonin (5-hydroxy-tryptamine)	Derived from tryptophan	Platelet granules. Released during blood clotting	A neurotransmitter in the central nervous system. Its ability to cause leakage from the blood vessels derives from its effect on the endothelial cells which become partially detached from each other
Kinins	Small basic peptides	Kallikreins (arginine esterases) act on kininogens – large proteins in the plasma – to give kinins	Affect the movement of smooth muscle, increase vascular permeability and vasodilation and induce pain. Bradykinin is a 9 amino acid peptide derived from a serum α_2 macroglobulin precursor. It causes slow, sustained contraction of smooth muscles, including those of the bronchi and vessels; increased vascular permeability; increased secretion by mucous glands, including those of the bronchi, and stimulation of pain fibres. It also activates phospholipase A_2, which stimulates arachidonic acid metabolism
Eosinophil chemotactic factors	Tetra-peptides	Mast cell granules	Attract eosinophils to the site of inflammation and may play a role in activation of the cells
Prosta-glandins and thromb-oxanes	Derived by cyclo-oxygenase metabolism of arachi-donic acid	Lung mast cells. Neutrophils, macrophages	Lung mast cells preferentially form PGD_2, a potent vaso-dilator. From neutrophils and macrophages, this pathway generates PGF_{2a}, a bronchoconstrictor, and PGE_1 and PGE_2, broncho- and vasodilators that regulate the tissue microenvironment. PGI_2 causes disaggregation of plate-lets; thromboxanes (TXA_2 and TXB_2) aggregate platelets and regulate blood coagulation and homeostasis
Leukotrienes	Metabolites of arachidonic acid	Antigen–antibody interactions; neutrophils	Leukotrienes are spasmogenic and involved in the continued bronchospasm of asthma. Also known as slow reacting substance of anaphylaxis (LTC_4, LTD_4, LTE_4). 5-Lipoxygenase generates 5-hydroxyeico-satetraenoic acid (5-HETE) which modulates cell motility and possibly glucose transport and LTB_4 which is a chemotactic agent comparable to C5a
Platelet-activating factors	Compounds derived from glycerol	IgE-containing ICs and by non-IgE reactions from basophils and alveolar macrophages	Released from platelets, granulocytes, monocytes, macrophages, mast cells and endothelial cells. Very potent, cause activation of neutrophils and monocytes resulting in the release of inflammatory mediators; induces lymphocyte proliferation and IL-2 secretion; platelet aggregation and thromboxane release

Table 3.7 The role of complement activation in inflammation

Proteins	Product of activation	Activity
C3, 4, 5	C3a, 4a, 5a	Anaphylatoxins which have intense effects on muscles and blood flow. At its worst extreme, anaphylaxis may result in death. Cause smooth muscle contraction, degranulation of mast cells and basophils leading to release of histamine and other vasoactive substances that induce capillary leakage. C5a is the most potent anaphylatoxin
C3, 5	C3a, 5a	C3a and C5a have important immunoregulatory effects on T cell function, either stimulating or inhibiting aspects of cell-mediated immunity
C5	C5a	C5a is a potent chemotactic agent for neutrophils and monocytes. It increases neutrophil adherence and causes aggregation; stimulates neutrophil oxidative metabolism and the production of toxic oxygen species; triggers lysosomal enzyme release from phagocytes

mediators also affect the expression of certain molecules on the endothelial cells lining the capillaries. These **adhesion molecules** (Table 3.8) promote binding to the endothelium of white blood cells, which express the corresponding ligands, thus allowing them to move over the surface of the vessel wall in a process known as **rolling**. The cells extend pseudopodia between the endothelial cells and secrete chemicals to dissolve the basement membrane allowing them to squeeze out of the capillaries into the tissues. This migration is known as **diapedesis**.

Once in the tissues, cells detect certain molecules that have diffused away from the site of infection/damage and move to that site by a process known as **chemotaxis**. The diffusion of these **chemotaxins** follows the usual laws (the molecules moving from a site of high concentration to one of low concentration), thus establishing a gradient, which the cells are thought to detect via surface receptors. One explanation proposed for the movement of cells up the gradient suggests that engagement of these receptors on a particular area of the cell surface stimulates pseudopod formation in that area and hence movement. As the concentration increases and more receptors are engaged, it is thought that their re-expression is downregulated, meaning that the migratory signals cease and the movement of the cell ceases. A number of molecules can act as chemotactic agents, including C3a and C5a. The latter attracts both neutrophils and monocytes, but neutrophils predominate in acute inflammation, due to their larger number in the circulation. In addition, a large family of structurally and functionally proinflammatory cytokines known as **chemokines** have been identified. Once cells have reached the site of tissue injury, they are capable of phagocytosing any debris or pathogens that may be present.

Table 3.8   Adhesion molecules, expression and function

Adhesion molecule pair	Cellular expression	Function in inflammation
Integrins	Leukocytes. Different integrins on different leukocytes providing specificity for binding to different types of CAMs on endothelium	Integrins are activated by chemokines (e.g. MCP-1, IL-8) allowing binding to ICAMs. Causes flattening of leukocytes on endothelium and subsequent extravasation
Intercellular adhesion molecules (ICAM-1, 2, 3, VCAM-1, MadCAM)	Endothelial cells	Corresponding ligands for integrins. Mediate cell binding and migration
Selectins (P-, L- and E-)	L-selectin: leukocytes P-selectin: found in preformed state in endothelial Weibel–Palade bodies and in alpha granules of platelets. Mobilised to cell surface in response to inflammatory signals E-selectin: endothelium	P&L-selectin mediate the initial interaction of leukocytes with endothelium – "rolling" of leukocytes. This is followed by stronger interaction, involving E-selectin, leading to extravasation to sites of inflammation
GlyCAM-1, CD34, MadCAM-1	GlyCAM-1: peripheral and mesenteric lymph node high endothelial venules CD34: variety of non-lymphoid tissues; capillaries of peripheral lymph nodes MadCAM 1: mucosal lymph node high endothelial venules	Ligands for L-selectin. Enable leukocyte migration into lymphoid tissues and inflammatory foci
P-selectin glycoprotein ligand (PSGL)	Myeloid cells, neutrophils and lymphocytes	Ligand for P&E-selectin. Mediates "rolling" of leukocytes on endothelium

3.3.3   CHEMOKINES

Chemokines are small proteins, which comprise the largest family of human cytokines (Table 3.9). They are defined by the presence of four cysteine residues and are classified according to the sequence of amino acids involving the first two of these residues. Thus, there are two major families (CC and CXC) and two minor subfamilies within this group.

Upon binding to their specific receptors, these molecules stimulate the migration and activation of a variety of cells including neutrophils, monocytes, lymphocytes and fibroblasts. Recently, it has been shown that Th_1 and Th_2 lymphocytes express a distinct range of chemokine receptors, suggesting that recruitment in inflammation may be selective and influenced by the type of chemokine produced (Table 3.10).

Table 3.9 Some characteristics of chemokines

Chemokine	Major sources/ inducers/ effects	Description
Interleukin 8	Sources	Produced by many cells including monocytes, lymphocytes, granulocytes, fibroblasts, endothelial cells, hepatocytes, keratinocytes
	Inducers	IL-1 and tumour necrosis factor
	Effects	Inflammatory cytokine which acts as a neutrophil chemoattractive and activating factor. It also attracts basophils and a subpopulation of lymphocytes. It is a potent angiogenic factor. It is a chemoattractive and activating factor for T cells
Macrophage inflammatory proteins 1α and 1β (MIP-1)	Sources	Monocytes/macrophages, T cells and B cells
	Inducers	Lipopolysaccharide (LPS; monocytes and macrophages), antibody to CD3 or phytohaemagglutinin (PHA) and phorbol myristate acetate (T cells), *S. aureus* Cowan strain (B cells)
	Effects	*In vitro*, stimulates chemokinesis and H_2O_2 production by neutrophils (human); acts as a prostaglandin-independent endogenous pyrogen (rabbit); MIP-1α is a stem cell inhibitor (mouse), an activity that may be antagonised by MIP-1β
Monocyte chemo-attractant protein (MCP)	Sources	PHA-stimulated peripheral blood mononuclear cells, fibroblasts, endothelial cells, certain tumour cells and monocytes
	Inducers	Some cells (e.g. certain tumour cells) express it constitutively, endothelial cells produce it after IL-1, TNF or LPS stimulation. Conflicting evidence exists over the production by monocytes, i.e. whether it is constitutive or induced
	Effects	Monocyte chemotaxis; enhances monocyte killing of certain tumour cell lines
RANTES	Sources	T lymphocytes
	Inducers	May be constitutively expressed and enhanced on stimulation with Ag or PHA
	Effects	Monocytic but not neutrophil chemoattractant. Also attractant for T cells. Shows subset specificity and migrating T cells are particularly enriched for CD4+ cells bearing markers which are thought to identify memory cells

Table 3.10 Chemokine receptor expression by T cell subsets

T cell subset	Chemokine receptor	Ligands
Th₁	CXCR3	IP-10 and mIg
	CCR5	RANTES, MIP-1α, 1β
Th₂	CCR3	Eotaxin, RANTES, MCP-2, 3, 4
	CCR4	TARC, RANTES, MCP-1, MIP-1α

- *Inflammation is a complex series of biochemical and cellular events leading to the five cardinal signs of heat, pain, swelling, redness and ultimately loss of function.*
- *It involves the concerted action of the immune, clotting, fibrinolytic and kinin systems.*
- *A range of chemicals such as prostaglandins and leukotrienes are released by cells and affect immune cells and others contributing to a proinflammatory state.*
- *Chemical mediators released affect vascular permeability, smooth muscle contraction and the secretion of cytokines. This leads to upregulation of cell surface antigens (adhesion molecules) encouraging migration of inflammatory cells from the circulation to the periphery.*
- *Chemokines encourage the migration of cells into the tissues by interacting with their receptors expressed on the surface of the cells.*

3.4   HAEMOSTASIS AND THROMBOSIS

During inflammation, cells are stimulated leading to the production of phospholipase A2 (PLA2), which converts the membrane lipid alkyl acyl glycero-3-phosphocholine into arachidonic acid and the **lyso-platelet-activating factor** (PAF). This precursor is acetylated converting it into active platelet activating factor which has a diverse range of effects including the aggregation and degranulation of platelets and neutrophils.

Usually, platelets do not adhere to each other or to normal endothelium but do so when the basement membrane or extracellular matrix is exposed as a result of endothelial damage. Platelet adhesion requires the secretion of von Willebrand factor (VWF) (found in the vessel wall and in plasma), which binds to the platelet surface receptor glycoprotein 1β. At the site of injury, platelets develop pseudopodia and express a receptor (formed by the association of glycoproteins IIb and IIIa), which binds fibrinogen and other adhesive proteins resulting in platelet aggregation. Collagen and thrombin (formed as a result of activation of the coagulation pathway) activate platelet phospholipase C, leading to the hydrolysis of inositol phospholipids, activation of protein kinase C, increased cytoplasmic calcium concentration and resulting in platelet activation. Activated platelets express P-selectin, allowing them to adhere to other cells such as monocytes, neutrophils and lymphocytes, thus providing a bridge between these cells and the damaged endothelium. In addition, they

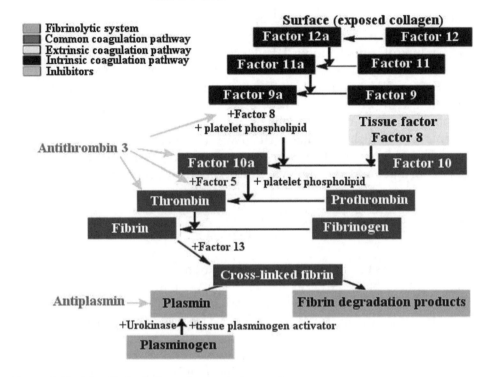

Figure 3.15 The fibrinolytic and coagulation pathways
The figure demonstrates the activation and inhibition of the fibrinolytic pathway and the extrinsic and intrinsic coagulation pathways.

secrete adenosine diphosphate, which can activate adherent platelets and recruit new platelets into the growing haemostatic plug. On the platelet surface, the membrane reorganises to expose phospholipids. These, along with Factor V secreted from platelet α granules, are required for the formation of enzyme/cofactor complexes, which play a key role in the coagulation pathways (Figure 3.15). Increased thrombin is generated, which converts fibrinogen to fibrin. The latter forms strands that radiate from aggregated platelets to help secure the haemostatic plug. Within the platelets, signals cause contraction of the actomyosin elements of the cytoskeleton resulting in the compression and consolidation of the haemostatic plug, securing it more tightly to the site of injury.

3.4.1 REGULATION OF COAGULATION

As a result of tissue damage and inflammation, blood coagulation occurs. However, as with other immune-related pathways, the clotting cascades are tightly regulated to prevent local thrombosis or disseminated intravascular coagulation (DIC). Regulatory mechanisms include the neutralisation of the enzymes and activated cofactors and clearance in the liver. In addition, there are specific inhibitors, which can regulate coagulation. These include tissue factor pathway inhibitor, antithrombin III (which inhibits thrombin, Factor Xa and IXa), α_2 macroglobulin, α_1 antiprotease, heparin cofactor II, protein C (which inhibits Factor VIIIa) and protein S (which inhibits Factor Va). Recently, the therapeutic use of protein C has been established in persons with toxic shock. Thrombin bound to thrombomodulin on endothelial cells cleaves a small peptide from protein C, which becomes an active serine protease. The latter in the presence of cofactors (protein S and procoagulant phospholipid) causes the proteolysis of Factors VIIIa and Va, destroying their procoagulant activity.

3.4.2 THE FIBRINOLYTIC SYSTEM

When injury occurs to the vasculature, coagulation is initiated. However, whilst it is important to block any leakage and ensure repair, it is vital to maintain circulation. This is achieved by the fibrinolytic system. Fibrin deposition activates this system and a balance is achieved between fibrin deposition and lysis, which maintains and restructures the haemostatic seal during vessel repair.

When fibrinogen is converted to fibrin, lysine residues become available on the molecule to which plasminogen can bind tightly by way of lysine-binding sites. Breakdown of fibrin is initiated by plasmin, a proteolytic enzyme derived from plasminogen as a result of the activity of plasminogen activators. **Tissue plasminogen activator (tPA)** is secreted by endothelial cells (amongst others) and when bound to fibrin in association with plasminogen is able to activate the latter. **Urokinase plasminogen activator (uPA)** exists in two molecular forms. The single-chain uPA is released by endothelial cells and activates plasminogen bound to fibrin. The double-chain form (which can activate plasminogen in solution as well as bound to fibrin) is produced when trace amounts of plasmin cleave the single-chain uPA. Clearly, these powerful mediators require regulation to ensure the desired balance between clot formation and remodelling. Thus, plasma contains plasminogen activator inhibitors (e.g. PAI-1 released from vascular endothelium and activated platelets) and plasmin inhibitors that slow fibrinolysis. The primary plasmin inhibitor is α_2 antiplasmin, which can rapidly inactivate free plasmin.

Thus, fibrinolysis is regulated by the rapid clearance and inactivation (by PAI-1) of plasminogen activators.

KEY POINTS FOR REVIEW

- *Platelet-activating factor promotes the aggregation and degranulation of platelets and neutrophils.*

- *Platelet adhesion requires the secretion of von Willebrand factor that binds to the surface glycoprotein 1β.*
- *Activated platelets bind to other cells and provide a bridge between them and the damaged endothelium.*
- *Fibrinogen is converted to fibrin forming strands which bind to platelets to secure the haemostatic plug.*
- *Coagulation must be tightly controlled to prevent thrombosis or disseminated intravascular coagulation.*
- *Regulation is achieved by cofactors and specific inhibitors.*
- *The haemostatic plug is remodelled by a balance between fibrin deposition and fibrinolysis.*
- *Fibrin is broken down by plasminogen, which is activated by the tissue plasminogen activator or the urokinase plasminogen activator.*
- *Fibrinolysis is regulated by the clearance and inactivation of plasminogen activators.*

BIBLIOGRAPHY

Anderson KV. (2000) Toll signaling pathways in the innate immune response. Curr Opin Immunol, 12; 13–19.

Ehlers MRW. (2000) CR3: a general purpose adhesion-recognition receptor essential for innate immunity. Microb Infect, 2; 289–294.

Febbraio M, Hajjar DP, Silverstein RL. (2001) CD36: a class B scavenger receptor involved in angiogenesis, atherosclerosis, inflammation, and lipid metabolism. J Clin Invest, 108; 785–791.

Fernandez EJ, Lolis E. (2002) Structure, function, and inhibition of chemokines. Ann Rev Pharmacol Toxicol, 42; 469–499.

Greenberg S, Grinstein S. (2000) Phagocytosis and innate immunity. Curr Opin Immunol, 14; 136–145.

Kraal G, van der Laan LJW, Outi Elomaa O, Tryggvason K. (2000) The macrophage receptor MARCO. Microb Infect, 2; 313–316.

Lindahl G, Sjöbring U, Johnsson E. (2000) Human complement regulators: a major target for pathogenic microorganisms. Curr Opin Immunol, 12; 44–51.

Matsushita M, Endo Y, Hamasaki N, Fujita T. (2001) Activation of the lectin complement pathway by ficolins. Int Immunopharm, 1; 359–363.

Platt N, Haworth R, Darley L, Gordon S. (2002) The many roles of the class A macrophage scavenger receptor. Int Rev Cytol, 212; 1–40.

Raj PA, Dentino AR. (2002) Current status of defensins and their role in innate and adaptive immunity. FEMS Microbiol Lett, 206; 9–18.

Shirai H, Murakami T, Yamada Y, Doi T, Hamakubo T, Kodama T. (1999) Structure and function of type I and II macrophage scavenger receptors. Mech Ageing Dev, 111; 107–121.

Teixeira MM, Almeida IC, Gazzinelli RT. (2002) Introduction: innate recognition of bacteria and protozoan parasites. Microb Infect, 4; 883–886.

Turner MW. (1996) Mannose-binding lectin: the pluripotent molecules of the innate immune system. Immunol Today, 17; 532–540.

NOW TEST YOURSELF!

1. Which of the following statements is FALSE? C1:
(a) Comprises three different types of molecule, C1q, C1r and C1s.
(b) Comprises one nonameric C1q molecule which binds the Fc portion of antibody in an immune complex.
(c) Enzymatic activity does not reside in the C1q molecule.
(d) Comprises one molecule of C1q and two each of the other components.
(e) When activated possesses an enzymatic site that will act on the next component in the pathway, C4.

2. C4:
(a) Has two chains, the largest of which is the beta chain.
(b) Has an alpha chain which is cleaved by C1q, causing the release of a small fragment called C4a.
(c) Is cleaved to give a large fragment, C4b, which binds to the target antigen via the formation of covalent amide or ester bonds.
(d) Is fragmented and, in the presence of calcium ions, C4b bound to the target antigen interacts with the next component of complement, C2.
(e) Is fragmented to give C4b which, with C2b, forms the C5 convertase of the classical pathway.

3. Which of the following statements concerning the alternative pathway of complement activation is FALSE?
(a) In the alternative pathway, C3 exists in two molecular forms: the native form which circulates in the serum, and a conformationally altered form in which the thiolester bond has been hydrolysed.
(b) The hydrolysed form of C3 can bind Factor D in the presence of magnesium ions.
(c) Factor D (a serine protease) cleaves Factor B to Bb.
(d) The alternative pathway C3 convertase is formed by the molecule C3bBb.
(e) The C5 convertase of the alternative pathway, $(C3b)_nBb$, is stabilised by properdin.

4. Which of the following components involved in the membrane attack complex is the first to interact with the lipids present in the membrane surrounding the immunogen?
(a) C5.
(b) C6.
(c) C7.
(d) C8.
(e) C9.

5.   Which of the following statements relating to the regulation of complement activation is FALSE?

(a)   Neither the classical nor the alternative pathway can be activated by antibody alone.

(b)   Relatively large amounts of specific antibody must be formed before complement activation can occur.

(c)   C1 inhibitor inhibits the activity of activated C1s and C1r by binding to their active sites.

(d)   C4 binding protein regulates the activity of C4b in the presence of Factor H, a protease which cleaves it.

(e)   Factor I in the presence of Factor H cleaves the alpha chain of hydrolysed C3 or C3b to form iC3b.

6.   Which of the following statements concerning phagocytes and phagocytosis is CORRECT?

(a)   Phagocytosis may be divided into a series of sequential stages that are in order of occurrence, ingestion, opsonisation and digestion.

(b)   Tissue macrophages are often the first cells to encounter and ingest a microorganism and are highly efficient at killing.

(c)   Neutrophils are the least efficient of the professional phagocytes.

(d)   Neutrophils are attracted to the site of infection by mediators, which may be released by macrophages.

(e)   Basophils, which also phagocytose, are efficient killers but are geared to killing extracellular pathogens.

7.   Which of the following statements concerning opsonins and opsonisation is INCORRECT?

(a)   An opsonin is something which coats a particle and makes it easier to phagocytose.

(b)   C3b may act as an opsonin. Both neutrophils and macrophages have receptors which bind C3b.

(c)   IgG acts as an opsonin and facilitates phagocytosis by binding to Fc gamma receptors on phagocytic cells.

(d)   Certain lipopolysaccharides or LPS-binding proteins act as "go-betweens" linking the particle and the phagocyte, allowing attachment and enhanced phagocytosis.

(e)   Receptors for IgG are always in an active state, whilst receptors for complement fragments are not. The former stimulate ingestion immediately.

8.   Upon stimulation, the phagocyte undergoes a respiratory burst which:

(a)   Is also known as the oxidative or metabolic burst and is characterised by a gradual increase in the consumption of oxygen by the cell.

(b)   Results in the production of non-toxic oxygen metabolites.

(c) Involves the action of a group of enzymes found in the cytoplasm and associated with the membrane of the phagosome known as the nicotinamide triphosphate oxidase.

(d) Results in the conversion of molecular oxygen to the superoxide anion, which is highly reactive and has an unpaired electron.

(e) Results in the production of free radicals. Addition of an electron to the superoxide anion produces superoxide; addition of a second electron converts it to peroxide.

9. Defensins:

(a) Accumulate as multimers in the membrane of target cells, forming cyclic peptides which form channels in the lipid bilayers.

(b) Are widely distributed, usually anionic and with a molecular mass of about 30–40 kDa.

(c) Are able to disrupt biological membranes, their richest source in humans being the lysosomes of macrophages.

(d) Have a double-stranded structure, and those from humans trimerise in crystalline form.

(e) Are a large number of small peptides which exhibit cytotoxicity to host cells.

10. The increased permeability of the blood vessels leads to the cardinal signs of inflammation, which are:

(a) Heat, redness and pain.

(b) Heat, redness, pain and swelling.

(c) Heat, pain, swelling and loss of function.

(d) Heat, redness, pain and loss of function.

(e) Heat, redness, pain, swelling and loss of function.

11. Which of the following systems is NOT involved in the inflammatory process?

(a) The immune system.

(b) The kallin system.

(c) The fibrinolytic system.

(d) The clotting system.

(e) The complement cascade.

12. Kinins are:

(a) Small, acidic peptides.

(b) Large, basic peptides.

(c) Derived from kininogens by the action of kallikreins, which are serine esterases.

(d) Peptides which affect the movement of smooth muscle, preventing vasodilation and causing pain.

(e) A group of peptides which include bradykinin, which is derived from a serum macroglobulin precursor and causes the slow, sustained contraction of smooth muscles.

13. Chemokines are:

(a) A large family of proinflammatory molecules which are not structurally related.

(b) A group of proinflammatory molecules which stimulate the migration and proliferation of a variety of cells.

(c) Molecules which stimulate cells such as neutrophils, monocytes, lymphocytes and fibroblasts.

(d) May attract both neutrophils and monocytes but the latter predominate in acute inflammation due to their capacity for replication.

(e) A small family of structurally related molecules which show distinct functions.

14. Which of the following is part of the intrinsic coagulation pathway?

(a) Factor Xa.

(b) Plasminogen.

(c) Factor XI.

(d) Thrombin.

(e) Tissue Factor VII.

15. Which of the following statements is INCORRECT?

(a) Factor XII may be activated by surface exposed collagen.

(b) Antithrombin III may inhibit the activity of Factor XIa.

(c) Tissue Factor VII may activate Factor X.

(d) Plasmin degrades cross-linked fibrin.

(e) Thrombin converts fibrinogen to fibrin.

4

THE ADAPTIVE IMMUNE RESPONSE

When the body is exposed to an antigen for the first time, a number of non-specific (or **innate**) mechanisms are brought into play to restrict its spread and the accompanying tissue damage. They do not require specific identification of the invader, merely the recognition that something foreign has entered the system. These mechanisms are very efficient and manage to prevent infection by many organisms. However, the latter have been particularly adept in evolving ways to avoid destruction by these non-specific defence systems and as a result, the host has developed more complex immune mechanisms which specifically recognise the invader and invoke reactions to destroy it. This **adaptive immunity** is characterised by the development of both T and B lymphocyte **memory cells**, which allow a more rapid and effective response on second exposure to the eliciting antigen.

The development of antigen-specific immunity largely depends on the ability of T cells to recognise antigen. This is a complex process since T cells cannot bind free antigen and must have it presented to them by products of the major histocompatibility gene complex (MHC) on the membranes of cells. T cells can only recognise antigen presented by self-MHC gene products.

In order for an antigen to associate with MHC gene products, it must be **processed** because only short peptides may associate with the antigen-binding regions of these molecules (see Section 2.2).

4.1 ANTIGEN PROCESSING AND PRESENTATION BY MHC GENE PRODUCTS

There are two major pathways of antigen processing and presentation which are not mutually exclusive but which depend partly on whether the antigen may

Immunology for Life Scientists, Second Edition. Lesley-Jane Eales.
© 2003 John Wiley & Sons, Ltd: ISBN 0 470 84523 6 (HB); 0 470 84524 4 (PB)

be classified as endogenous or exogenous. In general, peptides from exogenous antigens associate with MHC Class II molecules and those from endogenous antigens with products of the MHC Class I genes.

When T cells recognise antigen, the TCR–MHC–antigen complex is further stabilised by interaction between the CD4 or CD8 molecule and the MHC molecule. Antigen presented by Class II gene products are recognised by T cells which express the CD4 antigen. These are responsible generally for initiating a protective immune response. Antigens presented by Class I gene products are recognised by T cells which express the CD8 antigen and which may be capable of lysing the cell expressing the antigen.

4.1.1 GENERATION OF PEPTIDES PRESENTED BY MHC CLASS I MOLECULES

Most of the peptides presented by Class I molecules are derived from proteins present in the nucleus or the cytoplasm; although some have been shown to be derived from proteins in the mitochondria or endoplasmic reticulum (ER). In general, those peptides which associate with Class I molecules must be processed in the nucleus or cytoplasm by a highly controlled mechanism which allows only partial degradation and not complete reduction to constituent amino acids (Figure 4.1). This regulation is important since it has been shown that the amino acids surrounding the epitope to be presented may influence the breakdown of a particular protein. Proteins to be presented by MHC Class I molecules are degraded by a large, ATP-dependent, proteolytic complex called the **proteasome**. These are enzyme complexes found in the cytoplasm and nucleus. Under normal conditions, proteasomes comprise three catalytic subunits responsible for the proteolytic activity of the complex. However, in cells exposed to proinflammatory cytokines (i.e. interferon gamma) these subunits are replaced by others that appear to be more efficient at degrading endogenous proteins for presentation by MHC Class I molecules to cytotoxic T cells. This may be due in part to the interferon gamma-induced expression of the proteasome activator, PA28.

Breakdown products produced by the proteasome are transferred to the lumen of the ER by the peptide transporters, TAP1 and TAP2 (Transporter associated with Antigen Presentation). Evidence suggests that these molecules show some specificity in the peptides they transport.

Once inside the ER, peptides may be modified further by local proteases, which produce peptides of the correct size for binding to Class I molecules; the latter subsequently protecting these peptides from total degradation.

ASSEMBLY AND INTRACELLULAR TRANSPORT OF MHC CLASS I MOLECULES

Both the heavy and light chains of the MHC Class I molecules are synthesised in the ER. At physiological temperature, the Class I heterodimer is unstable but

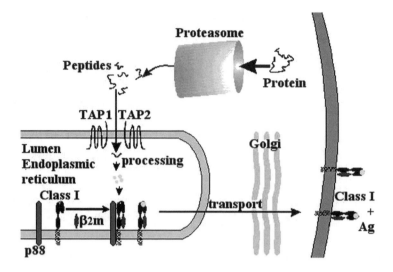

Figure 4.1   Endogenous pathway of antigen presentation
Most of the peptides presented by Class I molecules are derived from proteins present in the nucleus or the cytoplasm; although some have been shown to be derived from proteins in the mitochondria or endoplasmic reticulum (ER). The peptide must be processed in the nucleus or cytoplasm by a highly controlled mechanism which allows only partial degradation and not complete reduction to constituent amino acids.

is stabilised by the association of processed peptide. Other molecules, which transiently associate with the Class I heterodimer and are released upon binding of peptide, are thought to help Class I molecules achieve the correct folding upon synthesis.

In order for Class I-bound peptide to be presented on the cell surface, the heterotrimeric complex (Class I heavy chain, β_2 microglobulin and peptide) must be released from the ER. However, most Class I alleles only achieve limited assembly of the trimeric complex, which affects both the efficiency of the release and the rate of intracellular transport of the complex. Upon release from the ER, the Class I–peptide complexes are transported via the Golgi apparatus and the trans-Golgi reticulum to the cell surface.

4.1.2   GENERATION OF PEPTIDES PRESENTED BY MHC CLASS II MOLECULES

The products of the MHC Class II genes are expressed on a limited group of cells, which includes macrophages, B cells and dendritic cells. These cells endocytose or phagocytose extracellular foreign particles, which are processed and presented in association with MHC Class II molecules (Figure 4.2). After endocytosis, endosome–lysosome fusion occurs and degradation of the antigen

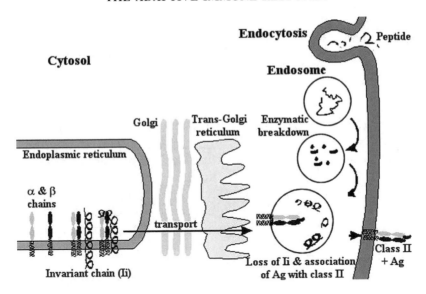

Figure 4.2   Exogenous pathway of antigen presentation
The products of the MHC Class II genes are expressed on cells capable of endocytosis and present antigens derived from an extracellular source. Fragments of an antigen, regardless of their degree of degradation, can bind to Class II molecules but require further processing by endosomal proteases to produce a minimal fragment which is protected from further degradation by the Class II molecule itself.

begins. Initially, the tertiary structure of a protein is destroyed by the reduction of disulphide bonds thus making it more accessible to other degradative enzymes which include the cathepsins B, D and E. Fragments of an antigen, regardless of their degree of degradation, can bind to Class II molecules but require further processing by endosomal proteases to produce a minimal fragment which is protected from further degradation by the Class II molecule itself. Distinct peptides bind with different affinities to the same Class II molecule.

ASSEMBLY AND INTRACELLULAR TRANSPORT OF MHC CLASS II MOLECULES

Class II molecules are structurally similar to Class I molecules. However, during assembly, they associate with a third molecule – the invariant chain. Thus, Class II molecules are assembled in the ER as a trimeric complex (composed of an α, a β and an invariant chain).

Since Class II molecules are assembled in the ER like Class I molecules, they could bind the same peptides theoretically. However, *in vitro* studies have shown that Class II molecules only bind peptide after removal of the invariant chain, which usually occurs beyond the ER. This suggests that the invariant chain may help to regulate peptide binding, although presentation of cytosolic or ER-derived peptides may occur.

The Class II-invariant chain trimers are exported in triplets. These nonamers are transported through the Golgi to the trans-Golgi reticulum where signals derived from the cytoplasmic tail of the invariant chain direct it towards the endocytic pathway of antigen processing. Having entered this pathway, they remain there for up to three hours before appearing at the cell surface. Proteases (e.g. **cathepsin B**) digest the invariant chain resulting in **Class II dimers loaded with invariant chain-derived peptides (CLIP)**. CLIP is removed from the Class II dimers through the action of **HLA-DM** (a product of the MHC Class II gene complex), which also facilitates the binding of processed peptides. This results in the formation of stable Class II–peptide complexes that are subsequently presented at the cell surface. This process is moderated by another Class II molecule, **HLA-DO**, which alters the peptide exchange function of HLA-DM. HLA-DO appears to facilitate the activity of HLA-DM only in acidic conditions such as those that occur after endosome–lysosome fusion.

KEY POINTS FOR REVIEW

- *T cells can only recognise antigen when it has been processed and presented by molecules coded for by the MHC.*
- *Antigen is taken up by antigen presenting cells and processed through the exogenous pathway leading to presentation by MHC Class II molecules.*
- *Antigen presenting cells include dendritic cells, macrophages and B lymphocytes.*
- *Antigen produced within the cell (e.g. viral antigens) are processed via the endogenous pathway and the peptides presented by molecules of MHC Class I molecules.*
- *All nucleated cells express Class I molecules and can therefore present antigen via the endogenous pathway.*
- *Peptides produced via the endogenous pathway are processed by a proteolytic complex called a proteasome.*
- *Class II molecules are produced along with the invariant chain in the endoplasmic reticulum.*
- *The invariant chain is removed in the endosome by cathepsin B and the remaining self-peptide is removed from the Class II dimers by HLA-DM.*
- *The action of HLA-DM is moderated in acidic conditions by HLA-DO.*

4.2   ANTIGEN PROCESSING AND PRESENTATION BY CD1

Amongst the molecules expressed on the surface of cells that may be antigenic, CD1 is of particular importance since it provides a link between the innate and specific immune responses. You have learnt about the products of the MHC gene complex that present antigens to antigen-specific lymphocytes and about the structures on lymphocytes capable of recognising antigens presented in this way (Section 2.3). However, there are a group of molecules – the glycolipids, which are presented by the molecule CD1.

4.2.1   STRUCTURE OF CD1

CD1 comprises a family of five genes that do not form part of the MHC complex and are separated into two groups on the basis of their sequence homology. Group 1 comprises CD1a, b, c and e whilst group 2 comprises CD1d.

CD1 proteins are found in non-covalent association with β_2 microglobulin, resulting in the formation of a structure similar to that seen in MHC Class I-β_2 microglobulin dimers.

Like MHC Class I molecules, the CD1 complex has an antigen-binding groove but in the case of CD1 it only has two pockets for anchoring antigenic residues and these are highly hydrophobic (i.e. likely to be attractive to lipid-containing molecules).

4.2.2   ANTIGEN PRESENTATION BY CD1

Recognition of the role of CD1 in antigen presentation is comparatively recent. Thus, much of the detail pertaining to this activity is still to be confirmed. However, currently it is thought that the fatty acid tails of glycolipids fit in the hydrophobic pockets of the binding groove and the polar residues of such molecules extend beyond the groove facilitating contact with T cell antigen receptors.

CD1a, b and c can present microbial lipid and glycolipid antigens such as mycolic acids and lipoarabinomannans (e.g. from mycobacteria). CD1d has been shown to present galactosylceramide suggesting that CD1 molecules have evolved to present lipids rather than peptides (although the group 2 CD1 molecules can also present hydrophobic peptides.

- *CD1 provides a link between the innate and specific immune responses.*
- *CD1 associates with β_2 microglobulin.*
- *CD1 has an antigen-binding groove with two hydrophobic pockets that attract lipid-containing molecules.*
- *CD1 can present mycolic acids and lipoarabinomannan from microbes.*

4.3 CELL-MEDIATED IMMUNITY

Stimulation of a specific immune response requires the recognition of antigen by T cells and B cells. Usually, although B cells can bind antigen directly, they require further signals provided by molecules on their surface binding to their respective ligands. These ligands may include surface antigens on other cells (e.g. CD40–CD154 ligation) or cytokines (e.g. IL-4–IL-4R). These signals may be provided by antigen-stimulated T cells. Indeed, T cell activation is also key to the cellular branch of specific immunity. Cell-mediated immunity includes all those specific immune responses in which antibody plays only a minor or subsidiary role. We will discuss these in the following sections.

4.3.1 ANTIGEN-SPECIFIC T CELL STIMULATION

Once processed and presented on the surface of cells in association with MHC molecules, antigenic peptides are able to stimulate T cells. The elicited responses may be influenced by a number of factors including the type of antigen, the route of entry and the type of antigen presenting cell to name but a few. The outcome of such antigenic stimulation will depend partly on the type of T cell that predominates in the response, i.e. Th_1 or Th_2, and on whether antigen-specific memory cells are present. In addition, some effector T cells have the capability of directly eliminating cells via cytotoxic action. These activities represent the role of T cells in immunity which is achieved by the secretion of chemical mediators, i.e. **cytokines**.

T CELL RESPONSES TO ANTIGEN STIMULATION

T cells in the periphery may be considered to be either naïve, memory or effector cells. Naïve cells are those that have not been stimulated by antigen since leaving the thymus. By contrast, memory cells are those which have had antigen presented to them at least once and have returned to a resting state from which they can be activated on subsequent exposure to the same antigen. This group of cells are considered to be long-lived. However, individual cells within this group may be short-lived and persistence may depend upon restimulation by antigen. Effector cells are those T cells that in response to presented antigen are able to carry out specialised functions such as the secretion of specific cytokines or the lysis of target cells. These cells derive from either naïve or memory cells several days after antigenic stimulation. They are short-lived, in a highly activated state but require further stimulation before they can perform their effector function. Studies in mice have shown that naïve cells only secrete interleukin 2 (IL-2) on initial stimulation whilst memory and effector cells may exhibit defined cytokine secretion profiles, e.g. Th_1 and Th_2 cytokine profiles. These profiles are less readily defined in humans but clearly do exist. Similar differential cytokine secretion profiles have been demonstrated for CD8 + T_{cyt} cells.

When a host is exposed to an antigen, depending on the site of entry, the antigen will be taken up by antigen presenting cells. However, antigen will also pass via the lymph to draining lymph nodes where it will be taken up by macrophages and dendritic cells. The latter have been clearly demonstrated to be most effective in presenting antigen to naïve T cells; a process which occurs with great efficiency in lymph nodes where T cells can enter from the blood or lymph and percolate through tissues rich in antigen presenting cells.

Interaction between a microorganism and an antigen presenting cell may lead to the production of certain cytokines. For example, the phagocytosis by macrophages of *Mycobacterium tuberculosis* stimulates the production of IL-12 (Table 4.1) by the macrophage, which encourages the subsequent development

Table 4.1 Characteristics of interleukin 12

Major cellular sources	IL-12 is a heterodimer made up of two chains: p35 and p40, and is produced by monocytes/macrophages, dendritic cells. B cells and PMNs can also produce it
Major inducers	Microorganisms, e.g. *S. aureus, M. tuberculosis, T. gondii, L. major* and the lipopolysaccharide from Gram-negative bacteria. Phagocyte interaction with inflammatory matrix molecules
Effects	Important in defence against intracellular pathogens. Induces IFNγ production by T and NK cells; enhances NK and ADCC activity; co-stimulates peripheral blood lymphocyte proliferation; stimulates proliferation and induces the differentiation of Th_1 cells
Cross-reactivity	Mouse IL-12 functions on human cells but NOT vice versa

Table 4.2	Characteristics of interleukin 10
Major cellular sources	Th$_0$ and Th$_2$ subsets of murine T cells, activated CD4+ and CD8+ human T cells, murine Ly-1+ B cells, monocytes and macrophages
Effects	Blocks activation of cytokine synthesis by Th$_1$ cells, activated monocytes and NK cells. Stimulates and/or enhances proliferation of B cells, thymocytes and mast cells and with TGFβ stimulates IgA production by human B cells
Cross-reactivity	Human IL-10 functions on murine cells but NOT vice versa

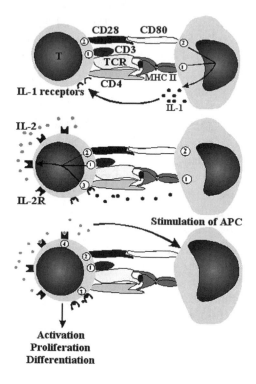

Figure 4.3   Molecular interactions leading to T cell activation
When a T cell recognises presented antigen, the interaction between the TCR–CD3–CD4 on the T cell and the antigen–MHC complex on the APC results in a number of vital events which ultimately lead to activation.

of a Th$_1$ response. Depending on the nature of the pathogen involved, macrophages may be induced to produce IL-10 (Table 4.2), which stimulates a Th$_2$ response, presumably through inhibiting the production of IL-12.

When a T cell recognises presented antigen, the interaction between the TCR–CD3–CD4 on the T cell and the antigen–MHC complex on the APC results in a number of vital events, which ultimately lead to activation (summarised in Figure 4.3). Other molecules, which include CD28, CTLA4, CD154 on T cells and CD80, CD86 and CD40 on antigen presenting cells, are

Table 4.3 Characteristics of interleukin 1	
Major cellular sources	IL-1 is a polypeptide which exists in two forms – IL-1α and IL-1β. Both bind to the same receptor and have the same functions. IL-1 is synthesised as a large precursor molecule which is processed at the cell membrane or extracellularly to give the mature, active proteins. It is produced by many cells but most importantly monocytes, activated macrophages, dendritic cells, T and B cells, NK cells and LGL. Mononuclear phagocytes produce mainly IL-1β
Major inducers	Endotoxin, muramyl dipeptide; interaction with T cells during antigen presentation
Effects	Induces fever, hypotension, neutrophilia and the acute phase response *in vivo*
Cross-reactivity	Both human and mouse IL-1 have cross-species activity

vital for this activation, ensuring the correct signalling within the T cells. As a result of interaction with the T cell, the antigen presenting cell is stimulated to secrete interleukin 1 (IL-1; Table 4.3). This binds to IL-1 receptors on the T cell and augments the stimulatory signal from the early activation events. This results in the production of **interleukin 2** and the expression of **IL-2 receptors**.

Interleukin 2 is a polypeptide, which is produced by, and acts on, T cells promoting their division (Table 4.4). It also acts on other cells of the immune system such as **natural killer** and **B cells**. Cytokines exert their effects by binding specific receptors on the membrane of their target cells.

There are three distinct receptors for IL-2, which differ in their affinity for the cytokine. The high-affinity receptor comprises three chains – the α, β and γ chains. The intermediate-affinity receptor comprises only the β and γ chains. The low-affinity receptor comprises the α chain alone. The IL-2 produced may act back on the cell that produced it (autocrine effect) enhancing its activation and proliferation, or it may diffuse away and affect other cells in the locality.

Table 4.4 Characteristics of interleukin 2	
Major cellular sources	IL-2 is produced by T cells. A single disulphide bond between residues 58 and 105 of the molecule is essential to its biological activity
Receptors	Exists in three molecular forms: low, intermediate and high affinity. Three constituent molecules: IL-2Rα, β and γ, and differential expression of these molecules gives rise to the different affinity receptors, i.e. IL-2Rα alone binds IL-2 with low affinity, IL-2Rβ and γ bind with intermediate affinity, and IL-Rα, β and γ bind with high affinity. The α chain appears to be vital for the assembly of the high-affinity receptor whilst the β chain is responsible for signalling to the cell that the receptor has been occupied, thus stimulating subsequent proliferation events. The γ chain helps stabilise the high-affinity receptor and helps in the cellular intake of IL-2
Effects	Stimulates growth and differentiation of T, B, NK and LAK cells, monocytes, macrophages and oligodendrocytes
Cross-reactivity	Human IL-2 acts on mouse cells but NOT vice versa

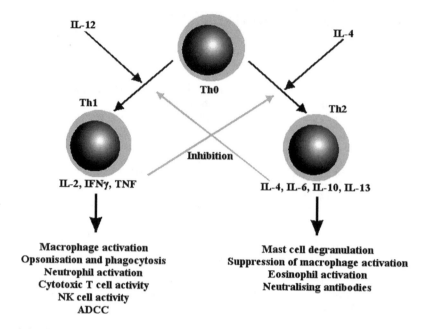

Figure 4.4   Cytokine secretion patterns of T helper subsets
Subsets of T cells have different patterns of cytokine production which stimulate different types of immune response. Th₁ cells produce cytokines which are responsible largely for the stimulation of cytotoxic effector cells and macrophage activities (known as cell-mediated immunity), i.e. IL-2, IFNγ, TNFα.

However, only those cells that have encountered antigen and thus are expressing IL-2 receptors are able to respond to this stimulus.

The interaction between IL-2 and its receptor initiates several intracellular signals, which ultimately help to cause the proliferation and differentiation of distinct subsets of effector T cells.

TH₀, TH₁ AND TH₂ CELLS

Subsets of T cells can be characterised by the different cytokines they produce, which influence the type of ensuing immune response (Figure 4.4).

Th₀ cells are naïve T cells that have not previously encountered antigen. They have a pattern of cytokine secretion, which is intermediate between those described for Th₁ and Th₂ cells, IL-2 being the most predominant. After stimulation, these cells may develop into Th₁ or Th₂ memory cells which on subsequent exposure to antigen respond more rapidly, producing cytokines that will stimulate an appropriate response (either cell-mediated or humoral) to ensure the rapid elimination of the stimulating antigen.

Th₁ cells produce cytokines (i.e. IL-2, TNFα and INFγ), which promote the differentiation and activation of T_cyt effector cells and the activation of

Table 4.5 Characteristics of interferon gamma

Major cellular sources	CD8+ and CD4+ T cells, NK cells
Effects	Regulates activation, growth and differentiation of T and B cells, macrophages, NK cells, endothelial cells and fibroblasts. Enhances MHC Class II and FcR expression on macrophages. Increases intracellular killing and ADCC activity. Weak anti-viral and anti-proliferative activity and promotes those activities of IFNα/β. Causes preferential production of mIgG$_2$A$^+$ B cells, counteracts effect of IL-4 on B cells. Inhibits proliferation of Th$_2$ cells

macrophages and natural killer cells (i.e. cell-mediated immune responses; Table 4.5).

By contrast, Th$_2$ cells produce cytokines that promote the proliferation and differentiation of B lymphocytes, i.e. IL-4, IL-5, IL-6 and IL-13 (Table 4.6) and influence the ability of B cells to switch production from one class of antibody to another (e.g. IgM to IgE).

IL-4 has an autocrine effect on Th$_2$ cells, specifically promoting their differentiation and proliferation. Characteristically, this results in the production of **IgG4** and **IgE** by human B cells.

Other cytokines are produced by both Th$_1$ and Th$_2$ cells but are produced in far greater quantities by Th$_1$ cells. These include granulocyte–macrophage colony-stimulating factor (GM-CSF; Table 4.7) and tumour necrosis factor (TNF).

Regulation of Th$_1$ and Th$_2$ responses: IL-2 is the chief growth-promoting factor for both Th$_1$ and Th$_2$ subsets. In addition, **IL-4** stimulates growth for a short time after encounter with antigen. At later stages, Th$_2$ cells still respond to both cytokines whilst Th$_1$ cells only respond to IL-2. As with naïve cells, **IL-1** is required as a co-stimulant after antigen presentation but only by Th$_2$ cells. As mentioned earlier, **IFNγ** can inhibit the growth of Th$_2$ cells by negating the effects of IL-4. In addition, Th$_2$ produced cytokines are able to inhibit the production of IFNγ by Th$_1$ cells and to suppress their growth. Thus, it appears that the outcome of a response to antigen depends on the balance of cytokines secreted (Figure 4.5). Initial responses may stimulate a Th$_1$-type response, but if the antigen is not cleared, a Th$_2$ response may develop. Such a change is observed in chronic *Mycobacterium tuberculosis* infections.

4.3.2 OTHER CELLS IN CELL-MEDIATED IMMUNITY

When an infection or tissue damage occurs, the complex molecular and cellular events involved in innate immunity attempt to resolve the situation and restore normal tissue function. If, however, the damage/infection persists, the specific

Table 4.6 Characteristics of Th$_2$-type cytokines

Cytokine	Sources/inducers	Effects
IL-4	Activated T cells, mast cells and bone marrow stromal cells	IL-4 causes the activation, proliferation and differentiation of B cells. It is a growth factor for T and mast cells. It exerts other effects on granulocyte, megakaryocyte and erythrocyte precursors and macrophages. IL-4 induces IgG$_1$ and IgE secretion by murine B cells; IgG$_4$ and IgE by human B cells. Receptors are found on B and T cells, macrophages, mast cells and myeloid cells. Their number increases on cell activation
IL-5	T cells, mast cells and eosinophils	Stimulates eosinophil colony formation and eosinophil differentiation. Also acts as growth and differentiation factor for mouse (but NOT human) B cells
IL-6	B cells, T cells, monocytes/ macrophages, bone marrow stromal cells; fibroblasts, keratinocytes, endothelial cells. Inducers: *S. aureus* Cowan strain 1, IL-4, IL-1, TNFα, LPS, IL-6, IFNγ, PMA, GM-CSF, CSF-1, viruses, adherence, C5a, TNF	Nuclear factor (NF)-IL6 binds to the IL-6 multiresponse element in the genome and is responsible for the induction of IL-6 in response to IL-1 and TNF. NF-IL6 binds to the regulatory region of IL-8, G-CSF, IL-1, immunoglobulin and the acute phase protein genes, indicating that it may interact with many genes involved in acute phase, immune and inflammatory responses
IL-13	Activated T cells	Inhibits production of inflammatory cytokines by LPS-stimulated monocytes (IL-1β; IL-6; TNFα; IL-8). Human and mouse IL-13: induce CD23 on human B cells, promote B cell proliferation in combination with anti-Ig or CD40 Abs; stimulate secretion of IgM, E and G$_4$. Prolongs survival of human monocytes and increases expression of MHC II and CD23. Human and mouse IL-13 have no known activity on mouse B cells

Table 4.7 Characteristics of granulocyte–macrophage colony-stimulating factor

Molecular weight	16.3 kDa (human); 16 kDa (murine). Two potential glycosylation sites and four cysteine residues. Disulphide bonding is important for biological activity
Major cellular sources	Activated lymphocytes, macrophages, fibroblasts and endothelial cells
Effects of GM-CSF	Promotes the growth and survival of haematopoietic progenitor cells; stimulates formation of granulocytes, macrophages, mixed granulocyte–macrophage colonies and, at higher concentrations, eosinophil colonies from pluripotent stem cells. GM-CSF is bound by neutrophils, eosinophils and monocytes

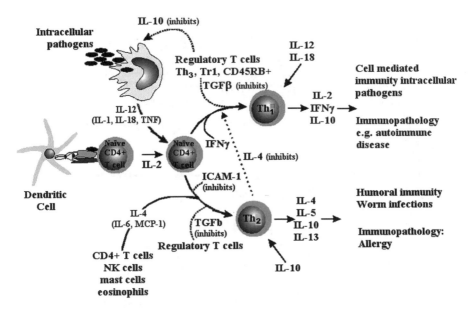

Figure 4.5   Regulation and outcome of Th₁ and Th₂ responses
The outcome of a response to antigen depends on the balance of cytokines secreted. Initial responses may stimulate a Th₁-type response, but if the antigen is not cleared, a Th₂ response may develop.

immune response is called into play. Numerous local influences will determine whether a Th₁- or a Th₂-type response is stimulated. Cytokines such as IL-12 and IL-18 will promote a Th₁ response. In reply, Th₁ cells will release cytokines that stimulate other cells involved in cell-mediated immunity. These cells, which include T_{cyt} and NK cells, and macrophages, are capable of destroying target cells either through cytotoxicity or by inducing apoptosis (Figure 4.6).

MECHANISMS OF TARGET CELL DEATH

The chemicals involved in inducing the death of target cells are usually found in the cytoplasmic granules of the effector cells. Exocytosis of these granules results in the release of chemicals such as perforin and granzymes. The latter may gain access to the target cell either through receptor-mediated endocytosis or via the pores formed by perforin in the target cell membrane. Once inside the cell, granzyme B is able to cleave and activate caspases, initiating the process of apoptosis. It also has an effect on caspase-independent and mitochondrial-dependent pathways resulting in cell death. In addition, the death of the target cell may be brought about by the action of other granzymes and cytoplasmic proteins.

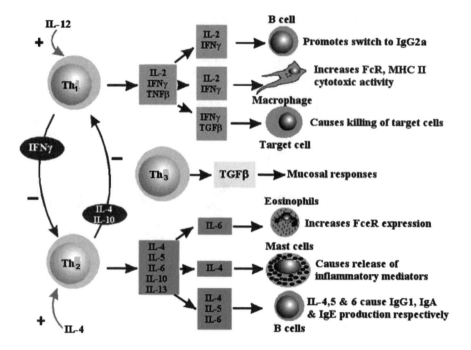

Figure 4.6   Influence of cytokines on the outcome of an immune response

CYTOTOXIC T CELLS

T cells capable of cytotoxic activity are usually CD8+ and recognise processed antigen presented by products of the MHC Class I genes. This means that CD8+ cells are important in recognising and destroying virally infected cells. They may also be involved in the destruction of cells containing obligate intracellular bacteria where endosomal, bacterial peptides escape into the cytoplasm and are directed to the MHC Class I presentation pathway (e.g. mycobacterial infection). Cytotoxicity may be achieved by the induction of apoptosis via the Fas–FasL pathway (Figure 4.7) or by the release of granzymes into the target cell through pores formed by perforin.

MACROPHAGES

Macrophages are able to phagocytose, process and present antigen to stimulate T cells. In return, the cytokines produced by the activated Th_1 cells are able to activate macrophages. This promotes respiratory burst activity leading to the production of bactericidal oxygen and nitrogen radicals. In addition, cytokines such as IFNγ increase surface antigen expression on macrophages thus increasing their capacity to present antigens (MHC Class II molecules),

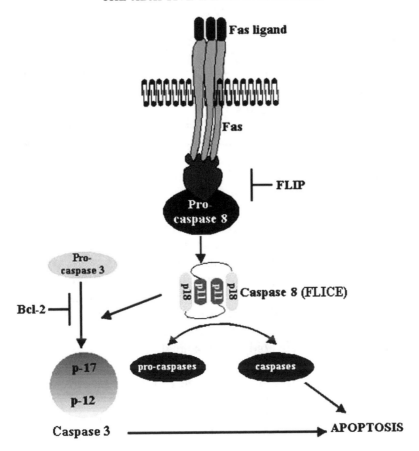

Figure 4.7 Fas/FasL intracellular signalling
When Fas binds Fas ligand, proteins are recruited to the Fas intracellular death domain forming a signalling complex which links activated Fas to pro-caspase 8 causing its activation. Activated caspase 8 (also known as Fas-linked IL-1b – converting enzyme-like protease (FLICE)) initiates the activation of other caspases leading to the induction of apoptosis. Fas activation is regulated by FLIP (FLICE-inhibitory protein) and in some cells by Bcl-2.

phagocytose microorganisms (scavenger receptors, FcR and CR1) and secrete enzymes, cytokines and complement components that promote Th_1 and NK cell activity and microbicidal activity.

Macrophages are capable, along with some NK cells and some T cells, of performing antibody-dependent cellular cytotoxicity (ADCC). Antibody (typically IgG_2) binds to its antigen on the surface of an infected cell. Effector cells with $Fc\gamma R$ are able to bind to the antibody. This ligation signals to the effector cell, which is then capable of destroying the antibody-coated target cell. This activity is upregulated by the production of Th_1-type cytokines since they enhance the expression of $Fc\gamma R$ on effector cells and promote the production of IgG_2 by antigen-stimulated B cells.

NK CELLS

As we have already discussed, NK cells have a number of receptors capable of recognising MHC Class I gene expression on target cells. Ligation of these receptors by MHC prevents the cytotoxic activity of the NK cell. Target cells lacking one or more of these Class I molecules, or only expressing them at very low levels, may be destroyed by the NK cells.

Also, NK cells were first identified for their ability to kill target cells in a non-MHC restricted fashion. This suggests that other receptor–ligand pairs may influence the activity of NK cells. Recently a group of molecules have been identified which have been classified as natural cytotoxicity receptors. These receptors (NKp46 and NKp30), when cross-linked, appear to trigger Ca^{2+} mobilisation, cytotoxicity and cytokine release from NK cells.

The importance of NK cells *in vivo* has always been difficult to determine. However, *in vitro*, these cells can be shown to lyse a range of transformed and virally infected cells. In addition, when incubated with IL-2, NK cells can lyse a range of cells previously resistant to their attack. Recent work has demonstrated the existence of a further NCR (NKp44) that is expressed only on IL-2 stimulated NK cells. This receptor appears to be directly related to the enhanced cytolytic activity of these stimulated NK cells.

NK T cells: T cells activated by **glycolipids** presented by group 1 CD1 proteins possess effector mechanisms that include IFNγ secretion, cytolysis and granulysin production leading to destruction of the cell bearing the processed antigen. Such cells have been described as **NK T cells**.

The killer cell immunoglobulin-like receptors (KIRs) and the lectin-like NK cell receptors NKG2A, NKG2C and NKG2E that form heterodimers with CD94 are also expressed on some T cells.

KIRs distinguish between MHC Class I molecules and usually contain cytoplasmic **immunoreceptor tyrosine-based inhibition motifs** (**ITIMs**) and therefore prevent cytotoxic activity. However, some members lack ITIMs and therefore promote cytotoxicity. About 5% of CD8+ T cells express one or more members of the KIR family, the inhibitory isoforms preventing antigen-mediated T_{cyt} activity. Expression of these molecules appears to be restricted to memory CD8+ T cells, which may derive from a distinct T cell subset with unique differentiation pathways and functional activities.

Less than 5% of circulating CD8+ T cells express the lectin-like NKG2A, 2C and 2E receptors. Only the NKG2A receptor is inhibitory, the others are stimulatory. *In vitro*, it has been shown that CD8+ T cells responding to TCR-dependent stimulation in the presence of TGFβ or IL-15 show *de novo* expression of NKG2A. This suggests that, in contrast to KIR, NKG3A induction is a general feature of many CD8+ T cell responses.

Another member of this group of receptors, NKG2D, is stimulatory. It is found on the majority of gdT cells and on peripheral blood CD8+ T cells. It is thought that NKG2D provides a co-stimulatory signal that enhances TCR-mediated antigen recognition.

- *Cell-mediated immunity involves all those specific immune responses in which antibody plays little or no part.*
- *T cells are naïve, memory or effector cells.*
- *Antigen presenting cells take up antigen, process it, and present it to T cells (usually in secondary lymphoid tissue).*
- *The outcome of the recognition of antigen MHC Class II by the TCR–CD3 complex depends upon additional stimuli derived from co-stimulatory molecules and their ligands.*
- *As a result of the interaction, the antigen presenting cell and the T cell produce a range of cytokines that promote T cell activation, proliferation and differentiation.*
- *Depending upon a range of factors, the prevailing response may be either Th_1 or Th_2.*
- *Th_1 and Th_2 subsets produce a range of cytokines that affect the type of ensuing immune response.*
- *Cell-mediated immunity involves the activity of T_{cyt} cells that are capable of destroying host cells bearing foreign antigens presented in the context of MHC Class I.*
- *Target cell death may be due to the activity of granzymes, perforin and/or Fas–FasL-induced apoptosis.*
- *NK T cells destroy cells bearing ligands presented by CD1.*
- *$\gamma\delta T$ cells and other CD8+ T cells express the NKG2D receptor enhancing antigen recognition.*
- *Cytokines produced by Th_1 cells stimulate macrophages to enhance their phagocytosis and bactericidal activity.*
- *NK cell activity is also enhanced by proinflammatory cytokines.*

4.4   B CELL ADAPTIVE IMMUNITY

The B cell response to an antigenic challenge results in the production of specific antibody. The type of antibody and the kinetics of its production depend on whether or not it is the first time that the host has seen the antigen (Figure 4.8). In a secondary response, not only is the response much more rapid and of much greater magnitude but also the antibodies show much **higher affinity** to the eliciting antigen. This change in antibody class and affinity is due to B cell maturation, differentiation and activation.

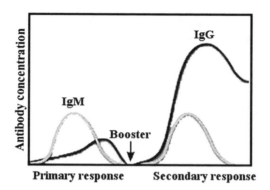

Figure 4.8   Primary and secondary antibody responses

Upon first exposure to an antigen, a lag phase occurs after which antibody of the IgM class which specifically recognises the eliciting antigen is produced. As the response continues, antigen-specific IgG is produced. This occurs much later in the response, reaches a plateau and then declines. Upon subsequent exposure to the antigen, a small IgM response occurs but a much larger IgG response develops very rapidly. Production continues to increase until a plateau is reached. This is at a much higher level than that observed in the primary response and declines only very slowly; returning to base levels over a period of months or even years depending on the eliciting antigen.

4.4.1   B CELL DIFFERENTIATION AND ANTIBODY PRODUCTION

Production of antigen-specific antibody by a B cell is the ultimate outcome of a complex, multistage differentiation. As mentioned in Section 1.1, B cells develop from stem cells in the bone marrow and are released into the blood stream as mature cells, which express antibody on their cell membrane (mIg$^+$ B cells). At a genetic level, maturation is dependent upon the rearrangement and expression of immunoglobulin heavy and light chain genes.

B cell activation is regulated by lymphokines binding to their receptors and the interaction of **cellular adhesion receptors** and their ligands. Once one set of signals has been received, the B cells express new or additional receptors, which allow the cells to migrate to distinct microenvironments where they receive additional signals. Within the secondary lymphoid tissues (e.g. spleen and lymph nodes), most B cells are organised in the primary follicles of B-dependent areas. These areas also harbour some T cells and follicular dendritic cells (FDC). After antigenic stimulation, germinal centres develop in these areas.

Some B cells are present in T areas where most of the T cells are organised in association with **interdigitating cells** (IDC). In addition, some B cells are present in the marginal zones of spleen where lymphocytes enter from the blood stream and which contain **marginal zone macrophages** and a subset of dendritic cells. Thus, within each area, lymphocytes can be associated with different populations of **accessory cells** (IDC, FDC or macrophages), which are thought to play different roles during the various stages of B cell responses.

Primary response (virgin) B cells are highly T cell-dependent, their activation being MHC Class II restricted and requiring direct contact with T cells and the cytokines they produce. By contrast, secondary (memory) B cells require fewer T cells and less antigen. This probably reflects the requirement for antigen presenting cells (such as macrophages and dendritic cells) to process and present antigen to virgin T cells. Once antigen-specific B cells exist, they bind antigen via their surface (Ig) receptors, process and present the antigen to memory T cells, which produce the cytokines required for B cell activation. Antigen uptake via the B cell antigen receptor occurs at much lower levels of antigen than by non-receptor mediated endocytosis (Figure 4.9).

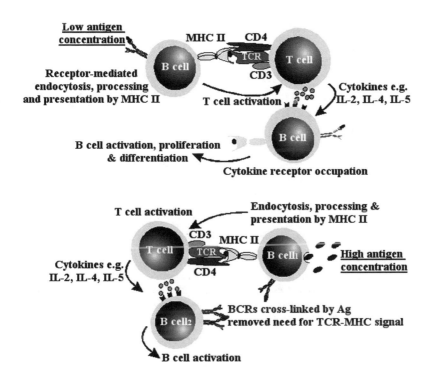

Figure 4.9   Antigen presentation by B cells
Antigen-specific B cells bind antigen via their surface (Ig) receptors, process and present the antigen to memory T cells which produce the cytokines required for B cell activation. Antigen uptake via the B cell antigen receptor occurs at much lower levels of antigen than by non-receptor mediated endocytosis.

The change from a primary to a secondary immune response is characterised not only by an alteration in the predominant antibody class, but also by antibody maturation. A series of complex, highly regulated events results in the transition from the production of low-affinity antibodies in the early primary response to high-affinity antibodies in the memory response. This maturation is dependent upon the occurrence of mutations in the H and L chain variable regions, the positive selection of advantageous mutants (which are given a considerable proliferative advantage over other cells) and the negative selection of those cells that have lost their capacity to recognise antigen. These selection processes, which are essential for the rapid development of the secondary response, depend on the ability of follicular dendritic cells within the germinal centres of the secondary lymphoid tissues to retain antibody–antigen complexes on their surface for long periods of time. Only activated B cells interact with these cells (since they do not express MHC Class II antigens) leading to their accumulation, differentiation and affinity maturation within the germinal centres.

CLASS SWITCHING

As the immune response to a T-dependent antigen matures, the predominant class of antibody changes from IgM to IgG, IgA or IgE. This may be explained by the **genetic switch hypothesis**, which proposes that in the primary repertoire, a given V region gene is brought close to the μ chain gene. After interaction with an antigen, this same V region gene is rearranged next to another heavy chain gene leading to a switch in the predominating antibody class, which is seen during the maturation of an immune response. The expression of the Cγ, α or ε gene is accompanied by the simultaneous repression of the Cμ gene.

> *Studies of serum antibody in a patient with multiple myeloma showed that the μ and γ chains had identical V region amino acid sequences. Since previous genetic studies had shown that constant domains of different heavy chains are synthesised by distinct structural genes, the myeloma protein studies suggested that heavy chain variable and constant regions are synthesised by different structural genes also. Thus, these experiments demonstrated that the different classes of antibody elicited by the same epitope had identical antigenic specificities and led to the determination that antibodies are the product of more than one gene.*

This "class switching" allows a cell to produce a different class of immunoglobulin (with different biological properties) whilst retaining the same specificity for antigen. In recent years, it has been demonstrated that T cells and their soluble products, lymphokines, regulate class switching.

Interleukin 4 has been shown to cause the switch to IgG_4 and IgE in humans. However, the switching process requires the presence of monocytes and physical interactions with T cells since isolated B cells and purified IL-4 do not show class switching. The physical contact with T cells is thought to require the *de novo* expression of a surface antigen on activated cells, which is the ligand for the **CD40** molecule expressed on B cells (**CD40L** or **CD154**). Indeed, antibodies to CD40 in association with IL-4 have been shown to negate the requirement for T cells in IgE switching.

The role of IFNγ in class switching has been clearly demonstrated in mice. This cytokine stimulates IgG_{2a} production in LPS-stimulated B cells. In addition, it stimulates the production of IgG_3 in B cells cultured with anti-Ig and IL-5. Despite this evidence in the murine model, there is no substantial evidence of a role for IFNγ in class switching in humans.

Finally, TGFβ has been shown to stimulate the switch to IgA production by pokeweed mitogen-stimulated human B cells. The switch also required T cell contact. However, the story cannot be that straightforward since IgA production is mostly restricted to cells in mucosa-associated lymphoid tissue, whilst TGFβ is produced in numerous tissues.

KEY POINTS FOR REVIEW

- *The B cell response to an antigen, i.e. the type of antibody produced and its kinetics, is dependent upon whether or not it is the first time that the antigen has been seen.*
- *Secondary responses are much greater and much more rapid than primary responses.*
- *In secondary responses, the antibody shows much higher affinity for the antigen.*
- *B cells bind antigen directly, but require interaction with T cells in the form of CD40–CD154 co-ligation to provide the intracellular signals for differentiation and proliferation.*
- *T-independent antigens may stimulate B cells without the need for T cell interaction but the cytokines produced by activated T cells are still necessary.*
- *Memory does not develop to T-independent antigens and so the antibody response is characteristically IgM in nature.*
- *Class switching (from IgM production to either IgG, A or E) requires T cell contact and specific cytokines.*

4.5 LYMPHOCYTE MEMORY

Generally, the rapidity of secondary responses is a reflection, in part, of an increase in the number of antigen-specific precursor cells. However, this precursor frequency must be carefully regulated in order to limit the response to that required to eliminate a pathogen without causing incidental damage to the host. In order to understand how this regulation works, we must consider the cellular responses that occur during a primary immune response. Briefly, antigen localises in the lymphoid tissues (particularly in the paracortex of the lymph nodes and the periarteriolar lymphocyte sheaths of the spleen) where T and B cell primary responses are initiated. Naïve lymphocytes recirculate through these areas and upon recognition of antigen, the reactive cells are stimulated by lymphokines and rapidly proliferate *in situ*. The level of proliferation is dependent upon the concentration of antigen and the affinity of the receptors on the responding cells. Having acquired specific effector functions and the associated homing/adhesion molecules, the proliferating cells are released into the circulation. These new surface molecules allow the cells to attach to, and pass through, capillary walls thus giving them access to tissues throughout the body. However, the primary response is usually short-lived, rapidly eliminating the stimulating antigen. The majority of the newly generated effector cells rapidly disappear probably due to exhaustive differentiation and the effects of prolonged TCR signalling that may lead to the activation of intracellular pathways, which induce a form of cell death known as apoptosis. Alternatively, effector cell death may be the result of a lack of growth-promoting lymphokines. This 'mass suicide' of effector cells may seem extravagant, but once the stimulating antigen is cleared, these cells are no longer required. Indeed, survival of these effectors could be deleterious, since the resulting response to antigen on second exposure would be excessive, leading to systemic shock. In addition, as more antigens were encountered, the increasing number of effector cells would eventually dilute out naïve cells, reducing the ability of the host to mount a primary response to a new pathogen. However, it would also be wasteful if the immune system did not learn from its experience and so, in most instances, a proportion of the antigen-reactive cells become long-lived memory cells.

The development of T cell memory does not seem to reflect a random survival of effector cells since, with CD8+ cells at least, memory cells appear to have high-affinity receptors. Since T cells do not undergo somatic hypermutation, this affinity maturation may be the result of selective survival of high-affinity cells. By contrast, the development of B cell memory is characterised by isotype switching and affinity maturation caused by somatic hypermutation. This occurs in the germinal centres of secondary lymphoid tissues; an environment

Table 4.8	Surface antigen expression on memory cells	
	Naïve T cells	Memory T cells
CD45R	High	Low
L-selectin	High	Low
CD44	Low	High

which appears to selectively promote the survival of high-affinity mutants. The survivors leave the germinal centres and become long-lived memory cells.

Recent evidence from studies in mice suggests that virgin and memory cells may be derived from different precursor cells which are distinguished by different levels of expression of the heat-stable antigen (HSA) marker.

Memory T cells may be distinguished from naïve cells by their **surface antigen expression** (Table 4.8) and by the **cytokines** they release after antigenic stimulation. In addition to the differential expression of those markers listed in Table 4.8, memory T cells express a range of surface antigens that are largely absent on naïve ones. It has been shown that human T cells with a phenotype typical of **memory** cells **divide much more rapidly** than those with a **naïve** T cell phenotype.

The ability of memory T cells to respond more quickly and strongly to antigen stimulation does not appear to be due to the expression of TCRs with increased affinity for antigen (i.e. T cells do not appear to exhibit **affinity maturation**) but rather to the increased expression of adhesion molecules such as CD2, LFA-1, LFA-3 and CD44 (ensuring enhanced interaction with antigen presenting cells) and expression of IL-2 receptors which allow more rapid response to secreted IL-2 after activation. Both CD4 + and CD8 + cells exhibit memory.

B cells also show phenotypic differences when they differentiate into memory cells. Naïve cells generally express mIgM (in association with mIgD) whilst memory cells generally express mIgG, mIgA or mIgE. Additionally, memory B cells, like T cells, express higher levels of CD44 than naïve B cells.

T and B memory cells are found throughout the secondary lymphoid tissues of the body. Experiments in animals have shown that lymphocytes rapidly recirculate through both the blood and lymph and that memory cells reside within this pool (although not all of them recirculate). Memory cells (particularly T cells) generally show decreased expression of L-selectin (the homing receptor for high endothelial venules in lymph nodes), suggesting that they may use a different recirculation pathway to naïve cells (such as via afferent lymphatic vessels).

Memory T cells are thought to be resting and need to be reactivated to an effector state. However, they also express many of the activation markers found on effector T cells, suggesting that memory cells may be engaged in low-grade responses to persisting antigens and thus are semi-activated. Although memory is often long-lasting, it can decay quite rapidly (i.e. within several weeks) depending on the priming conditions.

Evidence has shown that long-term memory cells are usually in G_0 – the resting stage of the cell cycle. However, both T and B memory cells remain CD44+ for long periods; CD8+ cells have been shown to remain CD44+ for 18 months after adoptive transfer without specific antigen. This suggests that memory cells may not be resting but in a semi-activated state due to low-grade stimulation via T or B cell antigen receptors. This signalling is enough to maintain the expression of CD44 (and other activation markers) but not enough to cause the cells to enter the cell cycle. It has been suggested that the low-grade stimulation may be provided by cross-reacting environmental antigens.

Experiments in animals have suggested that the maintenance of memory depends upon the persistence of antigen. How can the priming antigen persist in the tissues for prolonged periods?

When primed B lymphocytes were adoptively transferred in mice in the absence of antigen, memory responses decayed rapidly. In contrast to this, co-transfer with antigen led to the maintenance of memory. Recently, similar dependence on antigen persistence has been demonstrated for both CD8+ and CD4+ T memory cells.

Follicular dendritic cells are known to retain antigen on their surface for long periods. This antigen, if presented in association with MHC Class II products, can stimulate CD4+ cells. However, there is no evidence that these dendritic cells can present the same antigen in association with MHC Class I products to stimulate CD8+ cells. Thus, what is the explanation for CD8+ T cell memory? In the case of viral infections (which often elicit a CD8+ protective response), clearance of the organism in the primary response may be incomplete.

KEY POINTS FOR REVIEW

- *The primary response is usually short-lived and results in the rapid elimination of the stimulating antigen.*

- *Elimination of the effector cells is necessary since their persistence may lead to fatal shock on re-exposure to the antigen.*
- *T cells appear to show selective survival of those with high-affinity receptors.*
- *B cell memory is characterised by class switching and affinity maturation as a result of somatic mutation.*
- *Memory T cells may be distinguished from naïve cells by their surface antigen expression and the cytokines they produce.*
- *B memory cells express either IgG, A or E.*
- *Memory cells are found throughout the secondary lymphoid tissues and may recirculate round the periphery.*
- *Memory T cells may be resting or may be in a state of constant, low-grade activation.*

4.6   THE MUCOSAL IMMUNE RESPONSE

Most pathogenic organisms establish infection by attaching to, colonising and invading mucosal membranes, which line all the major internal surfaces of the body. Because they are moist, warm, and usually lubricated by nutrient-containing fluid, the mucosal membranes form an excellent environment for promoting the growth of bacteria. To limit infection, the large, complex, mucosal immune system has evolved which is anatomically and functionally distinct from that found elsewhere in the body. It comprises the gastrointestinal (GI) tract, upper and lower respiratory tracts and the urogenital tract. In addition, it may include the exocrine secretory glands such as the salivary, lachrymal, pancreatic and mammary glands.

4.6.1   STRUCTURE OF THE MUCOSAL IMMUNE SYSTEM

The largest part of the mucosal immune system comprises the immunological tissue in the GI tract, the surface area of which is about 400 square metres, approximately 200 times that of the skin. In evolution, the mucosal tissues were probably the first organs to require specific immune protection.

The lymphoid tissues of the mucosae comprise the largest part of the immune system with 60% of all T cells being found in the epithelium of the small intestine. These tissues are particularly important in protection owing to their proximity to antigen. They consist of very organised collections of cells where antigen exposure and initiation of the immune response occurs, and effector

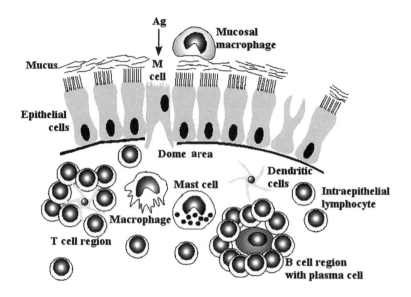

Figure 4.10   Mucosal immune responses
Antigen in the gut is transmitted via M cells into the submucosa where it is processed by dendritic cells or macrophages and presented to intra-epithelial lymphocytes. If the antigen acts as an allergen, upon second exposure mucosal mast cells will degranulate stimulating an acute inflammatory response – allergy.

cells scattered throughout the mucosae where they perform their functions (e.g. secretion of antibody).

ORGANISED MUCOSAL LYMPHOID TISSUE

The organised lymphoid tissue of the gut mucosa (e.g. Peyer's patches) forms aggregates, which are different from those of the systemic lymphoid system (Figure 4.10). The Peyer's patches have the anatomical appearance of classical secondary lymphoid organs, with clearly defined T and B cell-dependent areas in the submucosa. They are separated from the lumen of the intestine by a layer of cuboidal epithelial cells. This layer comprises lymphoid cells of all types and a population of specialised epithelial cells called M cells. These bind antigen and transport it through the cell in pinocytic vesicles. The antigen is released in an unaltered form into the sub-epithelial area. M cells do not express MHC Class II antigens and therefore are not capable of classical antigen presentation.

Dome area: The dome area, which lies beneath the epithelium, contains large numbers of antigen presenting cells. In addition, it contains many T cells most of which are CD4+, although a number lack both CD4 and CD8.

Follicular zone: Beneath the dome area is the follicular zone, which contains the germinal centres with undifferentiated, mIgD+, B cells. In addition, T cells are scattered throughout the zone but the majority of mucosal CD8+ T cells are found between the follicles. Unlike other germinal centre B cells, up to 40% are mIgA$^+$ but these leave before differentiating into plasma cells.

Diffuse lymphoid tissue: The villus/crypt units of the intestine contain large numbers of scattered lymphocytes, both in the epithelium itself (intra-epithelial lymphocytes) and in the deeper layer of the lamina propria. These cells provide immune protection throughout the length of the intestine.

INTRA-EPITHELIAL CELLS

Approximately 10–15% of the cells in the normal epithelium are lymphocytes, the majority of which are CD8$^+$ T cells. Interestingly, about 10% of the T cells express the $\gamma\delta$TCR.

Local production of cytokines such as TGFβ, IL-1, IL-6, IL-7, IL-8 and macrophage inhibitory protein-1 (MIP-1) can modulate the function of intra-epithelial lymphocytes. The latter express an integrin, which binds to E-cadherin expressed on enterocytes. Its expression is enhanced by TGFβ and it is thought that release of this cytokine by enterocytes encourages the migration and accumulation of T cells in the mucosa. However, the role of these lymphocytes in mucosal immunity is unclear. Most of the T cells show poor responses to mitogenic or antigenic stimulation *in vitro*. It has been suggested that the $\gamma\delta$ TCR$^+$ cells may act to downregulate local immune responses, thus ensuring that the majority of antigens from the gut are blocked from stimulating either a local or systemic immune response.

LEUKOCYTES IN THE LAMINA PROPRIA

The lamina propria lymphocytes comprise both B and T cells and lie beneath the epithelium. The majority of B cells are mIgA$^+$ but mIgM$^+$, mIgG$^+$ and mIgE$^+$ B cells are also found in decreasing concentrations. The T cells show increased expression of MHC Class II antigens and IL-2R and secrete cytokines in response to stimulation rather than proliferating, suggesting they are a type of memory T cell. These cells are found in close association with dendritic cells and macrophages.

The lamina propria also contains mast cell precursors, which rapidly differentiate into mature cells when stimulated. These cells are responsible for the inflammatory response to food allergens.

4.6.2   IMMUNOGLOBULINS AND MUCOSAL IMMUNITY

Uniquely, the B cells found in the follicles of the mucosae preferentially produce IgA. IgA production is dependent upon T cells, mucosal macrophages and stromal cells providing the signals required for isotype switching. IL-4, IL-5 and IL-6 have been implicated in this process but it has been shown that additional IgA-binding factors from $Fc\gamma R^+$ T cells are required for the terminal differentiation of IgA-secreting B cells.

PRODUCTION OF OTHER IMMUNOGLOBULINS IN THE MUCOSA

Patients with selective IgA deficiency have been shown to have mucosal protection provided by IgM, indicating a role for this antibody in mucosal immunity. In addition, during allergic reactions, IgE is found in the mucosae. However, in normal tissue, IgE-producing B cells are rare.

4.6.3 THE MUCOSAE AND THEIR ROLE IN IMMUNITY

The mucosal immune system is constantly exposed to antigens (derived from food or the normal microbial flora) to which an immune response would be inappropriate. However, its structure is such that these antigens are usually not exposed to the systemic immune system. In addition, a state of unresponsiveness or tolerance to such antigens may prevail. This may be due to antigen being presented by dendritic cells that lack the necessary co-stimulatory molecules, resulting in tolerance rather than immunity. In addition, antigens presented by epithelial cells appear to preferentially stimulate $CD8^+$ T cells, which have been implicated in down-regulating immune responses to mucosal antigens.

KEY POINTS FOR REVIEW

- *Most pathogenic organisms establish infection by attaching to, colonising and invading mucosal membranes.*
- *The largest part of the mucosal immune system comprises the immunological tissue in the GI tract.*
- *Effector cells are scattered throughout the mucosae where they perform their functions.*
- *The organised lymphoid tissue of the gut mucosa forms aggregates, which are different from those of the systemic lymphoid system.*
- *Antigen presenting cells are found in the dome area.*
- *The follicular zone contains the germinal centres with undifferentiated, $mIgD^+$, B cells.*
- *Intraepithelial lymphocytes comprise 10–15% of the epithelial cells, their activity being influenced by locally produced cytokines.*

- *Uniquely, the B cells found in the follicles of the mucosae preferentially produce IgA.*

4.7 TOLERANCE

In the preceding sections we have learnt how the immune system recognises and responds to antigen in order to provide a protective immune response. This response to non-self antigens is key to our survival. Generally, it is not beneficial for the immune system to recognise and react to self-antigens. Indeed, in most cases it is vital that the immune system tolerates 'self' and does not react to such antigens. How can we explain this **tolerance**; the fact that an antigen normally found in our own body does not elicit an immune response whilst one that is not, does? Why do we live quite happily with our own organs whilst one transplanted from someone else is rapidly rejected unless aggressive chemotherapy is employed? Originally, it was thought that all cells that showed reactivity to self-antigens were destroyed during development. However, there is a wide range of diseases in which the immune system does react to certain self-antigens. The existence of these **autoimmune diseases** suggests that the answer cannot be that simple and that self-reactive cells must survive. The reactivity of lymphocyte clones is determined at a genetic level and thus it stands to reason that due to certain events (such as **random, somatic mutation**) some self-reactive and therefore potentially damaging cells may develop.

Over the years, several areas of research have suggested the existence of a number of mechanisms by which tolerance is regulated. These mechanisms involve (1) the physical or functional neutralisation of self-reactive cells through **clonal deletion, clonal abortion** or **clonal anergy** or (2) the control of autoreactive lymphocytes through the normal regulatory mechanisms of the immune system, e.g. through **idiotypic networks** or **regulatory T cells**.

4.7.1 LYMPHOCYTE TOLERANCE

As you have already discovered, products of the major histocompatibility complex are found on the surface of all nucleated cells in the body. The structure of these molecules includes a cleft in which processed antigen is sited that may be presented to T cells (MHC Class I molecules to CD8$^+$ cells and Class II to CD4$^+$ cells). When processed foreign antigen is not available, peptides derived from the host's own proteins occupy these clefts. Since T cell antigen receptors are randomly generated, it is possible that a T cell would develop a receptor capable of recognising this processed self-peptide. If such development were uncontrolled, **self-reactive T cells** would be capable of initiating a response, which would destroy those host tissues in which the original antigen was expressed. The situation is even more problematic with B cells. As you have seen, the generation of antibody diversity is a random process due to recombination and somatic mutation. B cells, which recognise soluble, unprocessed antigen are capable (potentially) of generating antibodies that recognise any antigenic epitope. Antibodies recognising self-antigens could stimulate complement activation or antibody-dependent cellular cytotoxicity, leading to the destruction of the host's own tissues. Obviously, the capacity of T and B cells to react to self-antigens is detrimental to the host and a variety of mechanisms have developed to control or eliminate these self-reactive cells. This results in a state of non-responsiveness known as immunological tolerance. However, the efficiency of this process will depend on the mechanisms involved and the type of cell to be tolerised. The time required for the induction of tolerance, its duration and the level of antigen required to induce it will vary according to the type of cell involved, e.g. T or B lymphocyte.

INDUCTION TIME

Studies using cells from animals have given us an indication of the length of time required for the induction of tolerance in T and B cells. However, it must be remembered that tolerance can be induced *in vitro* much quicker than *in vivo* and that induction times will vary somewhat between species and even between individuals (Table 4.9).

Lymphocytes are very susceptible to the induction of tolerance during foetal development and the first few weeks of life, i.e. before the immune system reaches maturity.

Thus, immature B cells are particularly susceptible whilst both mature B cells and plasma cells are relatively resistant. This difference in susceptibility is thought to be due to the modulation of antibody on B cells. Membrane immunoglobulin (mIg) is aggregated by antigen and is either endocytosed or

Table 4.9   Time required for induction of tolerance in various cell types

Cell type	Antigen type	Time of induction
Splenic or thymic T cells	T-dependent	Within hours of challenge
Adult splenic B cells	T-dependent	Within 4 days of challenge
Mature bone marrow B cells	T-dependent	Within 15 days of challenge
B cells	T-independent	Quicker than T-dependent antigens due to higher avidity for BCR

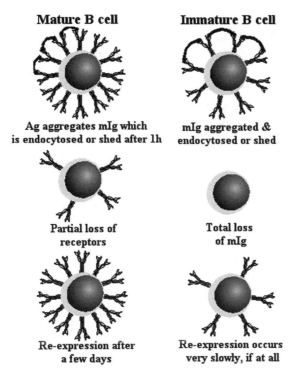

Figure 4.11   B cell tolerance
In mature B cells, mIg may be aggregated by antigen and removed from the cell surface in about an hour and is re-expressed after a few days although the process is rarely complete. By contrast, in immature B cells, this loss of mIg is more rapid, usually complete and re-expression may take a very long time, if it occurs at all.

shed from the cell surface. Until the mIg can be regenerated (or re-expressed), the cell is unable to respond to further antigenic stimuli, i.e. the organism is tolerant to the antigen. In mature B cells, the mIg is aggregated and removed from the cell surface in about an hour and is re-expressed after a few days. In addition, the process is rarely complete. By contrast, in immature B cells, this loss of mIg is more rapid, usually complete and re-expression may take a very long time, if it occurs at all (Figure 4.11). Thus, tolerance is much easier to establish in immature B cells.

ANTIGEN DOSE

The level of antigen required to tolerise B cells is usually 100 to 1000 times greater than that needed for T cells (**high zone tolerance**). However, the required dose may be reduced if the B cell binds the tolerogen with high avidity. The dose of the antigen required will also vary according to the maturity of the cells. In addition, the level of antigen required to induce B cell tolerance in neonates is approximately 100-fold less than that in adults. This is probably due to the lower concentration of mIg requiring cross-linking by antigen.

In addition to high zone tolerance, some weak immunogens may be given at very low levels and result in **low zone tolerance**. However, this form of tolerance has limitations in that it is usually only partially effective, only affecting some cells and is maintained by a subpopulation of T cells. These cells suppress the activity of the potentially autoreactive B cells. It is thought that the extremely low levels of antigen selectively activate these T regulatory cells (T_{reg}); T helper cells require much higher doses of antigen in order to be activated.

ANTIGEN PERSISTENCE

Generally, antigen must be present continually to maintain tolerance. Thus, tolerance which follows a single injection of an antigen which is only removed and digested slowly is more persistent than that induced by antigens which are rapidly cleared from the system.

SPECIFICITY

When tolerance is induced, the host fails to respond to a particular antigenic determinant. Thus, if the determinant is a common one, which appears in a number of different antigens, the host will be tolerant to that antigenic determinant in all the antigens in which it is expressed. If the determinant is the major immunogenic determinant (i.e. it is the determinant which is primarily responsible for eliciting an immune response to those antigens), then the host will be tolerant to a range of antigens (Figure 4.12). If however the antigens express other immunogenic determinants, then the host will be able to respond to them and clear the antigen from the system.

DURATION

It is difficult to envisage how, if a self-reactive cell has been deleted, self-reactivity can re-emerge. Self-reactivity is determined by the specificity of the TCR or BCR. Since these receptors are generated by recombination events between several genes and by somatic mutation, the new cells being produced by the bone marrow may, by chance, develop further self-reactive receptors. Thus, when tolerance is due to clonal deletion, recovery is related to the time required to regenerate mature lymphocytes from the stem cell population. However, if tolerance is caused by blockade of antibody-forming cells, this is rapidly lost by removal of the antigen. In general, T cell tolerance is more persistent than B cell tolerance.

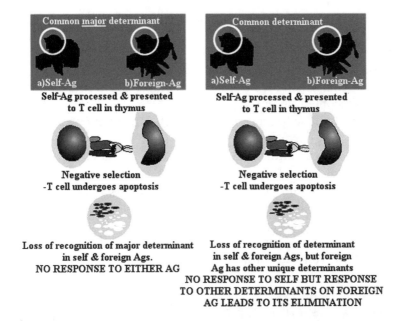

Figure 4.12   Effect of tolerance to a major immunogenic determinant
When tolerance is induced, the host fails to respond to a particular antigenic determinant. Thus, if the determinant is a common one which appears in a number of different antigens, the host will be tolerant to that antigenic determinant in all the antigens. If the determinant is the major immunogenic determinant then the host will be tolerant to a range of antigens.

ROUTE OF ADMINISTRATION

We have already mentioned how the dose of an antigen may affect tolerance induction. In addition, the route of administration may influence which cells become tolerised to a particular dose. For example, a given dose of an antigen may induce tolerance in both B and T cells when given internally. However, when applied to the skin, the same dose may induce an antibody response but fail to stimulate a cell-mediated response. In such a situation, the T cells responsible for the stimulation of a delayed-type hypersensitivity response are tolerised whilst other T cells and B cells are not. This implies that not only do B and T cells show differences in susceptibility to tolerance induction, but also subpopulations of T cells are differentially affected (in this case it is likely that Th_1-type cells are tolerised whilst Th_2-type cells are not).

TISSUE SPECIFICITY

Some tissues in the body exhibit surface antigens, which are peculiar to that tissue. In addition, the expression of certain antigens is associated with the stage of development or maturation of a particular cell. Although blood cells derive from the bone marrow, they may express antigens associated with their mature status that are not expressed on the immature precursors in the bone marrow. Thus, an animal (A) tolerised by the neonatal injection of bone marrow haemopoietic cells from another strain (B) may not be tolerant to an injection of blood from B. This is due to the host recognising foreign antigens on the strain B mature blood cells, which are not expressed on the strain B haemopoietic cells to which it has become tolerant.

Since the majority of self-reactive T and B cells are eliminated in the primary lymphoid tissues (the thymus and bone marrow respectively), lymphocytes capable of recognising an antigen whose expression is limited to a tissue distinct from these will escape destruction. In the periphery, these potentially autoreactive cells must be controlled to prevent disease. If the antigen is expressed in an immunologically privileged site (i.e. immunological cells do not normally have access to it), e.g. the brain, the autoreactive cells are unlikely to cause disease unless tissue damage (e.g. due to virus infection) causes the release of the antigen or recruitment of immunologically active cells to the site.

4.7.2 MECHANISMS OF TOLERANCE INDUCTION

The interaction between an antigen and its specific cell surface receptor may result either in the activation and differentiation of the cell (positive selection) or in its inactivation or even death (negative selection). Positive selection usually results in a cell leaving G_0 and entering the cell cycle giving rise to a clone of increasingly differentiated effector cells, e.g. cytotoxic T cells and plasma cells. This process is known as **clonal selection**. By contrast, when an antigen–receptor interaction results in negative selection leading to cell death, it is known as **clonal deletion** (Figure 4.13). Although only a single cell is destroyed, the host has lost the potential to develop the clone of cells that would recognise the epitope in question. When the self-reactive cell is not killed but made functionally inactive the outcome is known as **clonal anergy**.

The theory of clonal deletion was proposed first by Burnett to explain the lack of self-reactivity in the immune system. This suggested that all cells bearing receptors which recognise self-antigen were destroyed, thus preventing the development of an autoimmune response. Death usually results from the induction of apoptosis (often referred to as cellular suicide or programmed cell death) in the self-reactive cells.

An autoimmune response is one directed against antigens expressed by the host's own tissues (auto) which leads to tissue damage. If the antigen is restricted to one particular organ or tissue (e.g. the thyroid), the resulting signs and symptoms are typical of a disease affecting that organ. However, if the antigen is expressed in several tissues or organs, the signs and symptoms will be more generalised.

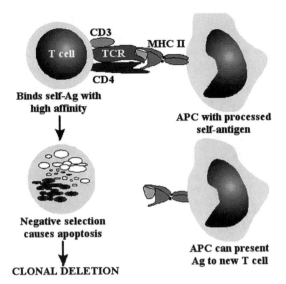

Figure 4.13   Clonal deletion
T cells capable of recognising self-antigens are deleted in the thymus during their differentiation. Negative selection ensures that most potentially damaging self-reactive T cells are identified and effectively neutralised by ensuring that they come in contact with a mixture of self-antigens within the thymic environment. The elimination of self-reactive T cells is thought to be dependent upon the avidity with which the T cell binds the antigen. T cells expressing receptors which bind antigens with only low affinity may escape elimination and pass into the periphery.

Since immunological activation depends on the concentration of the antigen and the level of receptor expression, some self-reactive cells may not be activated by the local antigen concentration or may not express high enough levels of receptor molecules under normal circumstances. Such cells would not be subject to negative selection but also would not normally cause disease. However, should circumstances change, i.e. an increase in local antigen concentration due to tissue damage, the cell may be activated and autoimmune damage would result. This type of non-reactivity has been called **clonal ignorance**.

B cell tolerance has been described as "the absence of a measurable antibody response to an antigenic challenge". In order that tolerance might be established, antigen must bind the BCR. However, in only a few cases does this interaction lead to tolerance rather than to activation and antibody formation.

CLONAL DELETION

Clonal deletion has been demonstrated to be responsible for the elimination of lymphocytes reactive with cell surface-bound self-antigen. Even antigens which have low affinity for the BCR or TCR can induce deletion. However, T cells which express TCR that bind with self-antigen with low affinity may escape deletion in the thymus. With B cells, deletion can occur in the bone marrow or after the cells leave the bone marrow. Clonal deletion of autoreactive T cells in the thymus is clearly influenced by thymic epithelial cells. It is easy to induce tolerance through clonal deletion in the embryo or in neonatal life, but not in the adult. This is thought to be due to mature T cells preventing the deposition of the antigen in the adult thymus.

T cells capable of recognising self-antigens are deleted in the thymus during their differentiation. Positive selection within the thymus ensures that all mature T cells are able to recognise the proteins coded for by the major histocompatibility complex (MHC) on all cells of the body. On the other hand, negative selection ensures that most potentially damaging self-reactive T cells are identified and effectively neutralised by ensuring that they come in contact with a mixture of self-antigens within the thymic environment. The elimination of self-reactive T cells is thought to be dependent upon the avidity with which the T cell binds the antigen. T cells expressing receptors, which bind antigens with only low affinity, may escape elimination and pass into the periphery.

CLONAL ANERGY

T cells may exhibit tolerance to self-antigens in the periphery through clonal anergy. This may result from defective antigen presentation or a lack of co-stimulatory signals from the antigen presenting cell.

B cells may also exhibit clonal anergy, its nature depending upon the type of antigen involved.

T-dependent antigens: The mechanisms controlling B cell tolerance to T-dependent antigens are difficult to define since T helper cells may recognise determinants on the antigen enabling them to trigger B cells. Thus, tolerance to these antigens can only be induced if the host lacks functional T cells or the T cells are effectively tolerant to determinants on the antigen.

The response of B cells to T-dependent antigens is dependent upon signals received from antigen-specific T cells. If this T cell help is not provided, the B cell cannot respond and is functionally deleted. This results in clonal anergy.

T-independent antigens: B cells may be tolerised to a variety of T-independent antigens, which generally are slowly metabolised *in vivo* and tend to promote relatively long-lasting tolerance. The degree of tolerance and its persistence is dependent on the dose of antigen injected.

To act as effective tolerogens, T-independent antigens are required in higher doses than T-dependent antigens. B cells show differences in sensitivity to tolerance induction depending on their mIg class. Thus, T-independent antigens induce tolerance in B cells in the following order: $mIgE^+ > mIgG^+ > mIgM^+$.

Usually, antigens that do not require T cell help in order to stimulate B cells are large molecules made of repeating subunits and have a high number of identical antigenic determinants. Such molecules are capable of cross-linking a

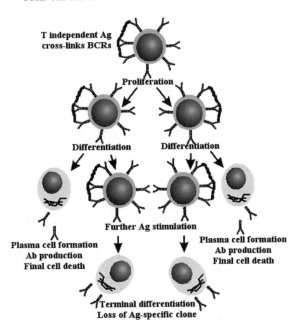

Figure 4.14 Clonal exhaustion
Repeated challenge with immunising doses of a T-independent antigen may cause clonal exhaustion of B cells. This type of antigen usually stimulates mIgM$^+$ cells and does not cause the formation of memory cells. The stimulated cells differentiate into antibody-producing cells which are only short-lived and after each challenge, fewer cells remain which are capable of responding, until eventually all reactive cells are exhausted.

large number of antigen-specific receptors on B cells, and in this way may eliminate the need for T cell help. If such a T-independent antigen is present in too high a concentration or is present in a non-immunogenic form, abnormal intracellular signals are produced which fail to trigger proliferation and differentiation of the B cells, i.e. they are functionally deleted or clonally anergic.

CLONAL EXHAUSTION

Repeated challenge with immunising doses of a T-independent antigen may cause clonal exhaustion. This type of antigen usually stimulates mIgM$^+$ cells and does not cause the formation of memory cells. The stimulated cells differentiate into antibody-producing cells which are only short-lived and after each challenge, fewer cells remain that are capable of responding, until eventually all reactive cells are exhausted (Figure 4.14). When self-antigens are the stimulating agent, their continued presence ensures clonal exhaustion. With non-self antigens, removal of the agent will allow clonal recovery over an extended period of time.

CLONAL ABORTION

If immature B cells developing in the primary lymphoid tissues (e.g. the bone marrow) are exposed to extremely low levels of specific antigen for the first time, normal maturation is inhibited and the cell is unable to respond appropriately upon subsequent challenge. This type of tolerance is known as clonal abortion and is easily induced.

ANTIBODY FORMING CELL (AFC) BLOCKADE

Although it is very difficult to tolerise antibody forming cells, very large doses of T-independent antigens can sometimes be effective. The process is similar to that described above in that high concentrations of antigen blockade the antigen receptors of the antibody forming cell and in doing so interfere with antibody secretion.

4.7.3 MAINTENANCE OF TOLERANCE

A number of processes have been identified which regulate tolerance. With T cells, the initial step occurs in the thymus and is clonal deletion of T cells with receptors that recognise self-antigen with high affinity. However, due to their recognition of short linear arrays of amino acids, T cells have a limited repertoire (when compared to B cells) and so the threshold of clonal deletion must be set low enough to ensure that a wide repertoire of T cells is available in the periphery to combat foreign antigens. This means that T cells whose antigen receptors have an affinity for self-antigens below the threshold avoid clonal deletion, mature, and enter the circulation.

REGULATORY T CELLS

Cells that are not deleted in the thymus but which show some measure of self-recognition may be controlled by other tolerance-inducing mechanisms. These include altered signal transduction (resulting in clonal anergy) and alteration of the expression of co-receptor and accessory molecules resulting in reduced affinity of the antigen receptor. In addition, T regulatory cells have been implicated in this process. In years past suppressor, $CD8^+$ T cells were thought to inhibit the activation of self-reactive T cells. More recently, regulatory T cells have been identified (T_{reg}) that appear to control the activation of other T cells.

The majority of T_{reg} cells are **CD25+** (i.e. they express the IL-2 receptor). The way in which these cells prevent reactivity to self has not been clearly established. However, it is known that T_{reg} require direct contact with autoreactive T cells to exert their function. Although antigen recognition is required, T_{reg} effector function is antigen independent. In addition, these cells have been shown to modulate the activity of antigen presenting cells (possibly by downregulating the expression of the co-stimulatory molecules CD80 and CD86). T_{reg} cell activity is dependent upon TGFβ and IL-4. By preventing the activation of self-reactive T cells, they also prevent self-reactive B cell activation.

ANTIBODY-INDUCED TOLERANCE

As we discussed earlier, anti-idiotypic antibodies are specific for the antigen-binding sites which induced their formation. If these stimulating **idiotopes** are part of the immunoglobulin molecules on the surface of a B cell, the anti-idiotypes will cause the mIg to be cross-linked. This may lead to tolerance if the appropriate concentration of anti-idiotype is present. The effect of such tolerance is to prevent the B cell from responding to its eliciting antigen. It is thought that this mechanism is involved in the "switching-off" of an immune response.

4.7.4   MECHANISMS INVOLVED IN THE DEVELOPMENT OF INCOMPLETE TOLERANCE

Tolerance induction may involve the deletion of only some aspects of the immune response, which results in incomplete tolerance. For example, if T cell tolerance is induced to an antigen, B cells may still be able to respond. If the T cells are only tolerant to a single antigenic determinant on the antigen, help for B cells may be provided by T cells reacting to other determinants on the antigen (Figure 4.15).

KEY POINTS FOR REVIEW

- *The majority of antigen-specific cells do not recognise self-antigens, those that do so are either eliminated or prevented from responding. This state of lack of responsiveness to self is known as tolerance.*
- *Tolerance may be achieved by a range of central or peripheral mechanisms.*
- *Tolerance may be maintained through idiotypic networks or regulatory T cells.*
- *Immature B cells are much more susceptible to tolerance induction than mature B or plasma cells.*

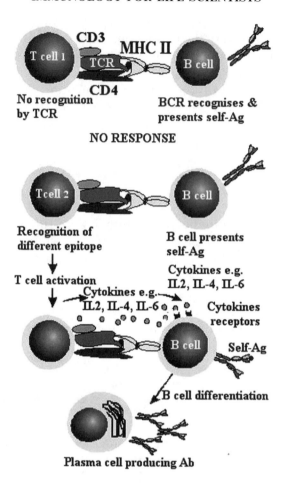

Figure 4.15   Induction of partial tolerance
Tolerance induction may involve the deletion of only some aspects of the immune response which results in incomplete tolerance. If T cells are only tolerant to a single antigenic determinant on an antigen, help for B cells may be provided by T cells reacting to other determinants on the antigen.

- *B cells require much higher doses of antigen than T cells for tolerance induction.*
- *Low zone tolerance is dependent upon a subpopulation of T cells (probably T_{reg} cells), which are activated at very low doses of antigen and suppress the activity of other cells.*
- *Usually, antigen must be continuously present to maintain tolerance.*
- *Tolerance is to a particular antigenic determinant, which may be expressed in one or more antigens. The host will be tolerant to the determinant regardless of the antigen by which it is expressed.*

- *When tolerance is due to clonal deletion, recovery is dependent upon the time required to regenerate mature lymphocytes from stem cells.*
- *Tolerance may depend on the route of administration of the antigen.*
- *The majority of self-reactive T and B cells are eliminated in the thymus or bone marrow respectively.*
- *The mechanism of B cell tolerance induction will vary depending in part on whether the antigen concerned is T cell-dependent or -independent.*
- *Maintenance of tolerance may be dependent upon idiotypic networks and the activity of T regulatory cells.*

BIBLIOGRAPHY

Alfonso C, Liljedahl M, Winqvist O, Surh CD, Peterson PA, Fung-Leung WP, Karlsson L. (1999) The role of H2-O and HLA-DO in major histocompatibility complex class II-restricted antigen processing and presentation. Immunol Rev, 172; 255–266.

Barry M, Bleackley RC. (2002) Cytotoxic T lymphocytes: all roads lead to death. Nat Rev Immunol, 2; 401–409.

Branch Moody D, Besra GS. (2001) Glycolipid targets of CD1-mediated T-cell responses. Immunology, 104; 243–251.

Brocke P, Garbi N, Momburg F, Hammerling GJ. (2002) HLA-DM, HLA-DO and tapasin: functional similarities and differences. Curr Opin Immunol, 14; 22–29.

DeFranco AL. (2000) B cell activation 2000. Immunol Rev, 176; 5–9.

Diehl L, Den Boer AT, van der Voort EI, Melief CJ, Offringa R, Toes RE. (2000) The role of CD40 in peripheral T cell tolerance and immunity. J Mol Med, 78; 363–371.

Freihorst J, Ogra PL. (2001) Mucosal immunity and viral infections. Ann Med, 33; 172–177.

Guermonprez P, Valladeau J, Zitvogel L, Thery C, Amigorena S. (2002) Antigen presentation and T cell stimulation by dendritic cells. Ann Rev Immunol, 20; 621–667.

Hamzaoui N, Pringault E. (1998) Interaction of microorganisms, epithelium, and lymphoid cells of the mucosa-associated lymphoid tissue. Ann N Y Acad Sci, 859; 65–74.

Harty JT, Badovinac VP. (2002) Influence of effector molecules on the CD8+ T cell response to infection. Curr Opin Immunol, 14; 360–365.

Jacquemin MG, Vanzieleghem B, Saint-Remy JM. (2001) Mechanisms of B-cell tolerance. Adv Exp Med Biol, 489; 99–108.

Jayawardena-Wolf J, Bendelac A. (2001) CD1 and lipid antigens: intracellular pathways for antigen presentation. Curr Opin Immunol, 13; 109–113.

Karre K. (2002) NK cells, MHC Class I molecules and the missing self. Scand J Immunol, 55; 221–228.

Lechler R, Chai JG, Marelli-Berg F, Lombardi G. (2001) The contributions of T-cell anergy to peripheral T-cell tolerance. Immunology, 103; 262–269.

Li J-H, Rosen D, Sondel P, Berke G. (2002) Immune privilege and FasL: two ways to inactivate effector cytotoxic T lymphocytes by FasL expressing cells. Immunol, 105; 267–277.

Mackey MF, Barth RJ Jr, Noelle RJ. (1998) The role of CD40/CD154 interactions in the priming, differentiation, and effector function of helper and cytotoxic T cells. J Leukoc Biol, 63; 418–428.

McHugh RS, Shevach EM. (2002) The role of suppressor T cells in regulation of immune responses. J Allergy Clin Immunol, 110; 693–702.

McMahon CW, Raulet DH. (2001) Expression and function of NK cell receptors in CD8+ T cells. Curr Opin Immunol, 13; 465–470.

Metz DP, Bottomly K. (1999) Function and regulation of memory CD4 T cells. Immunol Res, 19; 127–141.

Miller JF. (2001) Immune self-tolerance mechanisms. Transplantation, 72; S5–S9.

Moretta A, Biassoni R, Bottino C, Mingari MC, Moretta L. (2000) Natural cytotoxicity receptors that trigger human NK-cell mediated cytolysis. Immunol Today, 21; 228–234.

Moretta L, Biassoni R, Bottino C, Mingari MC, Moretta A. (2002) Natural killer cells: a mystery no more. Scand J Immunol, 55; 229–232.

Pieters J. (2000) MHC class II-restricted antigen processing and presentation. Adv Immunol, 75; 159–208.

Sakaguchi S, Sakaguchi N, Yamazaki S, Sakihama T, Shimizu J, Itoh M, Kuniyasu Y, Nomura T, Toda M, Takahashi T. (2001) Immunologic tolerance maintained by CD25[1] CD4[1] regulatory T cells: their common role in controlling autoimmunity, tumor immunity, and transplantation tolerance. Immunol Rev, 182; 18–32.

Sijts A, Zaiss D, Kloetzel PM. (2001) The role of the ubiquitin–proteasome pathway in MHC class I antigen processing: implications for vaccine design. Curr Mol Med, 1; 665–676.

Silva CL, Bonato VLD, Karla M, Lima KM, Coelho-Castelo AAM, Faccioli LH, Sartori A, De Souza AO, Lea SC. (2001) Cytotoxic T cells and mycobacteria. FEMS Microbiol Lett, 197; 11–18.

Tsubata T, Honjo T. (2000) B cell tolerance and autoimmunity. Rev Immunogenet, 2; 18–25.

Tuma RA, Pamer EG. (2002) Homeostasis of naïve, effector and memory CD8 T cells. Curr Opin Immunol, 14; 348–353.

van Ginkel FW, Nguyen HH, McGhee JR. (2000) Vaccines for mucosal immunity to combat emerging infectious diseases. Emerg Infect Dis, 6; 123–132.

Wang J, Watanabe T. (1999) Expression and function of Fas during differentiation and activation of B cells. Int Rev Immunol, 18; 367–379.

Zarzaur BL, Kudsk KA. (2001) The mucosa-associated lymphoid tissue structure, function, and derangements. Shock, 15; 411–420.

NOW TEST YOURSELF!

1.   Which of the following is NOT a characteristic of interleukin 12?

(a) It is produced by B lymphoblastoid cells.

(b) Its production may be induced by microorganisms such as Toxoplasma gondii.

(c) It is important in defence against intracellular pathogens.

(d) It induces interferon gamma production by NK cells and T cells.

(e) It blocks activation of cytokine synthesis by Th$_1$ cells.

2.   Which of the following statements concerning the molecular and cellular events which occur after antigen presentation to T cells is INCORRECT?

(a) Once it is produced, any T cell may bind interleukin 2 and proliferate, regardless of whether or not it has recognised antigen or of its antigen-specificity.

(b) IL-1 binds IL-1 receptors on T cells, augmenting the stimulatory signal from the early activation events.

(c) The early activation events result in the production of a signal which stimulates the T cells to produce IL-2 and to express IL-2 receptors.

(d) IL-2 may act back on the cell which produced it (autocrine effect) or it may diffuse away and act on other cells, promoting their proliferation and differentiation.

(e) As a result of interaction with the T cell, the antigen presenting cell is stimulated to secrete IL-1.

3.   Subsets of T cells which show different patterns of cytokine production are generally accepted to exist in humans. Which of the following statements is FALSE?

(a) The recognised subsets of Th cells are Th_0, Th_1 and Th_2.

(b) Cytotoxic T cells do not show a similar pattern of subsets which may be defined by their cytokine secretion profiles.

(c) Th_1 cells produce cytokines which are responsible for the stimulation of cytotoxic effector cells and macrophage activities.

(d) Th_2 cells produce cytokines which promote the proliferation and differentiation of B cells.

(e) The cytokines produced by the different subsets of T helper cells stimulate different types of immune response.

4.   Granulocyte–macrophage colony-stimulating factor:

(a) Is produced by bone marrow quiescent lymphocytes, bone marrow stromal cells, fibroblasts and endothelial cells.

(b) Is a molecule that contains disulphide bonding but this is not vital for the biological function of the molecule.

(c) At low concentrations stimulates the formation of eosinophil colonies from pluripotent stem cells.

(d) Is bound by lymphocytes and monocytes.

(e) Promotes the growth and survival of haematopoietic progenitor cells.

5.   Which of the following statements concerning the regulation of Th_1 and Th_2 responses is INCORRECT?

(a) IL-2 is the chief growth-promoting factor for both Th_1 and Th_2 subsets.

(b) IL-4 stimulates growth of Th_1 and Th_2 cells for a short time after encounter with antigen.

(c) As with naïve cells, IL-1 is required as a co-stimulant after antigen presentation but only by Th$_1$ cells.

(d) IL-12 induces the differentiation of Th$_1$ cells, its production being inhibited by IL-10, which is produced by Th$_2$ cells.

(e) GM-CSF and tumour necrosis factor are produced by both Th$_1$ and Th$_2$ cells.

6. Which of the following is NOT typical of an antigen-specific antibody response?

(a) When first exposed to an antigen, a lag phase occurs during which no antigen-specific antibody is detected.

(b) The first antigen-specific antibody to be produced is IgM, which very quickly reaches a plateau.

(c) Antigen-specific IgG is produced some time after IgM, reaches a plateau and declines.

(d) Upon subsequent exposure to antigen, a small IgM response occurs.

(e) The secondary IgG response is much larger and very rapid. It reaches a much higher plateau level which declines very slowly, returning to base levels only after months or even years.

7. The B cell response to an antigenic challenge:

(a) Results in the production of non-specific antibody.

(b) Is independent of whether or not the host has seen the antigen previously.

(c) Is similar on first exposure to antigen to that seen on secondary or subsequent exposures.

(d) Results in the formation of antibodies, their affinity for the eliciting antigen increasing with secondary and subsequent exposure to the antigen.

(e) Results in changes in antibody class and affinity which are independent of cell maturation, differentiation and activation.

8. Which of the following statements concerning B cell differentiation and antibody production is INCORRECT?

(a) B cells develop from stem cells in the bone marrow and are released into the blood stream as mature cells.

(b) All circulating B cells express membrane IgG.

(c) B cell maturation can be classified by the rearrangement and expression of immunoglobulin heavy and light chain genes.

(d) The immune response to T-dependent antigens is characterised by a change in the predominating antibody class from IgM to IgG, IgA or IgE.

(e) Class switching is achieved by rearranging the V region gene, which is apposed to the mu chain gene. After secondary interaction with antigen, the same V region gene is rearranged next to a gamma, alpha or epsilon chain gene.

9. **B cell activation is regulated by the binding of lymphokines to their receptors and the interaction of cellular adhesion receptors. Which of the following statements is FALSE?**

(a) *Once one set of signals is received, B cells express new or additional receptors which allow them to migrate to distinct microenvironments.*

(b) *Within the secondary lymphoid tissues (e.g. spleen and lymph nodes) most B cells are organised within the primary follicles.*

(c) *After antigenic stimulation, germinal centres develop in the primary follicles.*

(d) *Different areas of the secondary lymphoid tissue contain different populations of accessory cells which are thought to play different roles during the various stages of B cell responses.*

(e) *Virgin B cells are dependent upon the cytokines produced by T cells, which means that their activation is MHC Class II restricted but does not require direct contact with T cells.*

10. **Why do memory B cells require fewer T cells and less antigen?**

(a) *Because they require antigen presenting cells to process and present antigen to T cells.*

(b) *Because they bind antigen directly and process and present it to T cells.*

(c) *Because memory B cells do not require T cell-derived cytokines for their activation.*

(d) *Because memory B cells can endocytose much lower levels of antigen than virgin cells.*

(e) *Because antigen cross-links surface receptors (which are expressed at a higher density on memory cells), such T cell binding is not necessary.*

11. **Generally, it is not beneficial for the immune system to recognise and react to self-antigens. Which of the following is NOT involved in the regulation of self-tolerance?**

(a) *Clonal deletion.*

(b) *Clonal abortion.*

(c) *Clonal anergy.*

(d) *Idiotypic networks.*

(e) *Allotypic networks.*

12. **Which of the following statements concerning the time required for the induction of tolerance is CORRECT?**

(a) *B cells are tolerised more quickly with a T-independent antigen than with a T-dependent antigen.*

(b) *Adult splenic B cells are tolerised within hours of challenge with a T-dependent antigen.*

(c) *Adult splenic B cells are tolerised within 1 day of challenge with a T-dependent antigen.*

(d) Mature bone marrow B cells are tolerised within 10 days of challenge with a T-dependent antigen.

(e) Splenic or thymic T cells are tolerised within minutes of challenge with a T-dependent antigen.

13. Which of the following does NOT influence the development and persistence of tolerance to an antigen?

(a) Antigen dose.

(b) Antigen persistence.

(c) The route of administration of the antigen.

(d) The ability of the antigen to be phagocytosed.

(e) Antigen complexity.

14. The intraepithelial lymphocytes:

(a) Can be induced to proliferate by stimulation of the CD2 molecule but not the T cell receptor.

(b) Are found below the basement membrane distributed amongst the cells comprising the connective tissue.

(c) Are phenotypically homogeneous.

(d) Typically are CD3+, CD2+ and CD4+.

(e) Along with germinal centre lymphocytes comprise the diffuse mucosal lymphoid tissue.

15. Which of the following statements concerning the mucosal production of IgA is INCORRECT?

(a) The production of IgA is one of the distinguishing characteristics of the mucosal immune response.

(b) B cells in the mucosal follicles preferentially produce IgA.

(c) T cells and possibly mucosal macrophages or stromal cells taken from mucosal tissues play a role in causing the switch to IgA production by B cells in vitro.

(d) Fc alpha receptor-positive T cells are thought to release IgA-binding factors which act on mIgA$^+$ B cells, thus providing a mechanism by which mucosal IgA production is switched off.

(e) Some T cells secrete IL-5 which, in concert with IL-6, preferentially stimulates the differentiation of mIgA$^+$ B cells.

5

ABNORMALITIES OF THE IMMUNE SYSTEM

The purpose of this chapter is to introduce you to a range of conditions, which may be described as abnormalities of the immune system. When an antigen is introduced into an individual, the immune response recognises it as foreign and eliminates the invader in the most appropriate way, i.e. it limits any potential spread and destroys the antigen efficiently. The response is controlled such that only those mechanisms required are brought into play and there is little resulting tissue damage. However, in certain individuals the response to particular antigens may result in extensive tissue damage. It is accompanied by a massive inflammatory response, which results in the signs and symptoms that are classified as **hypersensitivity**. Some people refer to this type of response as uncontrolled or harmful, but these are misnomers. It may be that in certain cases, e.g. in an infectious disease, the hypersensitivity response is vital to preventing the spread of the agent. Although tissue damage may result, the overall outcome is beneficial. However, in some instances, the outcome is definitely not beneficial. Under certain circumstances, the immune response recognises self-antigen resulting in tissue damage and **autoimmune disease**. A number of familiar diseases may be considered to be autoimmune in nature, e.g. rheumatoid arthritis and multiple sclerosis. This means that the majority of the tissue damage observed in these diseases (**pathology**) occurs as a result of the immune system failing to maintain **tolerance** to self. Usually in autoimmune diseases, the immunopathology may be the result of one or more hypersensitivity reactions.

5.1 HYPERSENSITIVITY

When an individual is exposed to an antigen, the outcome depends upon the strength of the immune response. At one extreme is immunity or resistance to the antigen and at the other is hypersensitivity, where the increased response to

Immunology for Life Scientists, Second Edition. Lesley-Jane Eales.
© 2003 John Wiley & Sons, Ltd: ISBN 0 470 84523 6 (HB); 0 470 84524 4 (PB)

the antigen results in tissue damage. The scientist Paul Richet adopted the term **anaphylaxis** to describe the reaction, which occurs in certain individuals to specific antigens. Phylaxis means protection, so anaphylaxis refers to the situation where damage occurs as a result of a protective response to a particular antigen. Thus, by these definitions, the terms hypersensitivity and anaphylaxis should be interchangeable. However, recently the use of the term anaphylaxis has been restricted to a very particular type of hypersensitivity response; the latter being a term used to describe any immunologic reaction where considerable tissue damage occurs.

Another type of hypersensitivity response is the allergic response. The term **allergy** (from the Greek *allos* and *ergon* meaning altered action) was used initially to describe the outcome of the response to an antigen on second exposure.

5.1.1 HYPERSENSITIVITY REACTIONS

In recent years, research has shown that hypersensitivity reactions occur following re-exposure of an individual to an antigen to which he/she has previously been sensitised. This is similar to immunisation where on second exposure to an antigen, the host mounts a stronger, more efficient protective immune response than on initial exposure. The difference between this reaction and a hypersensitivity response is that the secondary response in the latter is so great that it causes varying degrees of tissue damage resulting in the appearance of specific clinical signs and symptoms. Hypersensitivity can be caused by a wide range of antigens and may affect a number of different organs or tissues. In individuals where an antigen causes one particular type of hypersensitivity response – a **Type I** response – the antigen is known as an **allergen** (i.e. **allergy gen**erating) and the clinical signs and symptoms characterise an allergic response. Allergies affect an increasing number of individuals every year (currently 20% of the population) and are an important cause of morbidity and mortality.

Hypersensitivity reactions were originally classified according to the symptoms which could be recognised in an individual. However, in the 1950s, Gell and Coombs proposed a classificiation system that depended upon the underlying immunologic reactions. Although this classification is still widely used today, there is some debate over its validity particularly in relation to hypersensitivity seen in response to certain types of drugs.

5.1.2 TYPE I HYPERSENSITIVITY

Type I hypersensitivity reactions are becoming more common and you would recognise them as the signs and symptoms associated with allergic responses

Table 5.1 Examples of Type I hypersensitivity		
Examples	Causes	Symptoms
Allergic rhinitis (hay fever), bronchial asthma, atopic dermatitis	Varies between individuals, e.g. ragweed or grass pollen, house dust mites	Symptoms result from antibody-bearing mast cells releasing histamine and other vasoactive amines

(Table 5.1). Whilst the allergens (antigens) that stimulate these reactions are diverse, the outcome of exposure to any allergen is similar. What determines whether or not an individual will respond normally to an antigen is not fully understood. Clearly there is a genetic influence, since family studies have shown that if both parents are allergic an offspring has a 75% chance of being allergic. Only one parent being allergic reduces this to 50%. In addition, recent evidence suggests the cellular interactions involved in antigen recognition and initiation of the immune response may influence the outcome.

Type I reactions are also known as immediate hypersensitivity reactions since they may occur within seconds of exposure to the antigen. The early phase of the response (occurring up to 30 minutes post-allergen challenge) is manifest by local oedema, smooth muscle contraction, vasodilation and increased permeability of post-capillary venules. This is caused by IgE-mediated mast cell degranulation (Table 5.2). The later phase of the response which starts between 4 and 12 hours post-challenge involves the recruitment and activation of basophils, eosinophils and other cell types and may persist for up to two days.

REGULATION OF TYPE I HYPERSENSITIVITY

The signs and symptoms of allergy are the result of a massive inflammatory response (Section 3.3) initiated by the release of intracellular granules from basophils and mast cells (Figure 5.1). Stimulation of this release occurs as a

Table 5.2 Some pharmacological mediators in mast cell granules	
Chemical	Effect
Histamine	Increases vascular permeability and levels of cAMP
Heparin	Causes anticoagulation
Serotonin	Increases vascular permeability
Chymase	Proteolysis
Hyaluronidase	Increases vascular permeability
Eosinophil chemotactic factor	Attracts eosinophils
Neutrophil chemotactic factor	Attracts neutrophils

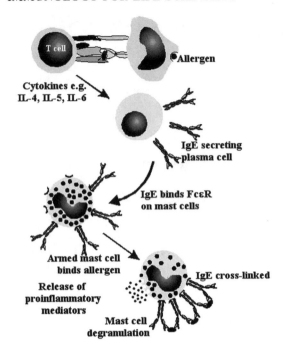

Figure 5.1 Type I hypersensitivity
Type I reactions are caused by the inflammatory mediators released from intracellular granules in basophils and mast cells, which occurs as a result of cross-linking cell-bound IgE.

result of cross-linking IgE bound to the cells via the IgE receptor (FcεR). The latter comprises three types of molecules, α, β and γ, that associate to form a tetramer (α, β, γ_2), which localises to special lipid-rich domains on the cell surface known as **lipid rafts**. The α chain contains the extracellular IgE-binding domain. The β and disulfide-linked γ chains are not expressed on the surface but are important in signalling the cell. Upon dimerisation of the tetramers (by multivalent antigen cross-linking the IgE associated with the FcεR), a series of intracellular signals are generated that ultimately result in mast cell degranulation. The earliest events involve phosphorylation of the FcεR β and γ chains on tyrosine residues. Such phosphorylation often occurs in proteins with a special 26 amino acid motif (called an **immunoreceptor tyrosine activation motif** or **ITAM**) consisting of six conserved amino acids (including two tyrosine residues). These ITAMs associate with **protein tyrosine kinases (PTKs)** of the Src family such as Lyn, activation of which leads to the phosphorylation of Tyr residues on both the γ and β subunits. Phosphorylation of these sites by Lyn increases the affinity of Syk for these chains. Syk is phosphorylated by Lyn resulting in mast cell activation. Human basophils also require Syk, expression of which can be induced by IL-3 (Table 5.3).

These early signalling events are controlled by regulatory proteins containing **immunotyrosine inhibition motifs (ITIMs)**. Signal regulatory protein α

Table 5.3 Characteristics of interleukin 3	
Molecular weight	5.1 kDa (human); 15.7 kDa (mouse). Two potential glycosylation sites and one disulphide bond
Major sources	Activated T cells, mast cells and eosinophils
Effects	Growth and differentiation of pluripotent stem cells; increased Syk expression
Cross-reactivity	Human and mouse IL-3, 29% homology. No cross-species reactivity

(SIRPα) recruits the protein tyrosine phosphatases SHP-1 and -2. These dephosphorylate ITAMs and thus switch off signal transduction and mast cell activation.

A lower affinity FcεR (FcεRII) shows antigenic similarity to a B cell surface antigen – CD23 – which in soluble form may represent an IgE binding factor.

HUMORAL EVENTS IN ALLERGY

Atopic diseases (allergies) are associated with elevated serum levels of both total and allergen-specific IgE. The factors that regulate the production of IgE in response to an antigenic stimulus will clearly determine the outcome of exposure to that antigen. Usually, the primary response (characterised by the production of antigen-specific IgM) is followed, on subsequent exposure, by a secondary response typically characterised by the production of antigen-specific IgG (or at mucosal surfaces, IgA). In certain individuals, antigen-specific IgE is produced after secondary exposure. This switch to IgE production is regulated through direct contact between T and B cells (via **CD40** and **CD154** (CD40L)) and the secretion of certain cytokines (particularly IL-4 and IL-13). The latter also affect other cells such as eosinophils, basophils and mast cells that, upon activation, produce cytokines (such as IL-4 and IL-5), which exacerbate the allergic response (Figure 5.2). These cytokines are vital to the differentiation, maturation and survival of effector cells (as shown for IL-5 and eosinophils). Thus, these cells modulate their own activity and perpetuate their participation in the allergic response. In addition, IL-4 provides a link between these effector cells and T cells, as it is vital for the development of a Th_2 response.

What determines whether or not an individual will produce IgE in response to a particular antigen? Experimental studies have suggested that antigens may deliver signals (via the TCR) that favour differentiation into Th_2 cells. Complexes, which bind the TCR with high avidity, appear to favour the development of Th_1-type responses. By contrast, weakly avid interactions favour the development of Th_2-type responses. The way in which the T cell, B cell and allergen interact influences the type of intracellular signals that are generated, leading to class switching in the B cell and causing the production of antigen-specific IgE.

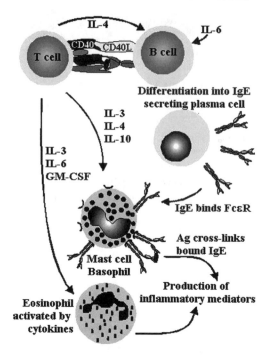

Figure 5.2   Cellular and molecular interactions leading to an allergic response
In certain individuals, antigen-specific IgE is produced after secondary exposure to an antigen. This switch to IgE production is regulated by T cells through direct contact with B cells and the secretion of certain cytokines. The latter also affect other cells such as eosinophils, basophils and mast cells, which, upon activation, produce cytokines (such as IL-4 and IL-5) that exacerbate the allergic response.

5.1.3 TYPE II HYPERSENSITIVITY

Under certain circumstances, an antibody (usually IgG or IgM) may recognise and bind to a normal or an altered cell surface antigen (Figure 5.3). Thus, the cell becomes part of an immune complex allowing activation of complement (via the classical pathway) and cell lysis. In addition, this leads to the formation of the anaphylatoxins C3a and C5a, which directly stimulate mast cells to release their granules leading to an inflammatory response. Alternatively, the cell may become the target of an antibody-dependent cell-mediated cytotoxicity (ADCC) reaction involving the action of macrophages, neutrophils and eosinophils attached to the antibody on the cell via their FcR. These reactions result in tissue damage. Examples of this type of hypersensitivity include erythroblastosis foetalis, myasthenia gravis (a disease characterised by the presence of antibodies to the acetyl choline receptor), and autoimmune haemolytic anaemia.

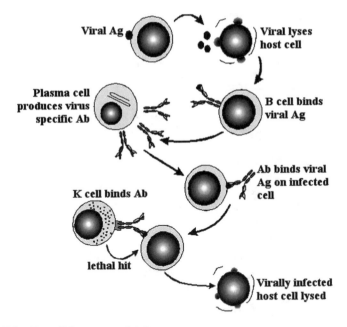

Figure 5.3 Type II hypersensitivity
Under certain circumstances, an antibody (usually IgG or IgM) may recognise and bind to a normal or an altered cell surface antigen. This may lead to complement activation and the release of inflammatory mediators resulting in tissue destruction.

 See the web site to find more information about autoimmune diseases and type II hypersensitivity

5.1.4 TYPE III HYPERSENSITIVITY

Type III hypersensitivity reactions are also the result of immune complex formation. Soluble antigen binds to specific antibody and may form large antigen/antibody lattices, which can activate complement (Figure 5.4). These complexes can also be deposited in organs, particularly those with filtering membranes such as the kidneys and the joints. This type of hypersensitivity is responsible for the damage caused by inflammation in the glomeruli of the kidneys (glomerulonephritis) in a disease called systemic lupus erythematosus caused by DNA anti-DNA immune complexes. The distinction between Type II and Type III hypersensitivity is that the immune complexes that initiate the inflammation in the former contain cell-associated antigens.

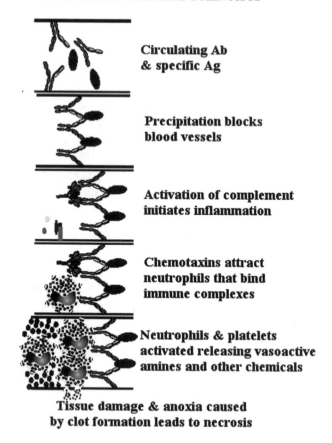

Circulating Ab
& specific Ag

Precipitation blocks
blood vessels

Activation of complement
initiates inflammation

Chemotaxins attract
neutrophils that bind
immune complexes

Neutrophils & platelets
activated releasing vasoactive
amines and other chemicals

Tissue damage & anoxia caused
by clot formation leads to necrosis

Figure 5.4   Type III hypersensitivity
Soluble antigen binds to specific antibody and may form large antigen/antibody lattices which can activate complement. These complexes can also be deposited in organs, particularly those with filtering membranes such as the kidneys and the joints.

5.1.5   TYPE IV HYPERSENSITIVITY

The final type of hypersensitivity is dependent upon the production of cytokines resulting from the interaction of T cells with each other or with cells such as macrophages and fibroblasts. These reactions take more than 24 hours to develop and thus are also known as delayed-type hypersensitivity (DTH) responses. These reactions are cell-mediated immune responses with which a large degree of pathology is associated. Characteristics of these reactions are summarised in Table 5.4. Since some pathology is always associated with cell-mediated immunity (e.g. destruction of virally infected cells by T_{cyt}), characterisation of a reaction as a hypersensitivity response is often a matter of degree.

Table 5.4 Summary of the characteristics of Type IV hypersensitivity responses

Type	Characteristics
Tuberculin-type	Macrophages; antigen is presented by APC such as dendritic cells and macrophages to CD4$^+$ cells that secrete cytokines, which recruit and activate macrophages. Th$_1$ cells are particularly important in these reactions
Granuloma	Macrophages and fibroblasts proliferate and produce collagen, which walls off the antigen. Giant cell formation occurs
Contact	Macrophages; response occurs in the skin; thought to be due to Langerhans cells presenting antigen to CD4$^+$ cells. CD8$^+$ cells play a role especially with haptens that modify MHC Class I antigens. Th$_2$ response may be involved

Classic DTH responses are characterised by the activity of Th$_1$ cells, which derive from precursor Th cells under the influence of IL-12 and IL-18 from macrophages. Th$_1$ (and NK) cells produce IFNγ, which activates macrophages accumulated at the site of infection/tissue damage. Activated macrophages secrete a range of proinflammatory mediators (including cytokines, chemokines, complement components, prostaglandins, reactive oxygen and nitrogen intermediates). Clearly, these events will be accompanied by the molecular and cellular reactions associated with inflammation and classical cell-mediated immunity. However, in DTH reactions, these processes lead to more severe pathological changes such as granulomatous inflammation, calcification, caseation, necrosis and cavity formation in the affected tissues.

In 1890, Robert Koch demonstrated that filtrates from cultures of Mycobacterium tuberculosis could stimulate an inflammatory response several hours after injection into animals infected with the organism but not in uninfected animals. This technique has been developed and skin testing using preparations from a range of organisms is commonplace in detecting infected individuals and in screening populations to determine prevalence of infection in specific communities.

TUBERCULIN-TYPE DTH

The classic delayed-type hypersensitivity reaction is seen in response to the purified protein derivative of tuberculin (PPD) from *Mycobacteria* spp. If PPD is injected intradermally in an individual who has been exposed to *Mycobacterium tuberculosis* previously, there is no immediate reaction. After about 10 hours, the site of injection becomes red (erythema) and swollen; the reaction reaching a maximum between 24 and 72 hours. These classic signs of inflammation take several days to subside.

Histologically, the site of such a reaction is infiltrated with T cells and large numbers of newly recruited monocyte-derived macrophages and mature macrophages. These cells are seen typically clustered around post-capillary venules. Deposition of fibrin is clearly evident and may be responsible for the solidity of the lesion.

The cell-mediated immune response is further enhanced in mycobacterial infection due to the presence of muramyl dipeptide (a component of the mycobacterial cell wall), which directly activates macrophages leading to the enhanced release of proinflammatory mediators.

GRANULOMA FORMATION

Infection with certain organisms (e.g. mycobacteria and schistosomes) is often associated with the formation of granulomata. These usually form as a result of the persistence of a non-degradable product (such as the bacterial cell wall) or as the result of a persistent DTH response.

In tuberculosis, there is an early accumulation of granulocytes in the tissues, which is rapidly followed by the formation of granulomata. Despite the name, it is accumulated mononuclear cells that form granulomata. The centre usually comprises macrophages, which differentiate into epithelioid cells. This is surrounded by lymphocytes, particularly T cells. Within these structures, T cells interact with macrophages allowing the destruction of the infecting organism. However, owing to the persistence of the cell wall, the stimulus for activation persists. This provides a stimulus for fibrin deposition (influenced by the production of transforming growth factor β), which eventually walls off the cellular mass, displacing (and often destroying) adjacent tissues. The structure may become calcified and the isolation of the cells leads to necrosis at the centre (caseation), which may result in the formation of a cavity within the tissue in which the granuloma formed.

Animal studies have shown that granulomata may develop in the absence of T cells but that CD4$^+$ T cells enhance the rate of development. Interestingly, it has been shown that knock-out mice lacking the adhesion molecule ICAM-1 do not show the pathology associated with tuberculosis infection but are able to kill the organisms, demonstrating a possible distinction between cell-mediated immunity and Type IV hypersensitivity.

CONTACT HYPERSENSITIVITY

Contact hypersensitivity is a cutaneous reaction involving the dendritic cells of the skin – Langerhans cells. Contact allergens bind to particular amino acids on proteins. Thus, the allergen (which normally alone may not stimulate an immune response) becomes a hapten on a carrier protein. This hapten is then seen by the immune system as an antigenic determinant on the larger protein. Langerhans cells are able to process these haptenated proteins and present antigen to T cells in the local cutaneous lymph nodes. Once activated, the T cells produce cytokines and chemokines that encourage the migration and activation of local macrophages initiating a local, cutaneous inflammatory response. Critical in the induction and initiation of the response are IL-12 (from Langerhans cells) and IL-4, IL-10 and IFNγ (from T cells).

Although considered to be a Type IV hypersensitivity response, contact hypersensitivity differs from classical DTH reactions in that it may be mediated by either CD4$^+$, or CD8$^+$, T cells (DTH is usually CD4$^+$ T cell-dependent). In addition, the contact response is not necessarily regulated by a Th$_1$ response, as is the case with DTH reactions. However, much of our understanding of contact hypersensitivity comes from studies with knock-out mice and so we have yet to obtain a true understanding of the cellular and molecular basis of the reaction in humans.

KEY POINTS FOR REVIEW

- *The outcome of the response to an immune stimulus may be resistance or, at the other extreme, hypersensitivity.*
- *In hypersensitivity, the increased immune response results in tissue damage.*
- *Hypersensitivity can be caused by a range of antigens, affecting different organs or tissues.*
- *Reactions are classified according to the underlying immunological reactions.*
- *Type I reactions involve cross-linking of IgE on tissue mast cells. The antigen involved is an allergen.*
- *Activation of mast cells through a network of intracellular signals results in the release of proinflammatory mediators that give rise to the signs and symptoms of allergy.*
- *The production of IgE requires T–B cell contact via CD40 and CD154 (CD40L).*
- *Type II hypersensitivity is stimulated by immune complexes containing altered or foreign cell surface antigens, whilst Type III involves immune complexes containing soluble antigens.*
- *Pathology is associated with complement activation and antibody-dependent cellular cytotoxicity.*
- *Type IV hypersensitivity includes those reactions that take more than 24 hours to develop (delayed-type) and involve the action of cytokines, T cells, NK cells, macrophages and fibroblasts.*
- *The classic delayed-type hypersensitivity reaction is seen in response to the purified protein derivative of tuberculin from Mycobacterium spp.*
- *With persistent stimuli, the inflammatory response may become chronic leading to granuloma formation.*

- *Contact hypersensitivity is a cutaneous Type IV response involving the action of dendritic cells.*

5.2   AUTOIMMUNITY AND AUTOIMMUNE DISEASES

Autoimmunity, as opposed to autoimmune disease, is vital to the development of a normal immune response. As we discussed previously, T cells recognise antigen only in association with self-MHC molecules; they will not respond if the antigen is presented by foreign MHC molecules, thus confirming that the reaction involves specific recognition of self molecules. This is an example of autoimmunity which is productive. A further example is the recognition of self-idiotypes by anti-idiotypic antibodies, which is essential for the diversification and regulation of immune responses. Apart from these instances, the immune system does not normally react to itself, i.e. it is tolerant to self.

Self-tolerance occurs early in foetal development and is vital for health and the normal functioning of the immune response; its breakdown resulting in autoimmune disease which may be debilitating or even fatal. How can such autoimmunity develop? One suggestion is that an antigen may be hidden from the immune system during development (e.g. an antigen within an organ which has little contact with immunologically active cells – an immunologically privileged site), thus preventing the development of tolerance to that antigen at the T or B cell level. If the antigen is exposed later in life as a result of some form of tissue damage, it will be foreign to the immune system and it will stimulate an (auto)immune response. This type of response may be a primary cause of, or a secondary complication in, a variety of human and animal diseases.

Many studies have demonstrated that self-reactive lymphocytes are part of the normal immunological repertoire and only a small fraction of these cells may be pathogenic; the remainder having a physiological role to play.

5.2.1   CAUSES OF AUTOIMMUNITY

Every day, the body is exposed to a number of factors, which alone, or in combination, under the correct conditions may initiate the development of an autoimmune disease. In addition, it is also a normal consequence of ageing and may be induced by certain drugs or microorganisms (especially viruses). The exact cause of most autoimmune diseases is largely unknown as are the factors that control the severity of the disease, the range of autoantigens or the target organs involved. However, a number of parameters are known to be generally

Table 5.5 Factors affecting the development of autoimmune disease

Agent	Effects/associated autoimmune disease
Genetic make-up	HLA-DR4 – rheumatoid arthritis HLA-DR2, 3 – SLE HLA-DQ3 – insulin-dependent diabetes mellitus
Viruses	e.g. Epstein–Barr virus
Hormones	Oestrogen aggravates autoimmune disease; androgens are immunosuppressive
Stress/trauma	Neurochemicals and hormones are involved in rapid onset of autoimmune disease in response to these agents

Pharmaceuticals
  Lithium
  Penicillin
  Penicillamine
 	
  α-Methyldopa
	
	Autoimmune thyroid disease
	Autoimmune haemolytic disease
	Myasthenia gravis, pemphigus, autoimmune thyroid disease, autoimmune haemolytic anaemia
	Autoimmune haemolytic anaemia, autoimmune hepatitis

Chemicals and organic solvents
  Hydrazine
  Vinyl chloride
  Silica dust
	
	Systemic lupus erythematosus
	Systemic sclerosis
	Systemic sclerosis

Heavy metals
  Gold
  Cadmium
  Mercury
	
	Immune-complex glomerulonephritis
	Immune-complex glomerulonephritis
	Immune-complex glomerulonephritis

Food additives *Tartrazine*	 Systemic lupus erythematosus

associated with autoimmune disease and these are discussed briefly in the following sections (Table 5.5).

GENETIC FACTORS IN AUTOIMMUNE DISEASE

The genetic make-up of the host may be a major determinant in the onset and development of autoimmune disease. Particularly relevant in this respect are those genes that control the size and type of immune response to an antigen, i.e. the MHC and antigen receptor genes.

It is well documented that organ-specific autoimmune diseases can show a familial association. However, within a family, the type of disease manifested may vary from one member to another. Recent evidence suggests that as little as a single mutation of one particular gene may switch the susceptibility for disease from one organ to another.

Several autoimmune diseases have been shown to be associated (at least loosely) with the expression of particular MHC and immunoglobulin allotypic genes. Individuals with seropositive rheumatoid arthritis (RA⁺) commonly express the product of the Class II gene DR4 whilst systemic lupus erythematosus (SLE) is associated with DR2 and DR3. Although these diseases are thought to be closely related, the distinct genetic association suggests that their pathology may be very different.

Modern developments in molecular biology have provided the potential for developing new types of treatment for autoimmune diseases such as gene therapy. However, further progress is required before it becomes the treatment of choice. First the genes involved in each disease must be isolated and characterised and delivery systems allowing efficient gene insertion in the target cells must be developed, as must the mechanisms to regulate expression of the introduced genes.

SEX-LINKED FACTORS IN AUTOIMMUNE DISEASE

Generally, women are much more susceptible than men to most connective tissue diseases which include autoimmune diseases. The incidence of the latter is demonstrably affected by both sex hormones and genes linked to the X, or Y, chromosomes. It is well known that many hormones affect the lymphoid system, the effect of gonadal hormones being particularly apparent. Indeed, it has been shown that elevated oestrogen levels exacerbate autoimmune disease whilst androgen has a protective, immunosuppressive role.

STRESS AND NEUROCHEMICALS IN AUTOIMMUNE DISEASE

Many instances are cited in clinical literature where patients have had a dramatic onset of autoimmune disease following trauma or extreme stress. Neurochemicals and hormones are thought to play a vital role in initiating disease under these circumstances.

CHEMICALS AND PHARMACEUTICALS IN AUTOIMMUNE DISEASE

With the worldwide explosion of manufacturing industry and pollution, an association between exposure to certain chemicals and the development of specific autoimmune diseases has been clearly established. These agents may interact with tissues resulting in the expression of modified self-antigens, which are the target for an autoimmune response. Similarly, pharmaceuticals may induce disease. For example, treatment with methyldopa has been associated with the development of autoimmune haemolytic anaemia.

VIRUSES IN AUTOIMMUNE DISEASE

Viruses have been found to be associated with the presence of autoimmune disease in humans and other animals. They may cause autoimmune disease by a number of different mechanisms including polyclonal activation of lymphocytes (e.g. Epstein–Barr virus), release of intracellular organelles due to destruction of

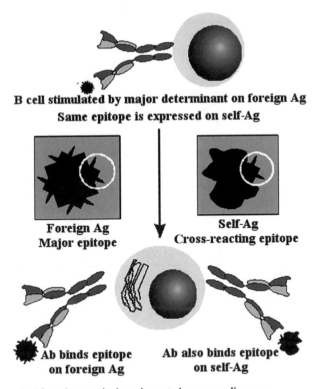

B cell stimulated by major determinant on foreign Ag
Same epitope is expressed on self-Ag

Foreign Ag
Major epitope

Self-Ag
Cross-reacting epitope

Ab binds epitope
on foreign Ag

Ab also binds epitope
on self-Ag

Figure 5.5 The role of antigen mimicry in autoimmune disease
If the major antigenic determinant of an infectious agent is similar antigenically to a self-antigen, then
the response elicited by the microorganism can result in an autoimmune response.

host cells, antigen mimicry (Figure 5.5; Table 5.6), induction of abnormal MHC
Class II antigen expression and functional impairment of immunologically
regulatory cells, e.g. T suppressor cells.

Role of Epstein–Barr virus in autoimmune disease: Epstein–Barr virus (EBV)
infects B cells and directly causes their activation. Although some autoreactive
B cells escape elimination in the bone marrow, they are usually prevented from
producing autoreactive antibody either by a lack of antigen-stimulated T cell
help or by T cell-mediated suppression. However, if a potentially autoreactive B
cell is infected by EBV it can proliferate and differentiate into a plasma cell
without the help of T cells. Infected cells from both healthy individuals and
patients with rheumatoid arthritis secrete polyclonal IgG and IgM anti-
immunoglobulin antibodies (rheumatoid factor) but B cells from patients
produce more, higher affinity antibody than those from normal persons.

ANTIGEN MIMICRY

More than a century ago, infectious diseases were associated with the onset of
autoimmune disease. Indeed, rheumatic fever, although uncommon now in the

Table 5.6   Examples of potential antigenic mimicry

Disease association	Potential antigen mimicry
Multiple sclerosis	Antibodies to measles virus cross-react with myelin basic protein
Myasthenia gravis	Antibodies to antigens from bacteria such as *E. coli, Proteus vulgaris, Klebsiella pneumoniae* are thought to cross-react with acetyl choline receptors
Systemic lupus erythematosus (SLE)	Antibodies to a variety of phospholipids and bacteria may cross-react with DNA
SLE and ankylosing spondylitis	Antibodies to *Klebsiella*-derived proteins show similarities to some anti-DNA antibodies
Rheumatoid arthritis	Epstein–Barr virus nuclear antigen shares an antigen found in synovial membranes
Coeliac disease	An adenovirus type 12 protein shows structural similarities to alpha gliadin in wheat

developed world thanks to the use of antibiotics, was associated with streptococcal infection. This association is thought to be due to the fact that antigens in the microorganism immunologically "look like" self-antigens. In this way, an immune response to the organism could lead to damage of self-tissue. At a molecular level we now know that this "antigen mimicry" is a common occurrence (Table 5.6). However, we lack hard evidence that such reactions actually cause autoimmune disease.

Perhaps the best evidence we have to date is that concerning the role of *Trypanosoma cruzi* in the cardiomyopathy associated with chronic Chagas' disease. Patients have an inflammatory infiltrate in their cardiac tissue and cross-reactive antigens have been demonstrated using sera from patients with Chagas' disease.

Recent developments demonstrating the flexibility of T cells' antigen recognition in relation to the amino acid sequence of the bound peptides have suggested that microbial peptides with relatively limited sequence homology to self-antigens can activate autoreactive T cells. In the same way, it has been suggested that unrelated infections could result in the presentation of antigens that could enhance (but not initiate) an autoimmune response by primed autoreactive cells. This would make it extremely difficult to prove that a particular autoimmune disease has a single aetiological infectious agent.

An infection may stimulate an autoimmune response either through the presentation of cross-reactive antigens or by the release of self-antigens. Depending upon the infectious agent, the outcome may be autoimmune; a response that would require the delivery of appropriate, co-stimulatory signals and the production of proinflammatory cytokines.

In susceptible A/J mice, infection with live, but not killed, CB3 virus causes autoimmune myocarditis. This implies that the inflammation caused by the live virus provides co-stimulatory signals that affect the immune outcome. In addition, when the less susceptible B10.A strain was co-treated with bacterial LPS and virus or cardiac myosin, the animals showed aggressive disease. This effect could be eliminated by injecting antibodies to either IL-1 or TNFα, which can block the activity of these cytokines. This suggests LPS was working by increasing the production of proinflammatory cytokines such as IL-1 and TNFα.

Thus the microorganism may provide an antigenic signal and a pro-inflammatory stimulus that would stimulate antigen presentation and co-stimulation, thus reducing the threshold at which T cell activation occurs. The latter may be protective or may be damaging or even autoimmune in nature.

5.2.2   CLASSIFICATION OF AUTOIMMUNE DISEASE

In the 1950s, Witebsky established the criteria for determining the aetiology of human diseases which were thought to be autoimmune. Witebsky's postulates were modelled on those of Koch and required the presence of autoantibody or a cell-mediated immune response to a self-antigen, which having been identified, could induce a similar disease in an experimental host mediated by the same immunological mechanism. Since these criteria were established, our knowledge of immunology has increased by leaps and bounds. However, they remain a good guide for identifying autoimmune diseases.

Clinically, autoimmune diseases have been divided into systemic or "non-organ-specific" and "organ-specific" diseases. However, this categorisation is not absolute. Many autoimmune diseases have both organ-specific and non-organ-specific complications. In addition, more than one type of disease may occur in the same individual.

The classical example of a non-organ-specific autoimmune disease is systemic lupus erythematosus (SLE) in which the autoimmune response is directed to a number of different tissue antigens. Such non-organ-specific diseases may develop as a result of an abnormal immune response to a single antigen, which is expressed in many tissues.

There are a wide range of organ-specific autoimmune diseases including Hashimoto's thyroiditis (the principal target organ being the thyroid) and insulin-dependent diabetes mellitus (pancreas).

5.2.3 IMMUNOPATHOLOGY OF AUTOIMMUNE DISEASES

Autoimmune diseases form a large, heterogeneous group with a wide variety of clinical signs and symptoms. Despite this disparity, the immunopathology of all these diseases may be considered to be the result of particular hypersensitivity reactions, each disease being the result of one or more type of response.

Type II hypersensitivity responses usually involve autoantibody that recognises either a normal (usually sequestered) or modified (by viruses or chemicals) cellular self-antigen (Figure 5.3). The resultant tissue damage gives rise to the signs and symptoms that are used in diagnosis of the disease. Autoantibodies may also interact with cellular receptors thus causing an abnormal expression of cellular activity, e.g. autoimmune haemolytic anaemia. In such a reaction, the autoantibody is not involved in an ADCC reaction.

Type III hypersensitivity reactions are seen in autoimmune diseases where the autoantibody binds to self-antigens free in tissue fluids or in the general circulation. The resulting complexes are free to circulate throughout the body. However, they may become quite large (depending on the relative concentrations of antibody and antigen) and therefore, insoluble. This results in their precipitation in the tissues and blood vessels. Particularly vulnerable are tissues with large filtering membranes such as the kidneys, joints and choroid plexus, where the presence of immune complexes results in the activation of the complement cascade and inflammatory sequelae (Figure 5.4). As a direct consequence, localised cell death occurs and the function of the organ or tissues involved may be lost due to blockage of blood vessels by clot formation (e.g. vasculitis in systemic lupus erythematosus).

T cells sensitised to self-antigens may cause tissue damage through the release of lymphokines, which either directly damage the tissues (e.g. TNF), or attract inflammatory cells to the site, resulting in tissue damage. These events initiated by self-reactive T cells result in the type of pathology typically associated with Type IV hypersensitivity.

5.2.4 THE IMMUNOLOGY OF AUTOIMMUNE DISEASE

Autoimmune diseases result from an abnormal immune response to self-antigens. In all these diseases, there is a breakdown of normal regulatory mechanisms and a lack of tolerance to the self-antigens concerned. The complex immunological responses that occur in these diseases are responsible for the resulting pathology and an understanding of these responses is vital for effective disease management.

Table 5.7 Target antigens involved in autoimmune diseases

Disease	Target antigens/potential target antigens
Myasthenia gravis	Acetyl choline receptor
Primary biliary cirrhosis	Mitochondrial enzymes of the 2-oxo-acid dehydrogenase family
Autoimmune thyroid disease	Thyroid-stimulating hormone receptor, thyroid peroxidase and thyroglobulin
Systemic lupus erythematosus	Double-stranded DNA

TARGET ANTIGENS

In many autoimmune diseases, the antigens that stimulate the disease or are the target of autoimmune attack are not clearly defined. There are some notable exceptions (Table 5.7).

One group of antigens, which have been implicated in the pathogenesis of a number of autoimmune diseases are the highly conserved heat shock proteins (hsp). When cells are stressed, heat shock proteins are produced preferentially and confer some protective effect on the stressed cells. They are so highly conserved that even bacteria produce these proteins and they show a high degree of homology to those produced by animals of various species. These proteins are grouped into families according to their molecular weight. Cell surface expression of hsp 90 is increased in about one-fifth of patients with systemic lupus erythematosus (particularly on B cells and $CD4^+$ T cells). By contrast, hsp 65 levels are increased in patients with rheumatoid arthritis.

NON-SPECIFIC IMMUNITY IN AUTOIMMUNE DISEASE

In recent years, it has been proposed that non-specific immune mechanisms (i.e. those that are not dependent upon specific recognition of antigen) are involved in the initiation of autoimmune diseases such as multiple sclerosis, rheumatoid arthritis, thyroiditis and diabetes. This model, the **REGA (remnant epitope generates autoantigen)** model, proposes that the disease is triggered by an agent that induces the production of disease-enhancing cytokines, which in turn stimulate the production of a range of other cytokines including chemokines for monocytes and neutrophils. These cytokines stimulate resident macrophages to produce proteinases and activate latent metalloproteinases, which cause the production of a large number of peptides from self-proteins such as myelin basic protein. This has been shown to lead directly to demyelination in multiple sclerosis. Once produced, the peptides may be processed and presented to T cells, suggesting that the specific cell-mediated autoimmunity develops at a relatively late stage of disease onset.

Further indirect evidence for a role of non-specific mechanisms in the development of autoimmunity is provided by the observation that cytokines, which suppress proteinase activity (e.g. IFNα and IFNβ), predominate in the remission phase of multiple sclerosis and rheumatoid arthritis.

MONONUCLEAR PHAGOCYTES IN NON-SPECIFIC IMMUNITY

Clearance, *in vivo*, of antibody-sensitised red blood cells is decreased in humans with autoimmune diseases. The persistence of immune complexes may contribute to the pathology observed and may be the result of defective phagocytic cell function or be the cause of it (by blocking Fc receptors). However, studies have shown that the number of Fcγ receptors on mononuclear cells is normal or increased in patients with systemic lupus erythematosus (a disease in which circulating immune complexes are typically present) and there is no correlation between the level of circulating immune complexes and the magnitude of the clearance defect.

Other receptors that are involved in phagocytosis include the C3b receptor, the expression of which is decreased in patients with systemic lupus erythematosus and rheumatoid arthritis. Regardless of what causes the change in expression of these opsonin receptors (both FcγR and C3R), the result is likely to manifest as a decrease in clearance of immune complexes leading to an increase in their deposition in tissues (such as the kidney), which may complicate the clinical course of the disease (e.g. glomerular nephritis).

MONONUCLEAR PHAGOCYTES IN SPECIFIC IMMUNITY

Changes in the cell surface expression of the MHC Class II gene product HLA-DR have been recorded in both non-organ and organ-specific autoimmune diseases. For example, epithelial cells in the thyroid of many patients with Graves' disease show high levels of HLA-DR; an antigen not usually found on normal thyroid epithelium. In addition, abnormal presentation of foreign antigens (resulting from an unusual association between an antigen such as a drug or microorganism and HLA-DR) has been implicated as a cause of systemic lupus erythematosus. Such an association would appear as an altered self-antigen, thus providing a new epitope that may be recognised, and reacted to, by Th cells. As a consequence, the latter produce lymphokines that stimulate the differentiation and proliferation of activated, self-reactive, B cells.

The mechanisms that cause the abnormal expression of DR antigens have not been definitively determined. It is known that interferon induces HLA-DR expression on epithelial cells and that viruses may induce the production of interferon. Thus, it has been suggested that such an infection could induce HLA-DR expression on thyroid epithelium allowing antigen presentation by cells not usually involved in this process. This may therefore increase the chance of unusual presentation of self-antigens and recognition by T cells leading to the development of autoimmune disease.

DENDRITIC CELLS IN AUTOIMMUNE DISEASE

There is a considerable body of evidence implicating dendritic cells in the pathology of autoimmune disease. Their number is elevated both in the serum and synovial fluid of patients with rheumatoid arthritis. Also, patients with multiple sclerosis have raised levels of circulating dendritic cells secreting proinflammatory cytokines. In diabetes, dendritic cells from people at high risk of the disease expressed low levels of co-stimulatory molecules affecting T cell responses.

Dendritic cells present antigen most effectively to naïve T cells. When dendritic cells are matured in the presence of proinflammatory cytokines, they are able to stimulate a Th_1-type response through the release of IL-12. If inflammatory conditions do not prevail, dendritic cells are able to tolerise T cells or prime Th_2-type responses. In autoimmune disease the balance between Th_1 and Th_2 cells and between effector and regulatory T cells may influence disease progression.

In addition to presentation, processing of antigen by dendritic cells may be influenced by cytokines. As a result, antigenic determinants that are usually hidden (cryptic) may be presented to T cells rather than major antigenic determinants. This type of epitope spreading is seen in autoimmune diseases.

Murine dendritic cells were shown to present to T cells the dominant, not the cryptic, antigenic determinant of hen egg lysozyme. However, when the dendritic cells were treated with IL-6, the responding T cells preferentially recognised the cryptic determinants.

ROLE OF T CELLS IN AUTOIMMUNE DISEASE

The thymus plays a vital role in the development of self-tolerance and thus abnormalities affecting the development or functioning of the thymus may contribute to the development of autoimmune diseases. For example, a variety of thymic abnormalities have been reported in systemic lupus erythematosus but it is unclear whether these are causative, or sequelae of the disease.

The TCR repertoire in autoimmune diseases: Evidence suggests that autoimmune disease is associated with restricted usage of particular TCR V region genes. In rheumatoid arthritis, studies have indicated that restriction of the TCR gene repertoire is limited to the genes of the junctional region of the TCR on $CD8^+$ cells.

Table 5.8   Mechanisms involved in the breakdown of T cell tolerance

Cause of abnormal self-antigen production	Effect
Abnormal synthesis or processing of self-antigen	Self-antigen with novel antigenic determinants
Drugs	e.g. Aspirin may combine with proteins in the tissues resulting in a new antigenic complex
Viruses or drugs	Novel association of different proteins (either self or viral) resulting in new antigenic determinants
Antigenic mimicry	Non-self, cross-reactive antigens stimulate T cells which may then recognise self-antigens

In myasthenia gravis, patients have increased expression of the $V\beta5.1$ (variable region gene 5.1 on the beta chain) and $V\beta8$ genes in the peripheral blood and on mature thymocytes but not on precursor thymic cells. This suggests that these patients may exhibit an altered thymic selection process.

T helper cells: Self-tolerance is maintained even though autoreactive B cells may be present. This is thought to be because T cell tolerance is long-lasting and therefore autoreactive B cells lack the T cell help they require. This T cell control may be demonstrated *in vitro* by the use of B cell mitogens or purified lymphokines, which eliminate the need for T cell help. *In vivo*, T cell maintenance of tolerance may be overcome in a number of ways (Table 5.8).

T regulatory cells: A subpopulation of T cells has been identified that plays a role in preventing organ-specific autoimmune diseases. These **T regulatory cells** (T_{reg}) tend to be in functional excess such that they prevent the development of T cell-mediated autoimmunity. It has been suggested that autoreactive T cells secrete IL-2 leading to an expansion of T_{reg} cells, which could then switch off the autoreactive cells.

A further group of regulatory T cells (**natural killer T cells – NKT**) are a minor subpopulation which play a key role in regulating the immune response through the rapid production of IL-4 and IFNγ. These cells have been shown to be deficient in persons with autoimmune, Type I diabetes. They are able to recognise lipid antigens in association with CD1 and respond by proliferation and the release of IL-4, IFNγ and IL-10, promoting a Th$_2$-type response and abrogating the autoreactive T cell response.

B CELLS IN AUTOIMMUNE DISEASE

Abnormal B cell activity is common in autoimmune diseases and is typified by the production of polyclonal antibodies, many of which react with self-antigens. Such autoantibody production may be a primary cause of disease or may result from abnormal T cell control. It may also affect the normal function of T cells thus causing an acceleration of the disease. In myasthenia gravis, antibodies to the muscle nicotinic acetyl choline receptor (AChR) are responsible for the majority of the clinical symptoms observed. Other antibodies, which recognise presynaptic membrane proteins or sarcoplasmic membrane proteins, are thought to play a role in the pathogenesis of the disease, particularly in patients lacking anti-AChR antibodies.

Abnormal B cell activity may be the result of genetic (e.g. certain autoreactive B cells may be extremely sensitive to selected stimuli due to their genetic make-up) or mitogenic (e.g. either endogenous or exogenous mitogens stimulate the formation of autoantibodies) factors, but both depend upon the presence of self-reactive B cells. However, such cells are normally eliminated during foetal development; their persistence results from the differences in tolerance induction in T and B cells. Self-antigens present in low concentrations may cause tolerance induction in T cells but fail to cause elimination of B cells which recognise them. These self-reactive B cells may be activated by substances that interact with them directly (e.g. T-independent antigens from bacteria and viruses) resulting in the production of autoantibodies. However, since such polyclonal stimulators usually induce the production of low-affinity IgM autoantibodies and the tissue damage seen in autoimmune diseases usually results from the action of IgG autoantibodies, it is unlikely that polyclonal activators alone can cause chronic disease.

B cell differentiation and proliferation: Resting B cells need at least three signals to stimulate their proliferation and differentiation into antibody-producing cells. Depending upon the type of antigen (T-dependent or T-independent) from which the signals come, they are: (i) recognition by T cells of antigen in association with HLA-DR on B cells or cross-linking of mIg on B cells by a T-independent antigen; (ii) recognition of antigen by mIg on B cells; (iii) association of T cell-derived lymphokines (e.g. interleukin 2, 4, 5, 6) with appropriate receptors on the B cells.

The pathology seen in autoimmune diseases may reflect abnormalities in B cell signal requirements, regulation of lymphokine production, or in B cell responses to lymphokines.

In myasthenia gravis (MG), anti-AChR antibodies are thought to cause pathology through the degradation of the receptor either by cross-linking or through complement-mediated lysis of post-synaptic membranes; they do not commonly affect signal transduction through blocking the cholinergic binding site. The antibodies produced usually do not recognise a single antigenic epitope and even those which do, do not show restricted gene usage. This suggests that MG is not the result of the escape from tolerance of a single self-reactive clone. Also, the poor correlation between anti-AChR antibody levels and disease progression suggests that only some clones are pathogenic.

These may result in hypergammaglobulinaemia (abnormally high serum levels of immunoglobulin), autoantibody production, preferential production of

Table 5.9   Lymphokine abnormalities in autoimmune diseases

Lymphokine	Disease
Defective IL-1 and IL-2 production	Systemic lupus erythematosus and rheumatoid arthritis
Elevated levels of IL-6	Rheumatoid, and juvenile chronic, arthritis
Qualitative and quantitative abnormalities in interferon	Systemic autoimmune diseases
High levels of acid labile IFNα	Systemic lupus erythematosus

pathogenic subclasses of autoantibodies, or a generalised autoimmune disease such as systemic lupus erythematosus.

CYTOKINE DEFECTS

As with all clinical studies in humans, data concerning lymphokine production in patients with autoimmune diseases is often controversial or inconclusive. Such studies may be influenced by a number of parameters including genetic, hormonal and diurnal factors, type of disease, other infectious or medical complications, therapy, etc. Thus, the relevance of abnormalities observed in serum lymphokine levels to the disease process is difficult to interpret, especially in organ-specific diseases where serum levels may not reflect those occurring within the affected tissues. Some accepted observations are listed in Table 5.9.

Clearly the key role of cytokines in the immune response establishes their role in autoimmune disease. However conflicting observations suggesting that inhibition of cytokine activity can lead to exacerbation or amelioration of existing disease makes it difficult to assign a particular role to these molecules. It has been suggested that the role of cytokines in dendritic cell differentiation may be key to their involvement in autoimmune disease.

CHEMOKINES IN AUTOIMMUNE DISEASE

Like other cytokines, chemokines have been implicated in the pathogenesis of autoimmune diseases. Some of the associations are detailed in Table 5.10.

KEY POINTS FOR REVIEW

- *Autoimmunity is vital to the development of a normal immune response.*
- *Apart from MHC and idiotypic recognition, the immune system does not normally react to self, i.e. it is self-tolerant.*
- *Breakdown of self-tolerance leads to autoimmune disease.*

Table 5.10   Some roles of chemokines and their receptors in autoimmune disease

Ligand/receptor	Disease association
CCL3, CCL4, CCL5, CXCL10	Elevated in multiple sclerosis. T cell responses to CCL5 and CCL3 increased
CCR2, CCR3, CCR5	CCR5 expression increased on T cells, macrophages and microglia from CNS tissue in multiple sclerosis
CCL2, CCL3, CCL4, CCL5, CXCL5, CXCL8, CXCL9, CXCL10	Increased in rheumatoid arthritis. CXCL5, CXCL8 may cause angiogenesis but CXCL9, CXCL10 are angiostatic
CXCR4 and its ligand CXCL12	In RA, CXCR4 is seen at high levels on memory T cells in the synovium but low levels on circulating T cells. CXCL12 produced through CD154/CD40 ligation on endothelial cells and T cells. May reduce T cell apoptosis
CXCL13 and its receptor CXCR5	CXCL13 is increased in synovial tissues in RA. CXCR5 is found on naïve B cells which may influence their accumulation in synovial tissues

- *There are a large number of factors affecting the development of autoimmune disease.*
- *Criteria for determining the aetiology of autoimmune diseases were proposed by Witebsky and were based on Koch's postulates.*
- *Autoimmune disease may be systemic (non-organ-specific) or organ-specific, but many diseases present a mixed picture.*
- *The pathology associated with autoimmune disease may be categorised according to the type of hypersensitivity reactions occurring.*
- *In many autoimmune diseases the target antigens for autoimmune attack have not been identified, although there are notable exceptions.*
- *A role for non-specific immunity in autoimmune disease has been proposed by the REGA model.*
- *A number of different immunological cells have been associated with the pathogenesis of autoimmune diseases.*
- *Cytokines and chemokines have been reported to be present in abnormal concentrations in a variety of autoimmune diseases. These observations suggest a pathogenetic linkage.*

5.3   IMMUNODEFICIENCY DISEASES

This section concerns those diseases which directly affect the normal functioning of the immune system. Immunodeficiency diseases were first described in the 1950s when the use of antibiotics and passive immunisation increased the survival of individuals with recurrent infections. Immunodeficiency diseases (IDs) are characterised by infections caused by organisms, which are easily overcome and eliminated in healthy persons. In addition, individuals with immunodeficiency diseases tend to contract infections very easily, have aggressive disease and respond poorly to therapy. The diseases can be broadly segregated into primary and acquired. Individuals are born with primary immunodeficiency diseases either as a result of genetic or developmental abnormalities. Acquired immunodeficiencies are those which result from infection or clinical treatment (iatrogenic immunodeficiency), e.g. damage to the immune system as a result of radiotherapy for cancer.

5.3.1 CLASSIFICATION OF IMMUNODEFICIENCY DISEASES

Immunodeficiency diseases fall into two principal categories – primary and acquired. The causes of primary immunodeficiency diseases may be congenital (due to developmental or genetic abnormalities occurring during pregnancy) or genetic (due to the inheritance of an abnormal gene from one or both parents; Table 5.11). Acquired immunodeficiency disease may result from exposure to chemicals, drugs, irradiation or microorganisms. In recent years, AIDS (the acquired immune deficiency syndrome) has received much attention, but other acquired diseases are becoming more common due to the use of chemo- and radiotherapy. These are known as **iatrogenic immunodeficiencies**, i.e. acquired as a result of treatment for another clinical condition. The resulting diseases may be classified according to which part of the immune system is affected, i.e. B cells, T cells, B and T cells, phagocytes, complement or a combination of these.

Table 5.11 Causes of immunodeficiency diseases

Cause	Example
Genetic	Autosomal recessive, autosomal dominant, X-linked, gene deletions and rearrangements
Biochemical and metabolic deficiencies	Adenosine deaminase deficiency
Vitamin or mineral deficiencies	Biotin, zinc
Developmental abnormalities	Cessation of development during embryogenesis
Autoimmune diseases	Antibodies or T cells with activity towards each other
Acquired immunodeficiency	Viral, transfusion-related, chronic infection, malnutrition, drug abuse, cancer, radiotherapy, chemotherapy, maternal alcoholism

Table 5.12   Clinical features associated with immunodeficiency

Clinical features

Chronic infection
Unusually frequent, recurrent infection
Failure to completely clear infection
Poor response to treatment
Skin rash
Diarrhoea
Stunted growth
Recurrent abscesses
Recurrent osteomyelitis
Signs and symptoms of autoimmune disease

5.3.2   PRIMARY IMMUNODEFICIENCY DISEASES

Primary immunodeficiency diseases are a diverse group of disorders, which arise from a range of genetic abnormalities. Many present with similar clinical signs and symptoms (Table 5.12). Some of these diseases (which may affect one or several parts of the immune system) are extremely rare and the precise underlying defect has not been defined. Examples of each of these diseases will be discussed below.

5.3.3   B CELL ABNORMALITIES

SELECTIVE IMMUNOGLOBULIN A DEFICIENCY

Selective IgA deficiency is the most common of the primary immunodeficiency diseases in the developed world, having an incidence of 1:600 individuals. Clinically it presents as a heterogeneous group of disorders, which include diseases affecting the gastrointestinal tract, allergic reactions, a diverse range of infections, and diseases that are autoimmune or genetic in origin. The clinical presentation of IgA deficiency is dependent upon the degree of abnormal B cell differentiation; the characteristic defect seen in classical IgA deficiency. This arrest in B cell development is thought to be due to abnormal immuno-regulatory signals since in patients with this disease, the genes coding for immunoglobulin molecules appear to be normal, as does their expression.

IgA-producing B cells have undergone somatic rearrangement such that the switch region immediately before the μ gene is joined to the one preceding the α gene and the sequences in between are removed. This process is influenced by **TGFβ1**. Patients with IgA deficiency appear to have a decrease in the recombination event (when compared with normal individuals), which may be due to the defective production of TGFβ1. However, the levels of mRNA coding for this cytokine in peripheral blood mononuclear cells isolated from patients with IgA deficiency have been shown to be the same as those in control subjects.

Genetic studies have suggested that the disease is related to the presence of a susceptibility gene in the Class II or Class III MHC gene region. The simultaneous change in IgG subclasses, exemplified by an absence of carbohydrate-specific IgG_2 or even a lack of serum IgG_2, IgG_4 and IgE, suggests that these patients have a block in switching to genes downstream of IgG_1.

X-LINKED AGAMMAGLOBULINAEMIA (XLA)

Newborn babies normally are unable to produce specific antibodies when exposed to an antigen. At this stage, a baby is protected by maternal antibodies, which have crossed the placenta. Later (7–9 months of age) normal babies begin to produce their own antibodies. Babies with X-linked agammaglobulinaemia (XLA) are unable to do so and present with recurrent bacterial infections. Individuals affected by this disease (the majority of which are male) usually have less than 10% of the normal level of serum IgG and less than 1% of the normal serum levels of IgA and IgM. Additionally, they have low levels of B, and plasma, cells. T cells in affected individuals seem to be normal. Thus, as might be expected, viral infections (which are largely controlled by T cells) are rarely life-threatening in patients with XLA.

As the name of the disease suggests, it is genetically based and the defect is inherited from the mother. In normal women, the active X chromosomes are derived equally from the mother and father. By contrast, in female carriers of a number of X-linked immunodeficiency disorders (including X-linked agamma-globulinaemia, X-linked severe combined immunodeficiency disease, and the Wiskott–Aldrich syndrome) all the active X chromosomes in the affected cell populations are those which carry the abnormal copy of the gene (allele).

Several studies suggest that the genetic defect in XLA affects B cell development at a number of different stages (Table 5.13). In addition, the cytoplasmic protein Bruton's tyrosine kinase (Btk) is mutated in XLA. Since several studies have shown such cytoplasmic kinases are essential for cell growth and differentiation and are involved in lymphocyte signal transduction, this mutated protein is likely to be involved in the developmental abnormalities seen in XLA. Indeed, the gene coding for Btk maps to the position (locus) q22 on the X chromosome, which has been identified as that involved in XLA. In addition, Btk is expressed in B but not T cells, which may explain why, despite the obvious B cell defect in these patients, T cells appear to be functionally, and phenotypically, normal. Interestingly, the abnormal gene is also expressed in the

Table 5.13   B cell abnormalities reported to be associated with XLA

B cell developmental abnormalities

Reduced pre-B cell proliferation, with fewer cells entering the S-phase of the cell cycle

Failure of pre-B cell to thrive

Inversion of bone marrow ratio of pro- and pre-B cells

Few, immature circulating B cells

myeloid cells of patients with XLA. However, these cells appear functionally normal.

Bruton's tyrosine kinase is intimately involved in signal transduction pathways regulating survival, activation, proliferation and differentiation of B cells. Following ligation of the B cell antigen receptor, Btk is activated by the tyrosine kinases Lyn and Syk resulting in calcium mobilisation mediated by phospholipase C2. Despite this knowledge, it is unclear how mutations in Btk affect downstream events leading to XLA.

CD40 LIGAND DEFICIENCY

X-linked hyper IgM syndrome (XHM) was first recognised in 1966 and is now known to be due to a defect in the gene coding for the CD40 ligand (CD154). CD154 is a surface antigen on T cells, which influences B cell antibody class switching through interaction with CD40 on the B cell surface.

Persons with CD40L deficiency have very low IgG and IgA levels and normal or raised serum IgM. Lymphocyte subpopulations and T cell function are apparently normal. Affected individuals are susceptible to bacterial infections such as *Pneumocystis carinii* and *Cryptosporidium parvum*.

CD40L also plays a role in T cell function since the T cell response to a range of antigens is defective in patients with CD40L deficiency.

X-LINKED LYMPHOPROLIFERATIVE DISEASE (DUNCAN'S SYNDROME)

A rare disorder, patients with X-linked lymphoproliferative disease (XLP) have a dysregulated response to Epstein–Barr virus (EBV). Usually, patients have fulminant, often fatal, acute, EBV infection, hypogammaglobulinaemia, B cell lymphoma, aplastic anaemia and vasculitis.

The gene responsible for XLP has been localised to Xq25 and codes for a protein known as the **signalling lymphocyte activating molecule associated protein** (SAP). The **signalling lymphocyte activating molecule** (SLAM) is found on the surface of T and B lymphocytes mediating binding between them and leading to their co-activation. SAP, which is mainly expressed in T cells, inhibits this reaction such that patients with XLP experience dysregulated T/B cell interactions leading to uncontrolled B cell proliferation.

5.3.4 T CELL ABNORMALITIES

There are a number of known primary T cell immunodeficiency syndromes, which include severe combined immunodeficiency syndrome, Di George syndrome, Wiskott–Aldrich syndrome, ataxia telangiectasia, defective expression of MHC Class II molecules, and defective expression of the CD3/TCR complex. The underlying defects for all these diseases vary, but the principal cell affected in all of them is the T cell.

CONGENITAL THYMIC APLASIA (DI GEORGE SYNDROME)

Congenital thymic aplasia is one of a group of diseases collectively known as the del22q11 syndrome, which is the most common chromosomal microdeletion syndrome in humans. The deletion concerned occurs in the proximal long arm of chromosome 22 and is characterised by a typically deleted region (TDR) comprising about 30 genes. Despite this apparent genetic commonality, Di George syndrome, velocardiofacial syndrome and conotruncal anomaly face syndrome, which comprise the del22q11 syndrome, have distinct clinical features. New animal models of the disease are providing insights into the precise genetic defects involved in these diseases. However, to date, it is unclear how this microdeletion on chromosome 22 gives rise to the immunological abnormalities described in patients with Di George syndrome. It is likely that the affected gene(s) are involved in the molecular pathways regulating neural crest development in the embryo. These cells ultimately give rise to organs such as the heart and thymus, defects in the latter potentially being responsible for the T cell defects observed in these patients.

   In contrast to many other immunodeficiency diseases, which become apparent after the loss of maternal antibodies, Di George syndrome is associated with symptoms that appear immediately after birth owing to defective T cell function. Affected babies have a range of abnormal clinical features (Table 5.14) and at birth will be lymphopenic (i.e. will have severely decreased numbers of lymphocytes) with very few circulating T cells. In addition, lymphocytes fail to proliferate in response to stimulation with mitogens (e.g. phytohaemagglutinin – PHA) or allogeneic cells. Thus,

Table 5.14 Clinical features associated with Di George syndrome

Clinical feature
Low-set ears with notched lobes
A fish-shaped mouth
Slanting eyes
Reduced parathyroid activity (hypoparathyroidism)
Congenital heart disease
Abnormalities of the thymus
Severely impaired cellular immunity

individuals with this disease must not be immunised with live, attenuated, viral vaccines due to the need for effective cell-mediated immunity to eliminate these organisms. Interestingly, the T cell defect in Di George syndrome may vary from reduced levels of functionally normal T cells to a complete lack of T cell immunity. This variability is probably related to the abnormal thymic development during the first trimester (0–12 weeks) of pregnancy, which is associated with this disease.

Although the primary defect in Di George syndrome is T cell-dependent, some patients have low immunoglobulin levels and fail to make specific antibody following immunisation.

WISKOTT–ALDRICH SYNDROME

Wiskott–Aldrich syndrome (WAS) is a rare X-linked recessive disease. Affected individuals suffer from immune dysregulation and microthrombocytopenia. They demonstrate a susceptibility to pyogenic, viral and opportunistic infection, and eczema. Immunologically, WAS is characterised by a progressive loss of T cells resulting in abnormal cell-mediated and DTH responses and abnormal antibody responses.

The genetic basis of the disease has been unravelled by the identification of a disease-specific protein – WASP (Wiskott–Aldrich syndrome protein). The WASP gene encodes a protein found solely in cells of haemopoietic origin. The WAS protein is involved in transporting signals from cell surface receptors to the cytoskeleton. Abnormalities in WASP lead to defects in the organisation of the cytoskeleton such that cellular motility (and therefore trafficking) is adversely affected.

5.3.5   T AND B CELL ABNORMALITIES

SEVERE COMBINED IMMUNODEFICIENCY DISEASE (SCID)

Severe combined immunodeficiency disease (SCID) affects one in every 80 000 live births. It is the most severe form of primary immunodeficiency with a number of different causes. Affected individuals have abnormalities affecting T, B and NK cells, which prevent the development of normal cell-mediated or humoral responses. One of the features of this disease is lymphopenia (severely reduced numbers of circulating lymphocytes), which is largely due to an extremely low number of T cells that may fail to express MHC gene products (see the section on Bare lymphocyte syndrome). Indeed, the severity of the T cell depletion is reflected in the fact that despite the overall lymphopenia, B cells may be increased in number. In addition, affected individuals generally have very low serum levels of all classes of immunoglobulin and fail to produce specific antibodies following immunisation or infection. At least eight types of SCID can be distinguished according to the clinical signs and symptoms and the inheritance pattern of the disease.

Due to the T cell abnormality, shortly after birth affected babies may develop disseminated yeast infections (usually caused by *Monilia* spp.), severe pneumonia (caused by *Pneumocystis carinii*) and recurrent infections caused by other opportunistic pathogens (organisms which, in healthy individuals, are normally prevented from causing disease by the immune system). Since these infections usually affect the skin and the pulmonary and gastrointestinal tracts, their prevalence in patients with SCID suggests that the defect also affects the immune mechanisms normally involved in surface and mucosal immunity. Since both the cell-mediated and humoral systems are affected, patients may die as a result of infection with common viruses such as varicella, herpes and cytomegalovirus. In addition, affected children often have chronic diarrhoea and malabsorption of nutrients from the gut, resulting in a failure to thrive.

The disease is inherited as an autosomal or X-linked, recessive trait. In recent years, clear progress has been made in identifying the genetic lesions leading to the different types of disease. We will consider some of the most common forms of SCID below.

X-LINKED SEVERE COMBINED IMMUNODEFICIENCY DISEASE (XSCID)

The most common form of SCID is X-linked SCID (XSCID), which accounts for 50–60% of all cases of the disease. It is characterised by a severe decrease in the numbers of circulating T and natural killer (NK) cells. B cells are usually normal or increased in number, although their functionality is affected by the lack of T cell help. Histologically, thymic tissue from these patients shows a lack of differentiation between the cortex and medulla, few thymocytes and no Hassal's corpuscles. In addition, the peripheral lymphoid organs are also hypoplastic.

The locus for the genetic defect associated with XSCID was mapped to Xq12–13.1 and this led to the identification in XSCID patients of mutations in the gene encoding the γ chain of the IL-2 receptor (IL-2R), which is found in this region. This γ chain is common to a number of other cytokine receptors (i.e. IL-4, 7, 9 and 15) and is the signal-transducing molecule for each of these cytokines (γc). Defects in this chain mean that these cytokines are unable to induce the cellular responses seen in normal cells as a result of binding to their respective receptors.

As a result of receptor ligation, a series of downstream molecular interactions occur resulting in the regulation of transcription of certain genes. The downstream interactions (signalling pathway) that occur after γc ligation comprise the Jak–STAT pathway. When IL-2, IL-4, IL-7, IL-9 or IL-15 bind to their respective receptors, the common gamma chain activates an enzyme known as the Janus family tyrosine kinase 3 (Jak-3). In addition, receptor-specific chains (namely IL-2Rβ (for IL-2 and IL-15), IL-4Rα, IL-7Rα and IL-9Rα) associate with Jak-1. Thus, since γc-dependent signalling is dependent on Jak-3, mutations in the gene encoding this protein would lead to identical defects to those seen in individuals with mutations in the γc gene. Thus, the defect in XSCID is defined as defective γc-dependent activation of Jak-3 and mutations in those genes encoding either γc or Jak-3 can result in disease.

Upon receptor–ligand interaction, Jak-3 binds to the intracellular tail of γc and is activated resulting in the phosphorylation of the STAT-5 protein. These phosphorylated proteins dimerise and translocate to the nucleus where they induce the transcription of a number of genes involved in cellular replication.

Immunologically, XSCID is characterised by the developmental failure of T and NK cells. IL-7 is known to regulate T cell development in the thymus. In humans, it does not appear to affect B cell development. Evidence has demonstrated that at least one cause of XSCID is abnormal IL-7Rα-dependent signalling. The NK cell abnormalities are probably due to defective IL-15 signalling. The other cytokines affected by the mutations identified in XSCID (namely in γc or Jak-3) do not appear to contribute to the abnormalities observed in the disease. This may be due to the fact that signalling via these receptors does not occur during normal T cell development prior to the key signalling required from IL-7.

SCID WITH ADENOSINE DEAMINASE DEFICIENCY (ADA-SCID)

ADA-SCID is inherited as an autosomal, recessive trait and accounts for 20% of the cases of SCID. The severe immune defect characteristic of this condition is a direct consequence of a deficiency in the enzyme adenosine deaminase (ADA), which is part of the salvage pathway of purine metabolism. ADA catalyses the conversion of adenosine (Ado) to inosine and deoxyadenosine (dAdo) to deoxyinosine. Individuals with ADA-SCID show severe T, B and NK lymphocytopaenia.

In ADA-deficient individuals, adenosine and dAdo accumulate intracellularly (as well as extracellularly) and become phosphorylated to deoxyATP (dATP), a compound that is toxic to lymphocytes and is normally not detected at high levels in mammalian cells. Although ADA is normally present in all cells of the body, its absence presents as a defect that characteristically affects the cells of the immune system alone. This is due to the fact that in most tissues, dATP is reversibly degraded into DADO. However, lymphocytes (particularly immature cells) have little ability so to do. dATP inhibits the activity of ribonucleotide reductase, an enzyme required for generation of the other deoxynucleotides. In their absence, DNA synthesis cannot proceed and thus cell division is inhibited.

THE BARE LYMPHOCYTE SYNDROME

Bare lymphocyte syndrome is a rare, primary immunodeficiency disease in which leukocytes fail to express MHC Class II antigens and show defective expression of MHC Class I antigens. As a consequence, affected individuals fail to mount an immune response to foreign antigens.

Symptoms start during the first year of life and affected individuals suffer from recurrent chest infections and chronic diarrhoea. The lack of T cell immunity means that patients may suffer from a range of viral infections (including meningitis and hepatitis) and autoimmune phenomena. Affected individuals do not have a great life expectancy – the mean age at death in one survey was 4 years – with the main cause of death being viral infection. Treatment by bone marrow transplantation has greatly improved the chances of long-term survival; success being affected by the presence of pre-existing viral infections.

5.3.6   ABNORMALITIES ASSOCIATED WITH PHAGOCYTIC CELLS

CHEDIAK–HIGASHI SYNDROME (CHS)

This is a rare disease arising from an autosomal-recessive trait principally affecting neutrophils. Affected individuals suffer from partial albinism, recurrent, pyogenic infections and have moderately reduced levels of circulating neutrophils (neutropenia), which contain characteristic giant lysosomes. These organelles contain enzymes and other constituents that are usually segregated in distinct cytoplasmic granules. Affected individuals undergo an accelerated phase of the disease characterised by a lymphocytic infiltrate associated with EBV infection. It has been suggested through analogies to other diseases that the accelerated phase may result from defective T_{cyt} activity. Indeed, CHS patients have decreased CTL killing due to an inability to secrete the giant granules that contain the lytic proteins granzyme A, granzyme B and perforin.

Several studies have demonstrated that CHS cells have defective antigen processing. CHS B cells show delayed or poor peptide loading and antigen presentation which may result from prolonged MHC II–HLA-DM intracellular association.

All the cellular defects observed in CHS patients are related to the formation and trafficking of intracellular vesicles. A model of the disease has been established in the Beige mouse which possesses a disease-specific cytosolic protein (the CHS:Beige protein). It has been suggested that this protein is involved in maintaining or possibly shuttling these vesicles to their proper location.

CHRONIC GRANULOMATOUS DISEASE (CGD)

The incidence of CGD varies geographically, being 1 in 200 000 in the USA. Several hundred cases have been reported since it was first described in the 1950s, but it is likely that it continues to be underdiagnosed. Affected individuals present with a variety of clinical features but all have a defect in the oxidative metabolism of phagocytic cells (i.e. neutrophils, monocytes, macrophages and eosinophils). A diagnosis of CGD is easily confirmed by the nitroblue tetrazolium reduction test or other tests of neutrophil oxidative metabolism.

Generally, patients with CGD suffer from recurrent infections (caused by bacteria and fungi) on epithelial surfaces in direct contact with the environment, and a range of other complications including chronic granulomatous inflammation, skin abscesses, hepatomegaly and pneumonia. A proportion of patients have diarrhoea and sepsis, which can cause a misdiagnosis of Crohn's disease.

Patients with the classic form of CGD develop serious infections usually within the first year of life. In most cases, infection is caused by catalase-positive bacteria, such as *Staphylococcus aureus* and the Gram-negative enterobacter-iaceae, *Salmonella* spp., *Klebsiella* spp., *Aerobacter* spp. and *Serratia* spp. However, infections with the fungi *Aspergillus* (usually *fumigatus*) and *Candida* sp. are also seen. Although severe, infection in CGD may be characterised initially only by malaise, low-grade fever and a mild leukocytosis (raised white cell count) or elevation in erythrocyte sedimentation rate. Organisms that produce H_2O_2 but are catalase-negative (e.g. *Streptococcus* sp., *Pneumococcus* sp., *Lactobacillus* sp.) are not major pathogens in CGD. This may be because the

H_2O_2 produced by the microbes within the phagosome acts with the host cell myeloperoxidase (MPO) resulting in bactericidal activity. Alternatively, O_2^- independent microbicidal mechanisms may be sufficient in CGD to kill certain pathogens.

The precise defect in CGD responsible for the decreased microbicidal activity of phagocytic cells has not been fully established. The electron transport chain involved in oxidative metabolism pumps electrons but not protons into the phagocytic vacuole leading to pH elevation. This alkalinisation fully activates neutral proteases, which kill bacteria. The formation of superoxide by the passage of electrons from NADPH to molecular O_2 is catalysed by the NAPDH oxidase. The latter consists of a membrane-bound flavocytochrome (b558) and four cytosolic factors, p47 phagocyte oxidase (p47phox), p67phox, p40phox and p21rac, which translocate to the membrane on activation of the cell by opsonised particles or soluble inflammatory mediators. Abnormalities in both of the subunits of the b558 and in the cytosolic factors p47phox, p67phox and p21rac2 have been identified in patients with CGD. The mutations are heterogeneous and were found to be unique to a particular family in 90% of cases.

A further consequence of the abnormal oxidative metabolism associated with CGD is that patients are predisposed to granuloma formation, occasionally resulting in throat, bowel or genitourinary tract obstruction. Normal neutrophils inactivate chemoattractants through the myeloperoxidase–hydrogen peroxide–halide system. The defect in oxidative metabolism in CGD leads to a lack of H_2O_2 production and thus a failure to inactivate chemoattractants. This is likely to lead to prolonged leukocyte recruitment. In addition, inefficient degradation of antigen may result in the chronic release of cytokines such as IFNγ that may stimulate the granulomatous process.

5.3.7 ABNORMALITIES OF THE COMPLEMENT PATHWAY

DEFICIENCIES OF COMPLEMENT COMPONENTS

Immunodeficiencies associated with defective complement activity generally behave as autosomal recessive traits. Affected individuals lack, or have reduced levels of, complement proteins caused by an abnormal gene. In heterozygous individuals (with one normal and one abnormal gene), reduced protein production occurs. However, since normal serum complement component concentrations vary greatly, it may not be possible to identify those individuals carrying an abnormal gene.

THE ALTERNATIVE PATHWAY

The alternative complement pathway is the immediate defence against microbial infection, allowing time for specific immunity to develop. Defects in this pathway may result in serious infection and affected individuals have frequent, severe, infections caused by organisms such as *Pneumococcus* spp., *Haemophilus influenzae* and *Staphylococcus* spp.

THE CLASSICAL PATHWAY

Genetic abnormalities, which affect the pre-C3 convertase part of the classical complement pathway, are not associated with repeated infections due to the activity of the alternative pathway. In contrast to this, deficiency of C3, which is common to both the classical and alternative pathways, results in severe, potentially fatal infections.

Deficiencies which involve C5 and subsequent complement components do not affect the patient's ability to control most infections since the opsonic and chemotactic activity of the earlier components is intact. However, individuals with such defects may suffer from repeated infections caused by *Neisseria* spp. and *Meningococcus* spp.; obviously, the lytic activity of the membrane attack complex is needed to eliminate these encapsulated organisms. However, defective C9 is not associated with uncontrollable infection. This is probably because the C5–C8 complex destabilises the membrane enough to mediate lysis of most infectious agents.

C1INH DEFICIENCY – HEREDITARY ANGIOEDEMA (HAE)

First described in the 1880s, hereditary angioedema (HAE) is an autosomal dominant disease that results from the lack of a protein that inhibits the action of the first component of complement (C1INH). This serine protease inhibitor is a member of the Serpin superfamily and is involved in the regulation of the coagulation, fibrinolytic and contact (or kinin-forming) systems. Lack of C1 inhibitor results in a range of severe symptoms (Table 5.15) and biochemical defects reflecting the importance of this protein.

Biochemically, the decreased level of C1 inhibitor leads to low serum levels of C2 and C4 due to the uncontrolled activation of C1. The central role played by C1 inhibitor in the control of the complement, clotting and kinin systems means that after an appropriate stimulus (trauma or stress) affected individuals undergo a massive inflammatory response. The implications of this may be seen in patients who have an oedematous reaction in their larynx. The swelling blocks the airway and, unless treated immediately, the patient will die. In order

Table 5.15   Clinical characteristics of hereditary angioedema

Clinical characteristics

Episodic, acute local oedema of the skin or mucosa affecting mainly the extremities, face, larynx and gut

Attacks (which are often associated with trauma or emotional stress) last from 24 to 72 hours

Attacks begin in childhood and increase in severity during adolescence

Frequency and severity of attacks decreases by the fifth or sixth decade of life Also in pregnant women particularly in the second and third trimesters

to prevent such attacks patients are treated with long-term androgen therapy. It is thought that this hormone may enhance the synthesis of C1 inhibitor by the liver.

Hereditary angioedema is classified as either Type I or Type II. Patients with Type I HAE (85% of affected individuals) have very low levels of C1 inhibitor (5 to 30% of normal plasma levels). In contrast to this, patients with Type II HAE have normal or elevated levels of C1 inhibitor. However, a large proportion of this protein is dysfunctional; only a very low level of the normal protein is present. It has been suggested that the two forms of the disease result from different genetic abnormalities. Type I HAE is thought to be due to a defect in a regulator gene whilst patients with Type II HAE most probably have a structural gene defect.

5.3.8   ACQUIRED IMMUNODEFICIENCIES

IATROGENIC IMMUNODEFICIENCIES

Iatrogenic immunodeficiencies are a consequence of our advances in patient care and therapy. They are a heterogeneous group of immunodeficiency diseases, the limits of which are difficult to delineate. However, they are all induced by the use of treatment regimes that result in temporary or permanent immunodeficiency (Table 5.16).

The incidence of iatrogenic immunodeficiencies is rapidly increasing as a consequence of the increase in chemotherapeutic treatment for cancer and leukaemia and the more widespread use of organ and bone marrow transplantation for treatment of terminal illnesses.

Since this form of acquired immunodeficiency results from therapeutic regimes, its occurrence depends upon the strength and/or duration of the therapy. However, presentation and outcome of the disease may also be affected by other factors (Table 5.17).

Table 5.16   Causes of iatrogenic immunodeficiency disease

Treatment	Treatment for
X- or gamma-irradiation	Cancer, leukaemia and immunologically mediated diseases
Corticosteroids or other immunosuppressive drugs	Cancer, leukaemia and immunologically mediated diseases; transplantation
Antibiotics	Infection; may indirectly cause proliferation of potentially harmful bacteria or fungi by altering the intestinal flora of the host; part of the innate immune system
Gold salts or other chemotherapeutic agents	Autoimmune diseases; may cause alterations in the haemopoietic system, producing anaemia, granulocytopenia, thrombocytopenia or immune deficiency

Table 5.17   Factors affecting the presentation and outcome of iatrogenic immunodeficiencies

Factors affecting presentation of disease	Example
The type of disease for which treatment is being given	Treatment of autoimmune diseases may lead to immunodeficiency
Reactivation of latent infections in the host	Treatment may eliminate immunoregulatory mechanisms which keep infections in check resulting in overwhelming and life-threatening infections
Allogeneic stimulation	Patients receiving blood transfusions or organ transplants who are therapeutically immunosuppressed may suffer from graft-versus-host disease caused by the immunologically active cells in the grafts
Exposure to infectious agents after development of immunodeficiency	Immunocompromised hosts are not able to fight off even common infections

5.3.9   THE ACQUIRED IMMUNODEFICIENCY SYNDROME (AIDS)

AIDS probably has become the most widely publicised infectious disease and, in the years since its first description, has been the subject of a mountain of both scientific and popular literature. It is not possible in a book like this to fully describe the extent of our knowledge of AIDS and its causative virus – the human immunodeficiency virus (HIV). The vast amount of research being performed in this area means that this section could be out of date before the book is published. Thus, it is my aim to introduce the topic at a fundamental level and to provide a number of references which cover in more depth the recent advances concerning the disease and virus.

The acquired immune deficiency syndrome was first identified as a result of a study at the Centers for Disease Control in Atlanta, Georgia. It was noticed

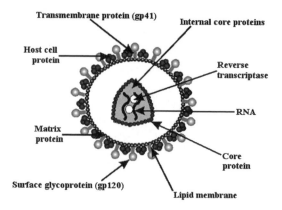

Figure 5.6   Structure of the human immunodeficiency virus

that a number of otherwise apparently healthy young men had died of opportunistic infections, which normally only kill individuals with some underlying, predisposing immunodeficiency. The types of infections that killed these individuals (and were found to be affecting others like them) would normally be controlled by cell-mediated immune mechanisms. Thus, further studies of affected individuals concentrated on examining their peripheral blood lymphocytes. These showed that the patients had decreased levels of circulating $CD4^+$ T cells. This led to a search for a causative agent, which could infect and destroy T cells. This led to the identification of a virus that eventually became known as the human immunodeficiency virus, or HIV.

THE HUMAN IMMUNODEFICIENCY VIRUS (HIV)

The human immunodeficiency virus has been classified as a Lentivirus due to its cone-shaped core, which contains the viral genetic code (ribonucleic acid – RNA) and an enzyme that allows the transcription of this viral RNA into deoxyribonucleic acid (DNA). The core is surrounded by an envelope, which consists of knobs made up of trimers or tetramers of the envelope glycoproteins (Figure 5.6). These glycoproteins are derived from a precursor molecule gp160, which is cleaved inside the cell to give the gp120 and gp41 proteins. The gp120 glycoprotein contains the virus receptor for cellular binding and the major neutralising sites. gp41 plays an important role in virus/cell and cell/cell fusion.

The genome of HIV is about 9.8 kb and the primary transcript produces a messenger RNA that is translated into the Gag and Pol proteins (Figure 5.7). The Gag proteins (p25, p17, p9 and p6) are derived from a precursor molecule, p55 and form the capsid (p25), the nucleocapsid (p17) and the core (p17) proteins of the virus. The Pol proteins derived from the Pol precursor molecule include the protease responsible for cleaving precursor proteins, the integrase

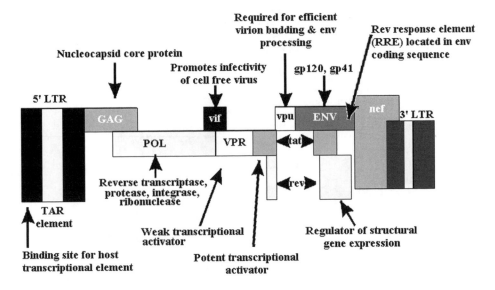

Figure 5.7 The HIV genome

involved in viral integration into the host cell genome and the reverse transcriptase (or RNA-dependent, DNA polymerase) that converts the viral RNA genome into DNA. In addition to these products, others are produced as a result of splicing mRNA. These include the product of the Rev gene (itself the result of mRNA splicing), which regulates the relative production of unspliced, singly or multiply spliced mRNAs. Other products of multiply spliced mRNA include a range of regulatory and accessory proteins, which control virus production (Table 5.18).

Table 5.18 Regulatory proteins of HIV	
Gene product	Effect
Tat (transactivating protein)	Binds the TAR (Tat responsive region) in the 3' portion of the viral long terminal repeat region (LTR) and is the main HIV replication-enhancing protein
Rev (regulator of viral expression)	Binds the Rev responsive element in the viral envelope mRNA and permits unspliced mRNA to leave the nucleus and enter the cytoplasm thus allowing the production of full-length viral proteins which are needed for infectious virus production
Nef (negative factor)	Has a variety of functions including downregulation of viral expression. It may cause this effect by interacting with the viral LTR or by interferring with Rev binding to the envelope mRNA
Vif, Vpr, Vpu/Vpx (accessory proteins)	These proteins are important in virus assembly and budding and in the infectivity and production of infectious virus

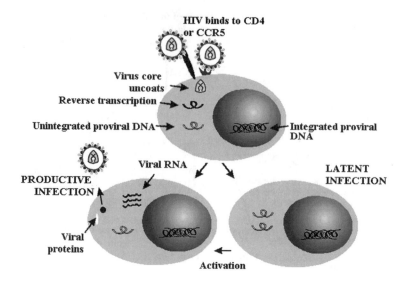

Figure 5.8　Mechanisms of virus replication

Attachment of HIV of the host cell is via the CD4, which is expressed on a subset of T cells and on some monocytes/macrophages. In order to infect cells, HIV binds to additional co-receptors, the two most common being the chemokine receptors CXCR4 on T cells and CCR5 on macrophages. Binding to CD4 and the co-receptors is thought to cause conformational changes in gp120, which along with cleavage of the envelope protein by cellular enzymes causes another change in the viral envelope leading to virus/cell fusion.

Once the virus has entered the cell, a sequence of events occurs, which results in the integration of the provirus into the host DNA. The virus genome is reverse transcribed by the viral RNA-dependent DNA polymerase, giving rise to a double-stranded DNA provirus that migrates to the nucleus of the cell and randomly integrates into the host genome (Figure 5.8). Replication of the virus appears to depend to some degree on the activation state and nature of the infected cells. T lymphocytes in the G_0 stage of the cell cycle undergo abortive infection whilst non-dividing macrophages are able to produce infectious virus. By contrast, T cells activated by antigen and a variety of lymphokines are permissive to virus infection; HIV undergoing integration and replication within approximately 24 hours.

Consequences of HIV infection: As a result of HIV infection, patients present with a number of immunological abnormalities affecting both B and T cell function. Antibody levels are typically elevated due to polyclonal activation of B cells but patients show an inability to respond to antigens to which they have been previously exposed. The most notable abnormality in these individuals is the gradual loss of $CD4^+$ cells. There are many explanations for the severe loss of $CD4^+$ cells, which cannot be explained merely by the

Table 5.19 The principal opportunistic infections and tumours in HIV infection

Classification	Opportunistic agent
Bacteria	Mycobacteria avium intracellulare
	Mycobacterium tuberculosis
	Salmonella spp.
Viruses	Cytomegalovirus
	Varicella zoster
	Herpes simplex
Fungi	Pneumocystis carinii
	Cryptococcus neoformans
	Candida
Parasites	Toxoplasma spp.
	Cryptosporidium spp.
	Leishmania spp.
Malignancies	Kaposi's sarcoma
	Burkitt's lymphoma

destruction of the cells as a result of virus replication. These abnormalities severely affect the ability of the individual to respond to infection, resulting in overwhelming infections from that the patients die. Some of the opportunistic infections and tumours that become life-threatening in the terminal stages of AIDS are listed in Table 5.19.

KEY POINTS FOR REVIEW

- *Immunodeficiency diseases may be primary or acquired.*
- *Primary ID may be due to congenital abnormalities or genetically inherited.*
- *Acquired ID may be due to exposure to chemical, physical or infectious agents.*
- *Primary IDs are a diverse group of diseases that often present with similar clinical signs and symptoms.*
- *They may affect any of the cells involved in immunity or indeed chemicals such as complement components.*
- *Selective IgA deficiency is the most common of the primary IDs and appears to involve abnormalities in switch/recombination events.*
- *In X-linked agammaglobulinaemia, newborn babies are unable to produce specific antibodies when exposed to antigen.*
- *XLA is linked to an abnormal cytoplasmic antigen, Bruton's tyrosine kinase.*
- *X-linked hyper IgM syndrome is caused by a defect in the gene coding for the CD40 ligand.*

- *T cell abnormalities include Di George and Wiskott–Aldrich syndromes.*
- *Some IDs have both T and B cell abnormalities such as severe combined immunodeficiency disease (SCID).*
- *SCID has many different clinical and immunological manifestations according to the nature of the abnormalities involved.*
- *Chediak–Higashi syndrome principally affects neutrophils. All the cellular defects are related to the formation and trafficking of intracellular vesicles.*
- *Patients with chronic granulomatous disease all have a defect in the oxidative metabolism of phagocytic cells.*
- *The precise defect in CGD is related to the passage of electrons from NADPH to molecular oxygen catalysed by NADPH oxidase.*
- *Abnormalities in the complement cascade affect individual components that may or may not result in severe infectious complications.*
- *Deficiency of the C1 inhibitor is the key pathological defect in hereditary angioedema.*
- *Iatrogenic immunodeficiency results from treatment regimes for a range of diseases, e.g. cancer and leukaemia.*
- *The acquired immunodeficiency syndrome is caused by infection with the human immunodeficiency virus.*
- *HIV binds to target cells using the CD4 molecule but infection requires the presence of co-receptors which include CXCR4 and CCR5, the chemokine receptors.*
- *HIV is a retrovirus containing a reverse transcriptase that allows proviral integration into the host genome.*
- *HIV infection leads to a range of immunological disorders leading to overwhelming infections and tumours.*

BIBLIOGRAPHY

Askin DF, Young, S. (2001) The thymus gland. Neonatal Netw, 20; 7–13.

Boros DL. (1999) T helper cell populations, cytokine dynamics, and pathology of the schistosome egg granuloma. Microbes Infect, 1; 511–516.

Carugati A, Pappalardo E, Zingale LC, Cicardi M. (2001) C1-inhibitor deficiency and angioedema. Molec Immunol, 38; 161–173.

Chinen J, Shearer WT. (2002) Molecular virology and immunology of HIV infection. J Allergy Clin Immunol, 110; 189–198.

Drakesmith H, Chain B, Beverley P. (2000) How can dendritic cells cause autoimmune disease? Immunol Today, 21; 214–217.

Ehlers S. (1999) Immunity to tuberculosis: a delicate balance between protection and pathology. FEMS Immuno Med Micro, 23; 149–158.

Epstein JA. (2001) Developing models of DiGeorge syndrome. Trends Genet, 17; S13–S17.

Fischer A. (2000) Severe combined immunodeficiencies (SCID). Clin Exp Immunol, 122; 143–149.

Fournie GJ, Mas M, Cautain B, Savignac M, Subra JF, Pelletier L, Saoudi A, Lagrange D, Calise M, Druet P. (2001) Induction of autoimmunity through bystander effects. Lessons from immunological disorders induced by heavy metals. J Autoimmun, 16; 319–326.

Geiszt M, Kapus A, bet Ligeti E. (2001) Chronic granulomatous disease: more than the lack of superoxide? J Leukoc Biol, 69; 191–196.

Godessart N, Kunkel SL. (2001) Chemokines in autoimmune disease. Curr Opin Immunol, 13; 670–675.

Goldblatt D, Thrasher AJ. (2000) Chronic granulomatous disease. Clin Exp Immunol, 122; 1–9.

Gorbachev AV, Fairchild RL. (2001) Induction and regulation of T-cell priming for contact hypersensitivity. Crit Rev Immunol, 21; 451–472.

Hammarstrom L, Vorechovsky I, Webster D. (2000) Selective IgA deficiency (SigAD) and common variable immunodeficiency (CVID). Clin Exp Immunol, 120; 225–231.

Hart PH. (2001) Regulation of the inflammatory response in asthma by mast cell products. Immunol Cell Biol, 79; 149–153.

Holgate ST. (2000) The role of mast cells and basophils in inflammation. Clin Exp All, 30; 28–32.

Jacques Descotes J, Choquet-Kastylevsky G. (2001) Gell and Coombs's classification: is it still valid? Toxicology, 158; 43–49.

Jones AM, Gaspar HB. (2000) Immunogenetics: changing the face of immunodeficiency. J Clin Pathol, 53; 60–65.

Kobayashi K, Kaneda K, Kasama T. (2001) Immunopathogenesis of delayed-type hypersensitivity. Microsc Res Tech, 53; 241–245.

Leonard WJ. (2000) X-linked severe combined immunodeficiency: from molecular cause to gene therapy within seven years. Molec Med Today, 6; 403–407.

Lindsay EA. (2001) Chromosomal microdeletions: dissecting del22q11 syndrome. Nat Rev Genet, 2; 858–868.

Mao C, Zhou M, Uckun FM. (2001) Crystal structure of Bruton's tyrosine kinase domain suggests a novel pathway for activation and provides insights into the molecular basis of X-linked agammaglobulinemia. J Biol Chem, 276; 41 435–41 443.

McVey Ward D, Griffiths GM, Stinchcombe JC, Kaplan J. (2000) Analysis of the lysosomal storage disease Chediak–Higashi syndrome. Traffic, 1; 816–822.

Oettgen HC. (2000) Regulation of the IgE isotype switch: new insights on cytokine signals and the functions of ε germline transcripts. Curr Opin Immunol, 12; 618–623.

Papiernik M. (2001) Natural CD4$^+$ CD25$^+$ regulatory T cells. Their role in the control of superantigen responses. Immunol Rev, 182; 180–189.

Ring GH, Lakkis FG. (1999) Breakdown of self-tolerance and the pathogenesis of autoimmunity. Semin Nephrol, 19; 25–33.

Rose NR. (2001) Infection, mimics and autoimmune disease. J Clin Invest, 107; 943–944.

Sharif S, Arreaza GA, Zucker P, Delovitch TL. (2002) Regulatory natural killer T cells protect against spontaneous and recurrent type 1 diabetes. Ann N Y Acad Sci, 958; 77–88.

Stephens LA, Mason D. (2001) Characterisation of thymus-derived regulatory T cells that protect against organ-specific autoimmune disease. Microbes Infect, 3; 905–910.

Stephens LA, Mottet C, Mason D, Powrie F. (2001) Human CD4$^+$CD25$^+$ thymocytes and peripheral T cells have immune suppressive activity in vitro. Eur J Immunol, 31; 1247–1254.

Watanabe H, Unger M, Tuvel B, Wang B, Sauder DN. (2002) Contact hypersensitivity: the mechanism of immune responses and T cell balance. J Interferon Cytokine Res, 22; 407–412.

http://www.the-scientist.com
You need to register to gain access to articles on this site, but it's free. Browse the "Hot Papers" archive for the following article(s):
Russo E. (2002) Scientists combine two approaches to thwart the spread of HIV. The Scientist, 16; 28–30.

NOW TEST YOURSELF!

1.   When an individual is exposed to an antigen, the outcome depends upon the strength of the immune response. Which of the following statements concerning hypersensitivity is INCORRECT?

(a) *The term anaphylaxis was first coined by Paul Richet and was used to describe the condition where damage results from a protective response to a particular antigen.*

(b) *An extreme response to an antigen is hypersensitivity, where the increased response results in tissue damage.*

(c) *The terms hypersensitivity and anaphylaxis are now used interchangeably.*

(d) *The allergic response is another type of hypersensitivity response.*

(e) *The term allergy was used initially to describe the outcome of a secondary exposure to antigen.*

2.   Which of the following describes a Type I hypersensitivity response?

(a) *A reaction caused by release of inflammatory mediators from mast cells and basophils as a result of cross-linking cell-bound IgE.*

(b) *A reaction resulting from antibody recognising and binding to a normal or altered cell surface antigen.*

(c) *A reaction resulting from immune complex formation between soluble antigen and specific antibody which may be deposited in organs and activate complement.*

(d) *A reaction which depends upon the activation of antigen-specific T cells.*

(e) *A reaction in which macrophages and fibroblasts proliferate and produce collagen which walls off the antigen.*

3.   Which of the following describes a Type III hypersensitivity response?

(a) *A reaction caused by release of inflammatory mediators from mast cells and basophils as a result of cross-linking cell-bound IgE.*

(b) *A reaction resulting from antibody recognising and binding to a normal or altered cell surface antigen.*

(c) *A reaction resulting from immune complex formation between soluble antigen and specific antibody which may be deposited in organs and activate complement.*

(d) *A reaction which depends upon the activation of antigen-specific T cells.*

(e) *A reaction in which macrophages and fibroblasts proliferate and produce collagen which walls off the antigen.*

4. Which of the following describes a Type II hypersensitivity response?

(a) *A reaction caused by release of inflammatory mediators from mast cells and basophils as a result of cross-linking cell-bound IgE.*

(b) *A reaction resulting from antibody recognising and binding to a normal or altered cell surface antigen.*

(c) *A reaction resulting from immune complex formation between soluble antigen and specific antibody which may be deposited in organs and activate complement.*

(d) *A reaction which depends upon the activation of antigen-specific T cells.*

(e) *A reaction in which macrophages and fibroblasts proliferate and produce collagen which walls off the antigen.*

5. Which of the following statements concerning the regulation of Type I hypersensitivity is CORRECT?

(a) *The switch to IgE production is regulated by Th_1 cells through direct contact with B cells and the secretion of certain cytokines.*

(b) *The production of IL-4 clearly favours the production of IgG rather than IgE by B cells.*

(c) *Antigens may deliver signals via the CD4 molecule which favour the differentiation of Th_2 cells.*

(d) *Complexes which bind the T cell antigen receptor with high avidity tend to favour the development of a Th_2-type response.*

(e) *Cell surface molecules on both the T and antigen presenting cells may influence the outcome of the TCR–MHC–allergen interaction.*

6. Which of the following statements concerning autoimmunity is CORRECT?

(a) *Autoimmunity is vital to the development of a normal immune response.*

(b) *T cells only recognise and respond to antigen when it is processed and presented in association with foreign MHC gene products.*

(c) *Autoimmune disease arises as a result of the development of self-tolerance.*

(d) *Autoimmunity may develop as a result of exposure in adult life to an antigen which was hidden from the immune system in the early stages of development.*

(e) *Self-tolerance develops within the first 6 months of life.*

7. The genetic make-up of the host may be a major determinant in the onset and development of autoimmune diseases. Which of the following statements is CORRECT?

(a) *The genes which control the magnitude and type of immune response (i.e. the MHC type Class II and Class III genes) are particularly relevant to the development of autoimmune disease.*

(b) Several autoimmune diseases have been associated with the expression of particular MHC and immunoglobulin isotypic genes.
(c) Seronegative rheumatoid arthritis has been associated with the expression of HLA-DR4.
(d) Systemic lupus erythematosus has been associated with the expression of the Class I gene, HLA-DR2.
(e) Insulin-dependent diabetes mellitus has been associated with the expression of HLA-DQ3.

8.   Which of the following statements is INCORRECT?
(a) Women are generally more susceptible to autoimmune disease than men.
(b) The incidence of autoimmune disease is clearly affected by sex hormones.
(c) The incidence of autoimmune disease is clearly affected by genes linked to the X, but not the Y, chromosome.
(d) Androgen has a protective, immunosuppressive role in autoimmune diseases.
(e) Increased levels of oestrogen exacerbate autoimmune disease.

9.   The REGA model of autoimmune disease has recently been proposed. Which of the following statements concerning this model is CORRECT?
(a) The acronym REGA stands for restricted epitope generating autoimmunity.
(b) The REGA model proposes that disease is triggered by the release of cytokines due to antigen-specific stimulation.
(c) Disease-enhancing cytokines stimulate the production of a range of other cytokines, which activate T and B cells leading to an antigen-specific response.
(d) Evidence for the role of non-specific immune mechanisms in autoimmunity includes the observation that cytokines that suppress proteinase activity predominate in the remission phase of rheumatoid arthritis.
(e) Resident macrophages are stimulated by the disease-enhancing cytokines and produce proteinases and activate latent metalloproteinases, which results in demyelination in rheumatoid arthritis.

10.   Which of the following statements concerning the classification of auto-immune disease is INCORRECT?
(a) Witebsky's postulates (which were modelled on those of Koch) require the presence of autoantibody or a cell-mediated immune response to a self-antigen.
(b) Clinically, autoimmune diseases have been divided into systemic or non-organ-specific and organ-specific.
(c) Systemic lupus erythematosus is a classical example of an organ-specific autoimmune disease.
(d) Non-organ-specific diseases may develop as a result of an abnormal immune response to a single antigen which is expressed in many tissues.

(e) Insulin-dependent diabetes mellitus is an example of an organ-specific autoimmune disease.

11. Which of the following is NOT a cause of primary immunodeficiency disease?

(a) Abnormalities caused by infection after birth.
(b) Developmental abnormalities.
(c) Genetic abnormalities.
(d) Inherited abnormalities.
(e) Congenital abnormalities.

12. Which of the following clinical features is not associated with immuno-deficiency?

(a) Chronic inflammation.
(b) Skin rashes.
(c) Diarrhoea.
(d) Signs and symptoms of autoimmune disease.
(e) Chronic infection.

13. Which of the following statements concerning IgA deficiency is UNTRUE?

(a) IgA deficiency is the most common of the primary immunodeficiency diseases.
(b) IgA deficiency presents as a heterogeneous group of disorders, including diseases affecting the gastrointestinal tract, allergies and autoimmune diseases.
(c) The clinical presentation of IgA deficiency depends upon the degree of abnormal B cell development.
(d) The arrest in B cell development in patients with IgA deficiency is thought to be due to abnormal immunoregulatory signals, since the genes coding for IgA in these individuals appear to be abnormal.
(e) Patients with IgA deficiency appear to have a decrease in switch recombination leading to IgA production.

14. Which of the following statements concerning infantile, X-linked agamma-globulinaemia is CORRECT?

(a) XLA presents immediately after birth.
(b) The majority of individuals affected by XLA are female.
(c) Patients with XLA present with recurrent bacterial, viral and fungal infections.
(d) Affected individuals usually have less than 10% of normal levels of serum IgG and less than 1% of normal levels of IgA and IgM.
(e) Patients with XLA have low levels of B and plasma cells as well as T cells.

15. Which of the following is NOT a B cell abnormality reported to be associated with X-linked agammaglobulinaemia?

(a) *Reduced pre-B cell proliferation.*
(b) *Failure of pre-B cells to thrive.*
(c) *Low levels of circulating immature B cells.*
(d) *Expression of Bruton's tyrosine kinase.*
(e) *Inversion of the pro- and pre-B cell ratio in the bone marrow.*

6

INFECTION, IMMUNITY, IMMUNOPATHOGENESIS

Having discussed how both the innate and specific immune responses develop, we will now examine how they act to prevent or overcome infection. Every day we are exposed to an enormous number of bacteria, viruses, fungi and parasites. However, most of us are usually quite healthy. Relatively few of these organisms cause infection but when they do so, they may cause tissue damage in the host. If these organisms are allowed to grow unchecked, they will cause the death of the host either directly or indirectly. However, most infections do not have such a terminal outcome and in people who are generally healthy, infection is usually confined and any tissue damage easily repaired. This "damage limitation" is brought about by the cellular and chemical components of the immune system acting together to limit the spread of the infection, kill the microorganisms, and repair the tissue damage.

The ability of different organisms to cause disease (their pathogenicity) varies greatly and is related to how easily they can be controlled by the immune system. This may depend on the evolutionary changes the organism has undergone to evade the immune response, or it may depend on the genetic make-up of the host.

> *The occurrence of pathological changes in some infectious diseases varies from individual to individual. Chlamydia trachomatis (which is a major cause of infection in the eyes and genital tract in humans) does not cause pathological changes in most people. However in some individuals, severe disease develops, leading to blindness and infertility.*

The immune system is designed to prevent infection but it may contribute to the clinical signs and symptoms of the disease, be solely responsible for the clinical disease, may help, or even increase, infection, or be affected by the pathogen leading to long-lasting immunosuppression. The purpose of this

Immunology for Life Scientists, Second Edition. Lesley-Jane Eales.
© 2003 John Wiley & Sons, Ltd: ISBN 0 470 84523 6 (HB); 0 470 84524 4 (PB)

chapter is to bring together all the information presented in the previous chapters to illustrate the role of the immune system during infection. We shall examine the relative contribution of both non-specific and specific defence mechanisms in overcoming infection and in causing the tissue damage that occurs in some cases.

6.1 THE INNATE IMMUNE SYSTEM IN INFECTION

In order for an organism to cause infection it must first overcome a number of physical barriers, which are often considered to be part of the innate immune system. These barriers – the skin, the respiratory epithelium, the gastrointestinal epithelium, etc. – are largely non-specific and non-immunologic, but play a vital role in host defence (Figure 6.1).

6.1.1 THE SKIN

The skin provides a horny, keratinised layer that is not easily breached and hence provides a very efficient barrier against microbial invasion. Its dry nature, the presence of competing microorganisms, and various chemical secretions, all combine to prevent colonisation by potentially pathogenic microorganisms. The skin and sweat have a number of substances which are inhibitory or toxic

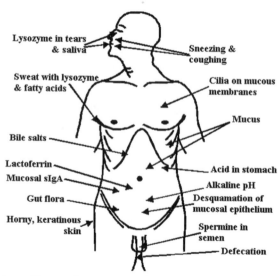

Figure 6.1   The body and innate immune mechanisms

to bacteria and fungi. These include a high content of fatty acids and the enzyme lysozyme.

6.1.2 THE MUCOSAE

Many pathogens cause infection by gaining entry to the body through the mucosal membranes lining the gut, lungs and urinogenital tracts. The epithelial cells, which make up these membranes, are coated with a mucus layer, which helps to prevent microorganisms attaching to the cell surface. Some mucous membranes have cilia, tiny, hair-like projections, movement of which wafts any organisms trapped in the mucus out of the body. This process may be accelerated by reflex actions such as coughing or sneezing, which propel entrapped organisms out of the body at great speed. In addition, infection may be limited by the short half-life of intestinal epithelial cells (approximately 30 hours). If invading microorganisms happen to attach to an epithelial cell as it is shed (**desquamation**), infection is prevented.

Various chemical substances secreted by the mucosae also aid in protection against infection. These include lactoferrin, an iron-binding protein that sequesters free iron such that the concentration falls below that necessary for bacterial growth.

6.1.3 PROTECTIVE CHEMICALS

LYSOZYME

Probably the most ubiquitous anti-bacterial substance formed at body surfaces is lysozyme. This enzyme is present in tears, saliva, sweat and many other mucosal secretions. It is bactericidal for many Gram-positive bacteria where it destroys the integrity of the cell wall by disrupting the N-acetyl muramic acid–N-acetyl glucosamine linkages. However, some organisms are resistant to the action of lysozyme and their cell walls may represent a problem to the immune system even after the organism has been killed.

The group A streptococcal cell wall is resistant to digestion by lysosomal enzymes and macrophages choked by it tend to accumulate at sites of infection. Lysosomal enzymes and other substances leak from these cells and cause local destruction of collagen and connective tissue. The macrophages eventually die or form giant cells, which may result in the formation of granulomas. Thus, the indigestible streptococcal material may cause chronic inflammatory lesions.

ALIMENTARY FLUIDS

The highly acidic content of the stomach is enough to kill most gastrointestinal pathogens. Organisms surviving this environment have to face the alkaline nature of the intestine. However, some organisms are able to utilise extremes of pH to their advantage and cause inflammatory diseases such as gastritis.

> *Helicobacter pylori excretes urease, which catalyses the hydrolysis of urea to yield ammonia and carbon dioxide, which may enable the survival of this acid-sensitive organism in the gastric mucosa. Ammonia generated by urea hydrolysis may produce severe cytotoxic effects within the gastric epithelium, the tissue damage leading to acute inflammation and the signs and symptoms of gastritis. In addition, the enzyme elicits a strong immune response during acute infection, suggesting that this antigen is readily available to the immune system and may stimulate a more chronic inflammatory response.*

COMPLEMENT

Complement (as described in Section 3.1) acts by inactivating microorganisms and enhancing phagocytosis. Breakdown products induce vasodilation and are chemoattractants. Thus, complement plays an important role in inflammation. Although the classical pathway generally requires the presence of immune complexes for its activation, the lectin and alternative complement pathways can be stimulated to kill some Gram-negative bacteria and to inactivate certain viruses in the absence of antibodies. Early in infection, prior to synthesis of specific antibodies, the ability of complement to non-specifically opsonise or kill certain bacteria may be critical to recovery from infections.

> *Certain fungi bind fragments of C3 which may allow attachment and phagocytosis by polymorphonuclear leukocytes, e.g. C3bi, C3d and C3dg, binding to Cryptococcus neoformans. However, whilst this is essential for the phagocytosis of encapsulated cryptococci, on its own, it is not sufficient since some species that bind to these fragments are resistant to phagocytosis. Other fungi may bind directly to complement receptors on the cell surface (e.g.* **Candida albicans***).*

DEFENSINS

The antimicrobial activity of defensins (described in Section 3.2) is thought to result from their ability to accumulate as multimers in the lipid bilayer of target cells in such a way that they form cyclic peptides. These form channels in lipid membranes, increasing membrane permeability by a charge or voltage-dependent mechanism. They are effective at very low levels (typically 10–100 μg/ml) against Gram-positive and Gram-negative bacteria, mycobacteria, fungi and enveloped viruses including HIV. Classical defensins permeabilise both outer and inner membranes of Gram-negative bacteria.

> *Defensins and other antimicrobial peptides are relatively ineffective against pathogenic strains of Salmonella typhimurium. Interestingly, strains in which mutations have occurred, that increase the susceptibility of these organisms to defensins in vitro, generally exhibit diminished virulence in a murine model.*

NATURAL ANTIBODIES

Antibodies found in the serum in the absence of an immune response are largely **natural antibodies**. The majority of these are of the IgM class. Natural antibody is produced by the B1 subset of B-lymphocytes in the apparent absence of antigenic stimulation. These B cells are long-lived and self-renewing and differ from the more usual B2 cells in their differentiation during foetal development and their compartmentalisation in the pleural and peritoneal cavities in adults. The repertoire of these cells is restricted (their variable regions are usually encoded by germ line V gene segments and during their early development they lack terminal deoxynucleotidyl transferase activity). They do not undergo somatic mutation, making affinity maturation impossible. Thus, a majority of natural antibodies is able to recognise a range of related antigens derived from highly conserved molecules such as nucleic acids, heat shock proteins, carbohydrates and phospholipids. Also, due to the lack of somatic mutation, they are generally of low affinity and prone to cross-reactivity. These antibodies provide a first line of defence against a range of common microorganisms since the pentameric structure of IgM makes it a powerful activator of complement.

> *Heat shock proteins (hsps) are a group of molecules found in both eukaryotes and prokaryotes, which exhibit an extremely high level of conservation. Hsp synthesis increases as a result of cellular stress, e.g. temperature fluctuations, viral infection, oxidative stress and fever. Peptides derived from these proteins are recognised by $\gamma\delta$T cells. Hsps may be released from damaged bacteria, stimulating T cells; this, because of the highly conserved nature of the proteins, may result in a breakdown of tolerance to self and the development of autoimmune phenomena. Infection with Chlamydia trachomatis may result in blindness and infertility. A chlamydial protein – HypB – that belongs to the 60 kDa Hsp family has been identified as the constituent that stimulates the immune response resulting in severe pathology.*

6.1.4 THE ROLE OF NORMAL BODY FLORA

Most body surfaces that are exposed to the environment are colonised by bacteria and fungi which are non-pathogenic or only weakly pathogenic. These are collectively known as the normal flora. These microorganisms compete for attachment sites with other potentially pathogenic organisms and prevent them colonising the body surfaces. In addition, they condition their local environment, which may make it unsuitable for the growth of pathogenic organisms whilst supporting the growth of the normal commensals. The normal flora clearly has a protective role to play since, if its balance is upset, e.g. in the gut by antibiotic treatment, patients become much more susceptible to infection by enteric pathogens such as *Shigella* sp. and *Salmonella* sp. The protection afforded by the normal flora may result from competition with potential pathogens for nutrients, for receptor sites on epithelial cells or may result from the secretion of toxic substances such as short-chain fatty acids, which are secreted by intestinal anaerobes.

KEY POINTS FOR REVIEW

- *The immune system is designed to prevent infection but may contribute to the clinical signs and symptoms of disease, be responsible for disease or may lead to immunosuppression.*
- *The innate system offers physical, chemical and physiological barriers to infection.*
- *The body has produced chemicals with potent antimicrobial activities – the defensins.*
- *The microbial flora that normally colonises the body surfaces may help prevent attachment by potential pathogens. Other mechanisms have evolved which also prevent attachment, e.g. sIgA.*

6.2 INFECTION – THE ROLE OF THE INNATE IMMUNE SYSTEM

In spite of the physical and chemical barriers described above, potentially pathogenic organisms may invade the body. This involves several steps, the first of which is attachment.

6.2.1 ATTACHMENT

Before organisms can invade the body, they must attach to a cell. If you think about the common forms of infection, most of them occur through mucosal surfaces and many bacteria are able to adhere to these surfaces using **pili**, proteinaceous projections, which bind to receptors on the cell surface. Similarly, viruses must bind to receptors on the surface of their target cells. Adherence may be prevented by IgA present in mucosal secretions. However, certain organisms can overcome this blockage by secreting enzymes that destroy the IgA (e.g. *Gonococcus* sp.).

Once an organism has successfully made an attachment and has invaded the body, the innate immune response involves the collaboration of cells (the polymorphonuclear leukocytes), serum proteins (complement, acute phase proteins, the clotting cascade, the kinin system) and a number of chemicals released from cells that affect the blood vessels (vasoactive amines). As a result of invasion and/or tissue damage, events occur that collectively form the inflammatory response (see Section 3.3).

One of the early events that occurs in an inflammatory response is the upregulation of adhesion molecules that promote cell–cell interactions including mediating extravasation of cells from the blood to the site of inflammation. Microbes may use adhesion molecules to facilitate cellular attachment and invasion. In many cases, this leads to increased tissue damage. For example, the adhesion of parasite-infected erythrocytes to brain endothelium may be a primary event in cerebral malaria in humans and is thought to involve CD36 and thrombospondin. In addition, ICAM-1 has been implicated in malaria, since its expression on vascular endothelium can be upregulated by TNF, and increased levels of this cytokine have been shown to correlate with disease severity.

These are designed to limit the infection/damage at the site of origin. However, the acute inflammatory response may not eliminate the organism and chronic inflammation may develop, which involves the specific immune response.

6.2.2 THE BODY'S RESPONSE TO INVASION – FEVER

An increase in body temperature (fever) in response to infection occurs in humans and many other animals. Although fever may be life-threatening to the host, it is beneficial in that many microorganisms are sensitive to even very small temperature rises. This will not necessarily kill the organisms but will slow their growth enough to allow the immune response to eliminate the infection. In addition, many of the protective responses in the host are more efficient at temperatures which are slightly greater than normal body temperature.

The precise causes of fever are legion and may depend on the type and site of infection. It is known that **exogenous pyrogens** derived from microorganisms stimulate the release of cytokines such as IL-1, IL-6 and TNF (known as **endogenous pyrogens**) into the blood. These are able to act on the central nervous system causing the release of prostaglandins which coordinate subsequent events leading to fever. However, more recently it has been shown that microorganisms may induce cytokine production at the level of the hypothalamus through binding (presumably) to Toll receptors.

6.2.3 CELLS INVOLVED IN INNATE IMMUNITY IN INFECTION

PHAGOCYTIC CELLS

Phagocytic cells include neutrophils and eosinophils (polymorphonuclear leukocytes), monocytes and macrophages (mononuclear leukocytes). These cells engulf organisms by phagocytosis (Section 3.2), a process that is enhanced by the presence of opsonins or by the presence of pattern recognition receptors. Phagocytes also mediate other functions through the secretion of cytokines and the action of enzymes.

Polymorphonuclear leukocytes are amongst the first cells at the site of infection and attack invading pathogens whilst producing chemotaxins to attract more polymorphs and mononuclear phagocytes. In addition, PMN products cause changes in host tissues, which are vital to the inflammatory process (e.g. vasodilation). Macrophages produce cytokines such as interleukin 1 (IL-1) and tumour necrosis factor (TNF; Table 6.1), which cause fever (and enhance the activity of inflammatory cells), vasodilation and generally augment the inflammatory process.

Engulfed organisms are enclosed in a phagosome, which fuses with a lysosome. This exposes the organisms to a variety of enzymes and chemicals derived from the lysosomal granules. These processes are designed to destroy the organisms. However, many have the means to avoid destruction in this manner.

*Some organisms have extracellular products, which inhibit phagocytosis (e.g. the polysaccharide capsules on Cryptococcus neoformans, Strep pneumoniae and **Haemophilus influenzae**), others resist killing or kill the phagocyte (e.g. leucocidin produced by* **Staphylococcus** *spp. causes the lysosome to release its contents into the cell cytoplasm which kills the phagocyte).*

Table 6.1 Characteristics of the tumour necrosis factors

Characteristic	Description
Molecular weight	TNFα has cysteine residues which form intra-chain disulphide bonds. It has a molecular weight of 17.4 kDa in man, 17.3 kDa in mice, TNFβ is a glycosylated molecule with molecular weight of 18.7 kDa in man and 18.6 kDa in mice. The genes for both are on chromosome 6 in humans and 17 in mice
Major cellular sources	TNFα is produced by activated monocytes and macrophages; by B cells, T cells, and fibroblasts whilst TNFβ is produced by activated T cells
Effects	TNFα regulates the growth and differentiation of many cell types. It is selectively cytotoxic for many transformed cells and mediates many of its effects in concert with other cytokines. Expressed as a Type II membrane protein. TNFβ has 35% homology with TNFα and binds to the same receptor. It is involved in inflammation and immune function and is cytotoxic or cytostatic for some tumours *in vitro*, causing haemorrhagic necrosis of certain tumours *in vivo*. It induces gene expression and stimulates fibroblast proliferation
Receptors	Both bind to the same high-affinity receptor. The degree of lysis is directly related to the amount of TNF bound to the cell. Receptor binding alone may not cause cell lysis; internalisation may be required. Not all cells binding TNF are lysed by it
Cross-reactivity	TNFα shows 79% homology in humans and mice and TNFβ 74%. There is significant cross-species activity

Phagocytes have been shown to be particularly important in the control of some fungal infections. Normal, healthy individuals rarely suffer from fungal infections since such organisms are poorly invasive and their spread is limited by the innate immune response until they are eliminated by the adaptive response. Neutrophils may be particularly involved in this control of fungal infections; they are thought to be primarily responsible for preventing the tissue invasion by, and the dissemination of, *Candida* spp.

In addition to neutrophils, monocytes/macrophages (mononuclear phagocytes – MNPs) are thought to be important in the clearance of fungi. They may be activated by lymphokines (produced by antigen-stimulated T cells), which enhance their ability to clear the fungi. Also, MNPs have been shown to express surface receptors that bind fungi, however, their role is unclear.

Eosinophils are particularly important in worm infections in the gut. Antigens released by the infecting worms cross-link Fc receptor-bound IgE on mast cells in the gut mucosa. This induces degranulation of the mast cells leading to the release of eosinophil chemotactic cytokine L (ECF-L), which induces extravasation of eosinophils. In addition, the release of IL-5 and GM-CSF by the gut mucosa stimulates the proliferation of eosinophils. Eosinophil granules contain a protein – eosinophil basic protein – which is particularly toxic to parasites such as *Schistosoma mansoni*. Also, since these cells have Fc receptors, they are able to kill worms by antibody-dependent cellular cytotoxicity (Figure 6.2).

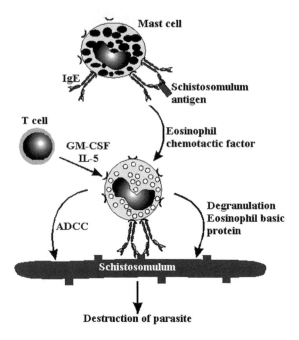

Figure 6.2   Elimination of parasites by eosinophils
Tissue mast cells activated by parasite-derived antigens cross-linking receptor-bound IgE release
eosinophil chemotactic factor, attracting these cells to the site of infection. Activated T cells release
GM-CSF and IL-5 that activate eosinophils. The latter degranulate, releasing the toxic eosinophil
basic protein. In addition, activated eosinophils are able to perform antibody-dependent cellular
cytotoxicity as a result of binding antibody attached to the surface of the parasite.

Macrophages activated by lymphokines such as interferon gamma may kill
parasites as a result of increased oxygen metabolism and increased FcR and
C3R expression. These cells play a vital role in the control of infections caused
by *Trypanosoma cruzi*, *Leishmania* spp., *Plasmodium* spp. and *Schistosoma
mansoni*. When parasites are not completely eliminated, **granulomata** form.
Antigens derived from the parasites stimulate T cells to release lymphokines,
which in turn stimulate macrophages. These cells release factors that enhance
fibrin deposition resulting in a meshwork, which traps inflammatory cells
behind a wall of fibroblasts (**fibrosis**).

NATURAL KILLER CELLS

Natural killer cells are non-adherent, non-phagocytic, large granular lymphocytes (Section 1.1). The granules show some similarity to those of mononuclear
phagocytes in that they contain β-glucuronidase. However, they lack
peroxidase. The principal characteristics of these cells are that they are able
to spontaneously destroy a range of target cells in a non-classical MHC-
restricted manner (Section 2.3; Table 6.2).

Table 6.2   Surface antigens expressed by NK cells

Marker	Distribution	Function
CD56	NK cells only	Function unknown. Thought to be NK cell-specific but some cells don't express it
CD2	T cells and NK cells	Sheep erythrocyte receptor; receptor for LFA1
CD8	Some T cells and NK cells	30–80% human NK cells have CD8 which recognises MHC Class I products
CD11a/CD18	Many leukocytes	LFA1 – the leukocyte functional antigen
CD11b/CD18	Many leukocytes	CR3
CD16	NK cells Neutrophils; macrophages	FcγRIII. In NK cells it is capable of mediating ADCC

NK cells are produced in the bone marrow, enter the circulation, and localise in the tissues. They can be triggered within a few minutes of encountering a target cell but can be activated by cytokines to exhibit even greater activity against a wider range of target cells. However, NK cells do not develop into memory cells or exhibit a secondary response.

Although typically thought to be involved in tissue surveillance and eliminating certain tumours, NK cells are capable also of killing some virally infected targets. These cells may be important in controlling or eliminating viruses even before they replicate and before the development of specific Tc cells.

The ability of a natural killer cell to destroy a target is dependent upon the outcome of the feedback from a range of activating and inhibitory receptors. Their activity was initially explained by the "missing self" hypothesis that suggested NK cells could recognise and destroy cells that did not express self-MHC Class I gene products. This led on to the observation that NK cells express receptors that may recognise ligands expressed on many cells but that inhibitory receptors that recognise specific self-MHC Class I gene products prevent the killing of normal, syngeneic cells. Thus, NK cells can kill foreign or altered-self targets but do not harm normal cells expressing self-MHC (Figure 6.3).

The role of altered self-MHC expression in NK cell-mediated killing may explain the ability of these cells to kill cells infected with certain viruses that may downregulate surface expression of MHC. It is common for NK cells to accumulate at the site of an infection. Indeed, viruses stimulate the production of interferon, which enhances NK cell activity, causing them to kill several targets one after the other and to do so more rapidly.

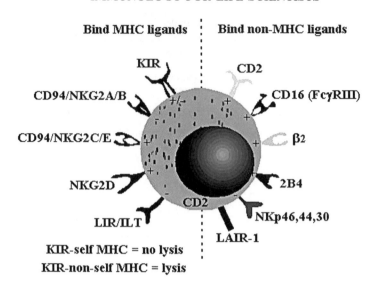

Figure 6.3   Receptors expressed by NK cells involved in recognition of target cells

> *A role for NK cells in recovery from infection has been shown for a number of viruses including human cytomegalovirus, Epstein–Barr virus, influenza virus, and paramyxoviruses such as mumps, measles and Sendai viruses.*

NK cells may also play a role in the destruction of pathogenic fungi. Studies have shown that they may lyse *Cryptococcus neoformans* in a similar way to that in which they cause the destruction of tumour cells except that attachment occurs more slowly (probably due to the formation of many, small microvilli at the site of attachment) and killing takes longer. By contrast, NK cells are not capable of killing *Candida* spp., indicating that the general role of these cells in controlling or eliminating fungal infections may be limited.

PLATELETS

Platelets from patients infected with *Schistosoma mansoni* are highly cytotoxic to the parasite *in vitro*. Normal platelets incubated with IgE-rich serum have the same effect, suggesting that the protective activity of platelets is mediated (at least in part) through their ability to bind IgE. Similarly, *in vitro* studies of trypanosomes have shown that they are rapidly lysed after contact with immune platelets. In addition, the lysis of sensitised *T. cruzi* promastigotes is dependent on the presence of the C3b receptor on platelets. These and other experiments have shown that platelets may be protective in parasitic infections through interaction with antibody and complement. However, even in the absence of serum, platelets have been shown to be as effective against *Toxoplasma gondii* as cytotoxic T cells.

6.2.4   INFLAMMATION AND IMMUNOPATHOLOGY

During an infection, there is inflammation, cellular infiltration of the tissues, and tissue damage (see Section 3.3). Such changes caused by the immune response are classed as immunopathological. These may be mild and play no part in the tissue damage of the disease or they may be severe causing disease or death. In all infections there is an immune response, which will contribute, to a greater or lesser extent, to the pathological changes associated with the infection.

The release of inflammatory mediators results in pain, swelling, redness, heat (cardinal signs of inflammation), release of enzymes and other factors from phagocytes, all of which may cause permanent tissue damage leading to loss of function of the affected part (another cardinal sign). Generally, inflammation is a major cause of the signs and symptoms of disease. Tissue damage causes cell death and the release of inflammatory mediators. In addition, bacteria may release factors that stimulate inflammation (e.g. endotoxin) and viruses may cause the release of inflammatory mediators from host cells. Thus, inflammation may be a direct or an indirect consequence of microbial infection and may account for the majority of detrimental changes in the tissues. Thus, many pathological changes may be considered to be a side-effect of the immune response to infection.

ENDOTOXIN

Endotoxins form part of the outer layer of the bacterial cell wall and may be released in soluble form during bacterial growth. The term endotoxin usually refers to the complex phospholipid–polysaccharide–protein macromolecules associated with the cell walls of Gram-negative bacteria such as *Salmonella* spp., *Shigella* spp., *Escherichia* spp. and *Neisseria* spp. The lipopolysaccharide (LPS) is the important component from a clinical point of view. The LPS of Gram-negative bacteria consists of three components, a core polysaccharide common to many Gram-negative bacteria, an O-specific polysaccharide which confers virulence and serological specificity on the macromolecule, and a lipid A component which is mainly responsible for the toxicity of the molecule (Figure 6.4). LPS is an important virulence factor and small changes in the O antigen, involving no more than changes in the sugar sequences in side-chains of the molecule, result in major changes in virulence.

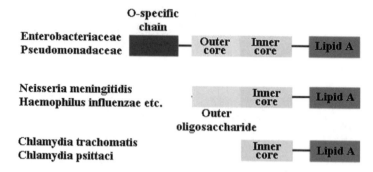

Figure 6.4   Structure of lipopolysaccharide

ENDOTOXIN-INDUCED INJURY

Endotoxin-mediated host injury, which clinically results in the sepsis syndrome or septic shock, is usually consequent to severe infection by Gram-negative bacteria such as *Meningococcus* spp. In this instance, much of the resulting disease is attributable to the host response to the endotoxin, not to direct injury by the endotoxin itself. LPS causes the release of vasoactive substances and activates both the alternative complement pathway and Factor XII (Hageman factor of the coagulation cascade). This latter capability sometimes results in the development of disseminated intravascular coagulation. With respect to the pathology associated with the sepsis syndrome, perhaps the most relevant effect of LPS is its ability to stimulate macrophages to release interleukin 1 (IL-1) and tumour necrosis factor (TNF). Endotoxins are also pyrogenic; LPS causes the release of IL-1 from macrophages, which acts on the hypothalamus to give a rapid elevation of body temperature.

KEY POINTS FOR REVIEW

- *Phagocytic cells play a key role in the innate response to infection.*
- *NK cells are involved in the destruction of certain virally infected cells and may help in the destruction of pathogenic fungi.*
- *Much of the immunopathology associated with infections derives from the immune response to the microbe. Often the inflammatory response is the chief culprit.*
- *In some instances, bacterial products cause a massive inflammatory response that leads to pathology and even death.*

6.3   INFECTION – THE ROLE OF THE SPECIFIC IMMUNE RESPONSE

In the same way that humoral and cell-mediated responses are known now to be closely interdependent, the distinction between specific and non-specific immune response to infection has become hard to define. For example, natural killer (NK) cells and macrophages play a role in innate immunity but they may be activated by lymphokines produced as a result of a specific immune response. In addition, Fc receptor-bearing phagocytic cells may act in an antigen-specific manner through binding antibody. When coated with specific antibody, virus-infected cells and other pathogens may be killed by antibody-dependent cellular cytotoxicity (ADCC) mediated by macrophages and killer cells.

If the inflammatory response is unable to eliminate an invading organism, the stimulus persists long enough to stimulate a specific immune response. The type of response that predominates is dependent largely on the type of organism causing the infection. Often both T cell and antibody responses are required to completely eliminate an invading pathogen.

6.3.1   INTRACELLULAR PATHOGENS AND FUNGI

Intracellular pathogens and fungi typically require a cell-mediated response for their elimination. This is demonstrated by the fact that such infections are common in patients infected with the human immunodeficiency virus (HIV), an organism that infects and impairs the activity of the main cells involved in cell-mediated immunity (i.e. $CD4^+$ T cells and macrophages). Although fungal infections are usually eliminated by cell-mediated immunity alone, some require more than this. For example, whilst chronic mucocandidiasis may be cured by effective cell-mediated immunity, recovery from systemic infection with *Candida* spp. requires the activity of granulocytes, cytokines from NK cells and others, complement and possibly humoral immunity. Thus, control of certain fungal infections requires the combined activity of the innate and specific immune responses.

6.3.2   PARASITIC INFECTIONS

In general, the immune response seems less well equipped to eliminate parasitic infections such as malaria, schistosomiasis and leishmaniasis, which present a major health problem, particularly in the Developing World. Over a long period of time, parasites have adapted such that, in general, infection tends to be chronic. As might be expected, cell-mediated immunity usually is more effective against intracellular parasites whilst antibody tends to play a major role in the elimination of extracellular stages. However, due to the complex developmental cycles of many parasites, one immunological mechanism may be more or less effective against a particular stage of a parasite's life cycle.

6.3.3   THE ROLE OF ANTIBODY IN IMMUNITY TO INFECTION

Antibody is particularly important in controlling disease caused by extracellular organisms. However, the methods of control exhibited by the different classes of antibody differ depending largely on the type of organism involved and its route of infection. Examples of the roles played by antibodies in immunity to infection are described below and summarised in Figure 6.5.

OPSONISATION

Specific antibodies bound to their target organisms may bind also to receptors on phagocytic cells (Fc receptors) but via their Fc portion rather than by the antigen-specific part (the F(ab)$_2$ fragment). This opsonisation increases the phagocytic efficiency of the cells, allowing the organism to be cleared more effectively. In addition, if the antibodies specifically bind flagellar antigens on

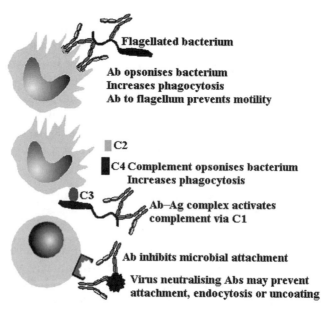

Figure 6.5   Biological activities of antibodies

certain bacteria (e.g. *Salmonella typhi*), they play a secondary role in that they immobilise the organism thus making it easier to capture.

COMPLEMENT ACTIVATION

Although antibodies alone may opsonise microorganisms, complement activation increases phagocytosis and killing still further. In addition, activation of the membrane attack complex (C5–C9) results in direct lysis of microorganisms. However, the type of organism may dictate how efficient the MAC is. Parasites may be directly damaged due to the activation of complement by antibody bound to the organism. However, bacteria show variability in their susceptibility to lysis. Gram-negative organisms are more easily lysed than Gram-positive. In addition, although the presence of a capsule is considered to protect microorganisms from immune attack, encapsulated organisms may be lysed by the MAC if the antibodies involved in activation of the complement pathway are directed against the capsular polysaccharides (e.g. *Neisseria meningitidis*).

The type of antibody involved may influence the role of complement in bacteriolysis. For example, IgM can only mediate killing of Gram-negative bacteria in the presence of complement.

INHIBITION OF ADHERENCE

Before an organism can cause infection, it has to become attached by binding to a receptor on the cell surface. In bacteria, this is often achieved through pili or fimbriae. Antibodies to these organelles may either directly inhibit attachment by blocking binding to the receptor on the cell or by sterically hindering such binding.

Similarly, antibodies may inhibit the attachment of viruses to their receptors on their target cells. Like bacteria, this inhibition may be direct, due to stearic hindrance or due to an allosteric effect.

In addition, as with bacteria and viruses, antibody may neutralise infection by parasites by preventing attachment to specific cellular receptors (e.g. *Plasmodium* spp.). In some infections, antibody is effective in preventing re-invasion of cells by blood-borne parasites (e.g. *Plasmodium falciparum*).

TOXIN NEUTRALISATION

Antibodies which bind exotoxins secreted by bacteria may neutralise their effect either by preventing their attachment to cellular receptors (e.g. the binding of cholera toxin to the ganglioside GM1) or by enhancing their clearance from the body (through cells with Fc receptors). Immunisation against tetanus works by inducing antibodies that react with the toxin; the latter causes the damage associated with infection.

VIRUS NEUTRALISATION

Virus neutralisation is a complex process, which varies depending upon the type of virus, the target cell, and the class of antibody. Since antibodies play an important part in limiting the infectivity of a virus, the level of circulating, neutralising, antibodies is often used as a measure of vaccine performance. Virus-neutralising antibodies may (as described for toxin neutralisation) inhibit virus–cell interaction, prevent endocytosis of the virus or prevent its uncoating inside the endosome. Neutralisation of enveloped viruses may be more effective in the presence of complement.

INHIBITION OF MICROBIAL ENZYME ACTIVITY

Some microorganisms secrete enzymes (or express them on their surface), which aid in infection (e.g. neuraminidase produced by influenza virus). Antibodies to these enzymes inhibit enzyme function and limit infection.

INHIBITION OF MICROBIAL GROWTH

Organism-specific antibodies may inhibit the growth of some prokaryotes (e.g. *Mycoplasma* spp.).

6.3.4 PATHOLOGY DUE TO SPECIFIC ANTIBODY

There are many examples of host injury, which occur as a result of the humoral immune response to a pathogen; some of these are shown in Table 6.3. The occurrence of cross-reactive antigens is quite frequent, and a number of microorganisms stimulate the production of antibodies, which are capable of reacting to host tissue components, giving rise to autoimmune damage. Typical examples of this include chorea and rheumatic fever.

POLYCLONAL B CELL ACTIVATION

Several infectious agents are thought to cause the polyclonal activation of B cells, which results in the production of antibodies that react with self-antigens. The latter include DNA, immunoglobulin, myofibrils and erythrocytes. Such autoantibodies have been demonstrated in patients

Table 6.3   Examples of injury caused by pathogen-stimulated antibody

Disease or clinical presentation	Infectious agent	Immune phenomena and pathology
Post-streptococcal glomerulonephritis	*Streptococcus* spp.	Immune complexes containing streptococcal antigens and IgG deposit in the kidney, activating complement and attracting inflammatory cells
Polyarteritis nodosa	Hepatitis B virus	Chronic antigen–antibody complex formation causes activation of complement and signs and symptoms of chronic inflammation
Chorea	*Streptococcus* spp.	Antibodies stimulated by the streptococcal infection react with neurons in the caudate and subthalamic nuclei of the brain
Rheumatic fever	Throat infection with group A *Streptococcus* spp.	Antibodies formed against streptococcal cell walls or membrane components also react with patient's heart muscle or valves, resulting in myocarditis

infected with trypanosomes, *Mycoplasma pneumoniae* and Epstein–Barr virus. Although it is unclear precisely what contribution these autoantibodies play in the pathology of each of these diseases, their production alone reflects a fundamental disturbance of the patients' normal immunoregulatory system, which is a pathological consequence of infection in itself.

IMMUNE COMPLEX FORMATION

When antigen–antibody reactions take place in the blood, the consequences are directly related to the size of the immune complexes formed and the relative proportions of antigen and antibody therein (Figure 6.6). In antibody excess, the antigen becomes coated with antibody and is removed rapidly by cells of the mononuclear phagocyte system (using Fc and complement receptors). At antibody–antigen equivalence, large lattices are formed, their size enabling their rapid clearance. By contrast, when antigen is present in large excess (such as at the start of an infection, few antibody molecules coat each antigen thus reducing the likelihood of clearance. However, there is usually only a very brief period before specific antibody levels in the blood rise, resulting in the formation of immune complexes that contain equivalent or greater levels of antibody. However, in some instances, small immune complexes persist and these continue to circulate in the blood and may become localised in small blood vessels, e.g. in the glomeruli of the kidneys, the choroid plexuses, the joints and the ciliary body of the eye. It is thought that factors such as local high blood pressure and turbulent flow (glomeruli) or the filtering function of vessels involved (choroid plexus, ciliary body) may influence the deposition of these small immune complexes. In the glomeruli, they pass through the endothelium and may localise beneath the basement membrane, although the smallest appear to pass through the basement membrane and enter the urine. This may be a normal mechanism for disposing of such complexes.

Immune complexes that localise in the kidney glomeruli can activate complement and induce an inflammatory response. This results in poly-morphonuclear leukocyte infiltration, glomerular basement membrane swelling, and albumin and red blood cells in the urine. This acute glomerulonephritis may be seen mainly in children as a post-infection complication with *Streptococcus* spp. When the immune system has eliminated the infection, immune complexes are no longer formed and any pathological changes are usually reversed, leading to complete recovery. However, repeated infection or the persistent deposition of complexes leads to irreversible damage. This happens in certain persistent infections in which microbial

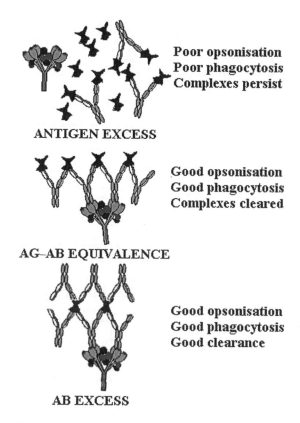

Poor opsonisation
Poor phagocytosis
Complexes persist

ANTIGEN EXCESS

Good opsonisation
Good phagocytosis
Complexes cleared

AG–AB EQUIVALENCE

Good opsonisation
Good phagocytosis
Good clearance

AB EXCESS

Figure 6.6   The influence of the structure of immune complexes on their clearance

antigens are released continuously into the blood but antibody responses are weak or of low affinity. In such cases, immune complexes localise in the glomeruli over a period of weeks, months or even years and ultimately cause impairment of their filtering function.

Circulating immune complexes may be deposited in other locations in the body and cause classical pathology. For example, immune complexes that localise in the joints lead to joint swelling and inflammation. The prodromal rashes seen in some viral infections and in hepatitis B are probably caused by immune complexes being deposited in the walls of small blood vessels in the skin. If the vascular changes are more marked (as is seen following streptococcal infections and in patients being treated for leprosy), they give rise to the condition called erythema nodosum in which there are tender, red nodules in the skin with deposits of antigen, antibody and complement in vessel walls.

When immune complexes are formed in the airways, the resulting inflammatory response causes wheezing and respiratory distress giving rise to the condition known as allergic alveolitis. Repeated inhalation of the antigen concerned leads to chronic, pathological changes, which result in fibrosis and respiratory disease, e.g. farmer's lung caused by the actinomycete *Micromonospora faeni* found in mouldy hay.

Immune complexes may be responsible for the pathology associated with a number of infectious diseases. Indeed, the fever, polyarthritis, skin rash and kidney damage seen in meningococcal meningitis and gonococcal septicaemia are indicative of immune complex deposition. In addition, the oedema and vasculitis of trypanosomiasis and the rashes of secondary syphilis may be a consequence of immune complex formation.

6.3.5 T CELL-MEDIATED IMMUNITY

Although T cells play a central and critical role in the generation of the immune response to invading microorganisms, their role is predominantly one of aiding and abetting other cells, rather than directly destroying the organisms themselves. Viruses are the major exception to this rule since cytotoxic T cells (T_{cyt}) are the major form of host defence against established viral infections.

Immune T cells are capable of secreting lymphokines (e.g. interferon gamma) that augment the activity of a range of cells including NK cells and macrophages, which are vital to recovery from infections with viruses such as *Herpes simplex*. A possible direct role for T cells in anti-bacterial defence has been suggested by studies showing specific lysis of *Listeria monocytogenes*-infected macrophages by sensitised T lymphocytes.

The role of T cells in fungal infection has been most extensively studied using Histoplasma capsulatum in mice. Animals treated with an antibody to remove T helper cells could not eliminate the fungus very efficiently. However, mice given T helper cells from genetically identical (syngeneic) mice resistant to H. capsulatum were able to clear the infection whilst those given normal Th or Ts/c cells from resistant mice, did not.

PARASITIC INFECTIONS

In parasitic infections, T_{cyt} cells do not appear to play a vital role in recovery from infections but other T cells are important in prolonging survival of the host, probably by affecting the proliferation of the parasite. Generally, the role of T cells in parasitic infections is to secrete cytokines in response to released antigens. These cytokines increase the activity of eosinophils, mast cells, macrophages and B cells. However, in some parasitic infections (e.g. *Trypanosoma cruzi*) patients with T_{cyt} cell activity present with more severe symptoms.

In worm infections, T cells can help to remove the organisms by producing factors which cause goblet cells to secrete more mucus.

VIRAL INFECTIONS

In virus infections, cytokines control antibody responses and influence the early (natural killer cell activation) and late (T_{cyt} cell activation and proliferation) protective responses. Since viruses replicate within host cells and virus proteins are expressed in the cell cytoplasm, they present a different challenge to the host immune system than extracellular microorganisms. Viral antigens are likely to be presented in the context of Class I MHC antigens initially and only later by Class II antigens after viral antigens have been produced and taken up from outside host cells. This results in an initial preferential stimulation of CD8$^+$ T cells.

TH$_1$ AND TH$_2$ CELLS

Studies of experimental bacterial and parasitic infections have demonstrated differential T cell responses, which are dependent on the type of organism eliciting the response. These responses are characterised generally as either Th$_1$ or Th$_2$. In a Th$_1$ response, IL-2, interferon gamma and tumour necrosis factor are produced. These are associated with macrophage activation (resulting in enhanced activity against intracellular pathogens and parasites) and stimulation of T_{cyt} activity. By contrast, a Th$_2$ response is associated with the secretion of

IL-4 and IL-5, which is instrumental in switching B cell immunoglobulin production to IgE and in promoting eosinophil activation; events that are important in nematode worm infections. Thus, the production of particular cytokines by T cells may be associated with the activation of different elements of the immune system; the type of response elicited being dependent upon the nature of the infecting organism.

CYTOTOXIC T CELL ACTIVITY

Once activated, Th_1 cells produce cytokines that favour the differentiation of cytotoxic effector and memory cells. These usually express the CD8 antigen but a few may express CD4. In order to express their cytolytic activity, the cytotoxic T cells must bind to their target cells (those which are to be lysed); a process which is temperature, energy and magnesium ion-dependent and requires an intact cytoskeleton in the effector T cell. In addition, it has been shown that a stable union between the effector and target cells is dependent upon a number of factors (Table 6.4).

Whilst cytotoxic T cells usually recognise specific processed antigens (which may be foreign or altered-self molecules) in association with MHC gene products on the surface of infected or transformed cells, some bind their target cells via antibodies (which are bound to specific antigens on the target cells) or lectins (compounds that bind sugar residues on cell surface molecules). However, regardless of the means by which effectors and targets become bound, the ultimate outcome of the union is highly variable. The cause of this variability is unknown, but appears to be dependent upon the effector:target cell ratio and the nature of the target cell. Thus, although the attachment between effector and target cells may be brief (the process follows first-order kinetics with a half-life of 1.4 minutes), the length of time required for cytolysis may vary from 5 minutes to 24 hours, and even at high effector:target cell ratios, may be only partial.

The complexity of the adhesion process is reflected structurally also. Studies of effector–target cell conjugates by transmission electron microscopy (TEM) revealed extensive folding of the plasma membrane at the site of contact. In this area, the cytoplasm of the T_{cyt} contained a network of fibrillar material but lacked cytoplasmic organelles such as ribosomes and granules. It has been proposed that after the initial period of conjugation, the lytic granules move back into the cytoplasmic projections allowing them to come into contact with that part of the T_{cyt} plasma membrane involved in target cell binding. Thereafter, the granules fuse with the membrane, releasing their lytic contents (such as perforin) into the junctional area between the effector and target cells. Once a lytic signal has been delivered, most T_{cyt} can dissociate from the target cell and attach to further targets at least twice before needing to be re-activated.

Table 6.4 Parameters affecting the stability of the union between effector and target cells
The union involves contact over a large area of both cells' membranes
Interaction between the TCR-CD8 (or CD4) and processed antigen presented by MHC Cass I molecules (or Class II) is required
A 'zipping-up' process involving a group of cell surface antigens called adhesion molecules stabilises the union (e.g. CD2, 28, 43 and leukocyte function antigen (LFA)-1 on the effector T cell and B7, CD22, ICAM-1 or 2 and LFA-3 on the target cell). Some of these molecules also provide co-stimulatory signals for T cell activation (e.g. CD2, 4, 8, 28 and LFA-1)

Table 6.5 Mechanisms involved in T cell-mediated cytolysis
Mechanisms of cytolysis
Pore formation in the target cell membrane caused by molecules secreted by the effector cells, e.g. perforin and granzymes. This leads to osmotic imbalance, leakage of cytoplasmic components and ultimate cytolysis
Programmed death or apoptosis of the target cell caused by initiation of intracellular signals leading to apoptosis caused by the engagement of certain cell surface receptors, e.g. Fas
Initiation of intracellular signals which lead to cell death caused by certain cytokines, e.g. TNF and IFNγ upon engagement of their specific cellular receptors

CYTOLYTIC MECHANISMS

Having been stimulated by cytokines produced by Th_1 cells, and having recognised and bound the target cell, the T_{cyt} effector cells must induce the lysis of the target. Experimental evidence suggests that several different mechanisms of cytolysis may occur (Table 6.5).

After conjugation with a target cell, the T_{cyt} delivers its "lethal hit", an event that requires continued interaction between the TCR/CD3 complex and processed antigen associated with autologous MHC molecules on the target cell. The signals or molecules which cause cytolysis are only delivered in the region where the effector and target cells are in close contact and only the target cell is affected (Figure 6.7). Once the "lethal hit" has been delivered, the target cell undergoes a number of changes, which do not require the further presence of the effector cell.

Perforin: The effector cell releases perforin monomers, which by binding to phosphorylcholine residues in the cell membrane, undergo aggregation leading to the formation of a hydrophilic channel not unlike that formed by the membrane attack complex of complement. This allows the development of an osmotic imbalance between the cell and its surroundings leading to cell lysis or necrosis. In addition, granzymes are released from the cytoplasmic granules of the T_{cyt} into the target cell via the perforin channel. These enzymes cause the activation of specific cellular components leading to the induction of apoptosis.

Apoptosis and necrosis are two forms of cell death which are quite distinct. During necrosis, the integrity of the cell membrane is destroyed leading to osmotic imbalance and cell lysis. By contrast, apoptosis is characterised by condensation of nuclear chromatin, ballooning of discrete areas of the cell membrane and fragmentation of the DNA. This causes the cell to shrink and eventually to fragment into membrane-bound apoptotic bodies. The initiation of apoptosis is dependent upon the appropriate signal being delivered to the target cell nucleus. Surface antigens such as Fas/FasL have been shown to be involved in the initiation of apoptosis. Both are anchored in the cytoplasm and are structurally related to the receptor for tumour necrosis factor alpha.

Apoptosis, which occurs as a result of T_{cyt} activity, is distinct from classical apoptosis since usually, the synthesis of relevant molecules by the target cell is not required. In addition, unlike classical apoptosis in which DNA fragmentation may require hours or days, that induced by cytotoxic T cells is detectable within minutes of effector–target cell interaction.

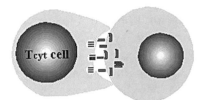

**T_cyt cell releases perforins causing
pores to form in target cell**

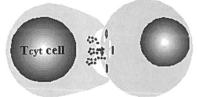

**T_cyt cell releases granzymes that enter
the pores in target cell and cause its lysis**

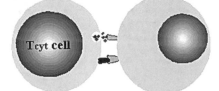

**T_cyt cell releases TNF or expresses Fas
which, after binding their receptors induces
target cell apoptosis**

Figure 6.7   Mechanisms of action of cytotoxic T cells

Fas/FasL: Fas is a molecule expressed on the surface of target cells which can bind to FasL on T_{cyt} cells. This ligation results in the induction of apoptosis in the target cell. This process has been proposed as a method by which the immune response is terminated. T cells expressing both Fas and FasL are induced to undergo apoptosis, thus eliminating an antigen-specific T cell response.

6.3.6 PATHOLOGY CAUSED BY THE CELL-MEDIATED IMMUNE RESPONSE

The mere expression of a cell-mediated immune response involves some degree of inflammation, lymphocyte infiltration, macrophage accumulation and activation and can therefore by itself cause pathological changes. This type of response predominates in the pathogenesis of tuberculosis, with mononuclear cell infiltration, degeneration of parasitised macrophages, and the formation of giant cells as central features. In chronic mycobacterial infection, the continuous release of microbial antigens leads to a chronic inflammatory response and the formation of granulomas. This particular pathological feature is also associated with a range of other chronic microbial and parasitic diseases including bacterial (leprosy and syphilis), chlamydial (lymphogranuloma inguinale), and fungal (coccidiomycosis) infections.

Mononuclear cells also cause pathological changes during a cell-mediated response by lysing host cells. When the latter are infected by a virus, antigens are expressed on their surfaces providing a target for cell-mediated responses. In this way, cell-mediated immunity may contribute to the pathology of hepatitis B infection and many herpes and poxvirus infections. In addition, the autoimmune damage associated with Chagas' disease may be due to the adsorption of antigens from *Trypanosoma cruzi* on uninfected host cells, allowing recognition by T_{cyt} or destruction by antibody-dependent cellular cytotoxicity.

Chagas' disease is caused by Trypanosoma cruzi and is transmitted by blood-sucking insects. The organisms spread throughout the body during the acute infection. Years later, a poorly understood chronic disease appears, involving the heart and the intestinal tract. These organs contain only small numbers of the parasite but show a loss of autonomic ganglion cells. It is thought the pathology arises as a result of an autoimmune reaction since a monoclonal antibody to T. cruzi has been obtained that cross-reacts with mammalian neurons.

One human virus infection in which a cell-mediated immune response appears to contribute greatly to the pathology of the disease is measles. This is evidenced by the fact that children with thymic aplasia suffer a fatal disease if they are infected with measles virus. Individuals with this particular immunodeficiency generally fail to develop antigen-specific T cell responses and cell-mediated immunity but have normal antibody responses. Thus, instead of the limited virus growth and respiratory disease seen in normal children, those with thymic aplasia show uncontrolled virus replication in the lung (despite specific antibody formation), resulting in giant cell pneumonia. In addition, the typical measles rash is absent. These studies indicate that the cell-mediated immune response is essential for regulation of virus growth and for the production of the characteristic skin lesions. Other studies have suggested that a similar conclusion can be drawn about the rashes in poxvirus infection.

Superantigens: The toxins of *Staphylococcus aureus* and *Streptococcus pyogenes* belong to a family of exotoxins which have a profound effect on the immune system. These bacterial superantigens promote cell-mediated immunity by stimulating T cell activation and recruitment to local sites of inflammation. The T cell-stimulating activity contributes to the pathogenesis of the respective diseases.

Superantigens stimulate both CD4+ and CD8+ T cells, as well as a fraction of T cells with antigen receptors, which are composed of gamma and delta chains ($T_{\gamma\delta}$). Stimulation is caused by cross-linking variable parts of the T cell antigen receptor and non-polymorphic parts of MHC Class II molecules on antigen presenting cells (Figure 6.8). For T cells with an antigen receptor composed of alpha and beta chains ($T_{\alpha\beta}$), the variable region of the β chain provides the site of attachment for the superantigen.

The T cell activation properties of superantigens have been implicated in a number of diseases where the consequence of this activation is pathogenetic. In allergy, superantigens induce the production of the proinflammatory cytokines interleukin 1 and tumour necrosis factor alpha, which enhance the expression of E-selectin. One ligand for E-selectin is cutaneous lymphocyte-associated antigen (CLA), which is found on T cells invading the skin in allergic individuals; its expression being induced by IL-12 presumably released by Langerhans cells or other antigen presenting cells upon stimulation with superantigen. Evidence

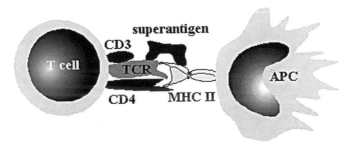

Figure 6.8 Superantigen stimulation of T cells
Unlike processed antigen presented to T cells, superantigens are able to bind to the relatively constant regions of the MHC and TCR, outside the normal antigen-presenting/binding regions. This brings the cells into close aposition, allowing the interaction of co-stimulatory molecules. This means that superantigens lead to polyclonal activation of T cells that does not depend upon their antigen specificity.

Table 6.6   Evidence of a role for superantigen in atopic dermatitis

Evidence:

Staphylococcus aureus isolated from skin lesions of patients with atopic dermatitis secrete large amounts of superantigen whilst those isolated from non-atopic (allergic) individuals do not

Skin colonisation by *Staph. aureus* can cause severe exacerbation of atopic dermatitis

Anti-*Staph. aureus* superantigen IgE has been found in patients undergoing exacerbation of atopic dermatitis due to *Staph. aureus* colonisation

Peripheral blood basophils 'armed' with anti-*Staph. aureus* superantigen IgE undergo degranulation and release histamine upon challenge *in vitro* with superantigen

that superantigens also influence antibody-mediated allergic responses is largely anecdotal but quite convincing (Table 6.6).

KEY POINTS FOR REVIEW

- *The type of specific immune response that occurs during infection is dependent upon the nature of the infecting agent.*
- *Extracellular organisms are largely controlled by antibody-enhanced functions such as phagocytosis and respiratory burst-mediated lysis and complement-mediated lysis.*
- *Antibody may act as an opsonin, activate complement, inhibit microbial attachment, neutralise toxins and viruses, and inhibit microbial growth and enzyme activity.*
- *Immune complex formation may lead to pathology via Type III hypersensitivity reactions.*
- *Intracellular organisms and viruses are largely controlled by cell-mediated immunity, i.e. T_{cyt} and NK cells, macrophage-mediated microbicidal activity and antibody-dependent cellular cytotoxicity.*
- *T cells may be activated in a non-specific manner by superantigens which may lead to autoimmune or hypersensitivity reactions.*

6.4   CYTOKINES IN IMMUNITY TO INFECTION

Apart from cytotoxic effector function, T cells play another important regulatory role in immunity to infection through the production of cytokines. These affect the activity of a wide range of cells, enhancing the function of some, inhibiting that of others. In particular, lymphokines activate macrophages; cells which play a vital role in host defence against many bacteria, fungi and parasites.

As described earlier, many extracellular bacteria are most effectively controlled by specific antibody production. The latter requires the activation of specific T cells that produce cytokines to promote the proliferation and differentiation of B cells and the switching of antibody class. We have previously discussed the effect of different cytokines on the proliferation of Th_1 and Th_2 subsets and there is clear evidence that recovery from certain infections is dependent upon the predominance of one of these subsets and the cytokines they produce, e.g. trypanosomiasis and Th_2 cells.

Intracellular infections are principally controlled by Th_1 responses. Products from bacteria and/or parasites stimulate IL-12 production (principally from macrophages) and thus, these early interactions initiate a Th_1 response. *In vivo*, IL-12 induces IFNγ production, enhances NK cell activation, and promotes protective responses.

The immune response to viral infections may be divided into separate stages, each being associated with a particular pattern of cytokine secretion. In the first stage, IFNα/β production causes the activation of NK cells (Table 6.7). This may be accompanied by IFNγ and/or IL-12 production.

The replication of viruses inside cells results in the production of a specialised cellular protein, interferon, which acts to limit the infection. Although most viruses stimulate interferon production, the amount produced depends on the virus. DNA viruses are poorer stimulators of interferon than RNA viruses (which include the paramyxoviruses, e.g. Sendai virus), which are the best. After production, interferon diffuses away from the site of infection, inducing an anti-viral state in neighbouring cells and preventing the synthesis of viral nucleic acids. These effects collectively inhibit growth and spread of the virus.

Interferon production is one of the earliest host responses to viral infection, which commences within the first 24 hours after invasion. Different types of interferon are produced depending upon the site of infection and the cells affected. If fibroblasts are among the infected cells, interferon-β is produced. If the site of infection is populated by leukocytes or if the virus spreads to the blood or lymphoid tissue, interferon-α is produced. Finally, if T lymphocytes are activated by antigen at the site of infection, interferon-γ is also produced. The combined action of these three interferons slows the infection down with interferons-α and -β exerting direct anti-viral effects and interferon-γ mainly enhancing the immune response (it activates macrophages, augments the activity of NK and T_{cyt} cells and increases the expression of MHC molecules on many cells).

Interferon is only effective for a short time and hence plays a major role in acute, short-term infections such as the common cold and influenza. It has no effect on viral multiplication in cells that are already infected.

The latter has potent immunoregulatory functions, which include augmentation of the activity of T_{cyt} and NK cells and enhancing the production of IFNγ, which has been shown to enhance Th_1 responses whilst inhibiting Th_2 responses.

Table 6.7   Characteristics of interferon alpha and beta

Characteristic	Type	Description
Types of interferon		Human interferons comprise: IFNαI (19.2–19.7 kDa), IFNαII (20.1 kDa), IFNβ (20 kDa) Murine interferons comprise: IFNα (19.1 kDa), IFNβ (19.7 kDa)
Major cellular sources	IFNα	Lymphocytes, monocytes and macrophages
	IFNβ	Fibroblasts and some epithelial cells
Effects	IFNα	Confers resistance to viruses on target cells, inhibits cell proliferation and regulates expression of MHC Class I antigens
	IFNβ	Related to IFNα; shares the same receptor and has very similar biological activities
Cross-reactivity	IFNα	IFNα shows about 40% homology between humans and mice and there is some species restriction depending on the particular molecule
	IFNβ	IFNβ shows about 48% homology in humans and mice; there is NO cross-species reactivity

Following the initial response to virus infection, T cells are activated resulting in the expansion of CD8$^+$ T cells and the production of antigen-specific, Class I restricted, T_{cyt} cells. The cytokines produced during this stage of the response include IL-2, IFNγ, IL-4 and/or IL-10, as well as biologically active TGFβ (Table 6.8). The role of these cytokines in the generation of active T_{cyt} cells is unclear since studies using IFNγ and IL-2-deficient mice indicate that these factors are not essential in this process. At this stage of the infection, it is interesting to note that NK cell activity is inhibited but B cells are stimulated. The latter appear to be vital in the final stages of the immune response to viral infection. Although resolution of infection appears to be dependent on T_{cyt} cell activity, termination of the immune response is related to antigen clearance, which is mediated by antibody.

The family of transforming growth factors known as beta are a group of proteins, which mediate diverse effects on a variety of cells such that TGFβ can be both immunosuppressive or immunoenhancing depending on the cell type involved. TGFβ inhibits the activation of macrophages by IFNγ and prevents the synthesis of reactive oxygen and nitrogen metabolites. Thus, the local production of this cytokine during intracellular infections, e.g. with bacteria or parasites, may be pathogenetic. In addition, TGFβ inhibits IL-2-dependent cytotoxic T lymphocyte responses but not by interfering with the binding of IL-2 to its receptor.

In recent years, another group of cytokines – the chemokines – have been shown to play an important role in the regulation of immunity to infection.

Table 6.8   Characteristics of the transforming growth factors

Characteristic	Description
Molecular weight	44.3 kDa (human TGFβ1); 47.8 kDa (human TGFβ2); 47.3 kDa (human TGFβ3)
Major cellular sources	Platelets contain TGFβ1 and β2. Most nucleated cell types and many tumours express TGFβ1, 2, 3 or combinations thereof
Effects	Involved in tissue remodelling, wound repair, development and haemato-poiesis. Inhibits cell growth. Switch factor for IgA
Cross-reactivity	TGFβ species show greater than 98% homology in humans and mice

CXCR4 and CCR5 have been shown to be key co-receptors for HIV infection and their ligands can inhibit this infection.

KEY POINTS FOR REVIEW

- *Immunity to infection may be regulated by cytokines produced by immune cells involved in the response.*
- *Intracellular infections are largely controlled by Th$_1$ responses, whilst extracellular infections are regulated by the production of Th$_2$-type cytokines.*
- *Chemokines have been demonstrated to play a role in the regulation of infectious disease particularly in HIV infection.*

BIBLIOGRAPHY

Behm CA, Ovington KS. (2000) The role of eosinophils in parasitic helminth infections: insights from genetically modified mice. Parasitol Today, 16; 202–209.

Boes M. (2000) Role of natural and immune IgM antibodies in immune responses. Molec Immunol, 37; 1141–1149.

Diks SH, van Deventer SJ, Peppelenbosch MP. (2001) Lipopolysaccharide recognition, internalisation, signalling and other cellular effects. J Endotoxin Res, 7; 335–348.

Garzino-Demo A, DeVico AL, Conant KE, Gallo RC. (2000) The role of chemokines in human immunodeficiency virus infection. Immunol Rev, 177; 79–87.

Llewelyn M, Cohen J. (2002) Superantigens: microbial agents that corrupt immunity. Lancet Infect Dis, 2; 156–162.

MacDonald AS, Araujo MI, Pearce EJ. (2002) Immunology of parasitic helminth infections. Infect Immunol, 70; 427–433.

Netea MG, Kullberg BJ, Van der Meer JW. (2000) Circulating cytokines as mediators of fever. Clin Infect Dis, 31; S178–S184.

Ochsenbein AF, Zinkernagel RM. (2000) Natural antibodies and complement link innate and acquired immunity. Immunol Today, 21; 624–630.

Ottenhoff TH, Verreck FA, Lichtenauer-Kaligis EG, Hoeve MA, Sanal O, van Dissel JT. (2002) Genetics, cytokines and human infectious disease: lessons from weakly pathogenic mycobacteria and salmonellae. Nat Genet, 32; 97–105.

Ryan JC, Naper C, Hayashi S, Daws MR. (2001) Physiologic functions of activating natural killer (NK) complex-encoded receptors on NK cells. Immunol Rev, 181; 126–137.

NOW TEST YOURSELF!

1. Which of the following statements concerning the role of cytokines in immunity to infection is INCORRECT?

(a) Many extracellular bacteria are most effectively controlled by specific antibody production which requires the production by T cells of cytokines which will promote switching of antibody classes.

(b) The early interaction between bacteria and/or parasites and macrophages stimulates the production of IL-10, leading to a Th_1 response.

(c) Intracellular infections are principally controlled by Th_1 responses and the cytokines produced by them.

(d) The response to virus infection may be divided into stages which are characterised by the different cytokines produced.

(e) Recovery from certain infections requires the production of cytokines by distinct T cell subsets, e.g. trypanosomiasis and Th_2 cells.

2. Endotoxins:

(a) Are produced in the cytoplasm of bacteria and are secreted.

(b) Refers to the phosphoprotein–polysaccharide complex associated with certain bacteria.

(c) Are usually associated with Gram-positive bacteria.

(d) Usually consist of a core polysaccharide, an O-specific polysaccharide and a lipid A component.

(e) Are an important virulence factor, and changes in the core polysaccharide result in major changes in virulence.

3. Which of the following statements is INCORRECT? Adhesion molecules:

(a) Promote cell-to-cell adhesion.

(b) May be used by microbes to facilitate attachment to host cells.

(c) May be used by microbes to facilitate invasion.

(d) Are involved in the attachment of parasitised red blood cells to brain endothelium.

(e) Have been implicated in the pathology of malaria. ICAM-1 expression on vascular endothelium is downregulated by tumour necrosis factor, and decreased levels of this cytokine have been shown to correlate with disease severity.

4.   Heat shock proteins:
(a) From a foreign source may stimulate T cells, which could cause the development of autoimmune phenomena.
(b) Exhibit a very low level of conservation between species.
(c) Are found in much lower concentrations in stressed cells.
(d) Are processed and presented to T cells expressing the alpha/beta T cell antigen receptor.
(e) Are a group of molecules found only in eukaryotes.

5.   There are many examples of host injury which occurs as a result of the humoral immune response to a pathogen. Which of the following statements is CORRECT?
(a) Immune complexes containing streptococcal antigens and IgG may deposit in the kidney, leading to the development of post-streptococcal glomerulo-nephritis.
(b) Polyarteritis nodosa is associated with the Epstein–Barr virus.
(c) Polyarteritis nodosa is caused by the release of interferons due to virus infection which leads to chronic inflammation and granuloma formation.
(d) Chorea is caused by antibodies to staphylococcal antigens which react with neurons in the caudate and subthalamic nuclei of the brain.
(e) Rheumatic fever is associated with Gram-negative bacilli, antibodies to which cross-react with patients' heart muscles or valves, causing myocarditis.

6.   In many instances of microbial infection, the resulting pathology is caused by the immune response, which may be classified as a hypersensitivity reaction. Which of the following statements is CORRECT?
(a) Type I hypersensitivity reactions may be the cause of some of the liver necrosis seen in hepatitis B and yellow fever.
(b) The haemolysis seen in malaria is caused in part by a Type III hypersensitivity response.
(c) The haemolytic anaemia associated with Mycoplasma pneumoniae infection is caused by a Type II hypersensitivity response.
(d) The arthus response which is seen as a consequence of some infections is a consequence of a Type I hypersensitivity response.
(e) Antigens absorbed from the gut combine with locally produced IgA and cause a severe Type III hypersensitivity response.

7. Which of the following statements concerning immune complexes is INCORRECT?
(a) The consequences of the presence of circulating immune complexes are directly related to the size of the complexes and the relative proportions of antibody and antigen.
(b) Immune complexes formed in antibody excess are rapidly cleared by the mononuclear phagocyte system.

(c) *Immune complexes formed when antibody and antigen are present in equal concentration form large lattices.*

(d) *Large lattices formed by antibody and antigen are rapidly cleared due to their size.*

(e) *Immune complexes formed when antigen is in excess are rapidly cleared by the mononuclear phagocyte system.*

8. Granuloma formation is associated with a number of infections. Infection with which of the following organisms is NOT classically associated with granuloma formation?

(a) *Mycobacterium spp.*

(b) *Actinomycete spp.*

(c) *Chlamydia spp.*

(d) *Treponema pallidum.*

(e) *Meningococcus spp.*

9. Which of the following statements concerning Chagas' disease is CORRECT?

(a) *Chagas' disease is caused by Schistosoma mansoni.*

(b) *The organs affected by chronic disease show only small numbers of organisms but a loss of autonomic ganglion cells.*

(c) *The organisms spread throughout the body asymptomatically.*

(d) *Chronic disease emerges years later, involving the lungs and liver.*

(e) *Chagas' disease is transmitted by aerosol.*

10. Which of the following statements concerning superantigens is INCORRECT?

(a) *Superantigens stimulate both $CD4^+$ and $CD8^+$ T cells.*

(b) *Superantigens stimulate T cells which express the gamma/delta TCR.*

(c) *Stimulation is caused by cross-linking variable parts of the TCR and polymorphic parts of the MHC Class II molecules on antigen presenting cells.*

(d) *The variable region of the beta chain of the TCR provides the attachment site for superantigens.*

(e) *The exotoxins of Staphylococcus aureus and Streptococcus pyogenes are superantigens.*

7

IMMUNITY AND THE MHC

We have already examined the role of molecules produced by the genes of the MHC in stimulating immune effector cells. The requirement for antigen to be presented by self-MHC for the stimulation of a protective immune response is well established. However, advances in modern medicine have meant that more and more commonly our immune systems are being exposed to foreign MHC gene products in the form of organ or tissue transplants. In addition, there is a very natural situation in which the female immune system potentially may be exposed to foreign MHC molecules – i.e. during pregnancy. Thus, this chapter is designed to look at these two situations and how the body reacts to the presence of foreign MHC gene products.

7.1 TRANSPLANTATION

The first successful human organ transplantation was a cadaveric renal graft (kidney transplant from a dead donor) carried out in 1954. Early operations were often unsuccessful due to fatal post-operative infections and rejection of the transplanted organ. However, by the 1960s the development of immuno-suppressive drugs such as prednisolone and azathioprine caused a significant reduction in rejection and mortality rates. This pioneering work led to the refinement of techniques that allowed the successful transplantation of hearts, livers, lungs and bone marrow. Although techniques differ according to the organ to be transplanted and its source, determining the suitability of donated tissue for a particular recipient depends on the key techniques of **tissue typing** and **cross-matching**. Despite these precautions, transplants fail and undergo **rejection**. Other transplantation techniques such as heart–lung and bowel are becoming more successful as we understand the nature of the rejection reaction and how to prevent or control it. Some of these more common transplantation protocols will be described in the following pages.

Immunology for Life Scientists, Second Edition. Lesley-Jane Eales.
© 2003 John Wiley & Sons, Ltd: ISBN 0 470 84523 6 (HB); 0 470 84524 4 (PB)

7.1.1 TISSUE TYPING

When a patient requires a transplant, s/he must be "tissue typed" so that a suitable (matching) organ may be found. This process involves ABO blood typing and human leukocyte antigen (HLA) typing.

In addition to being present on red blood cells, blood group antigens (the ABO antigens) are also expressed on the endothelium lining the blood vessels (vascular endothelium) of a graft. Thus, in order to prevent its rejection by the recipient's immune system, the blood type of the grafted kidney must be compatible with that of the recipient. If the organ and recipient are not matched, rapid rejection occurs due to the presence of natural antibodies directed against blood group antigens (isohaemagglutinins). These damage the vascular endothelium causing localised coagulation, reduced blood circulation through the transplanted organ and anoxia (oxygen lack). The outcome is widespread cytotoxicity, massive tissue damage and rapid organ rejection.

When a suitable organ is obtained, the degree of haplotype matching (i.e. identity between the recipient and donor for major human leukocyte antigens) must be determined.

7.1.2 CROSS-MATCHING

Previous exposure to alloantigens (for example in women who have had multiple pregnancies or persons who have had multiple blood transfusions) can lead to the development of HLA-specific antibodies, which may cause rejection of subsequent grafts bearing those antigens (particularly important in related-donor transplantation). In addition, patients receiving a second transplant (owing to previous rejection) are likely to have pre-formed HLA-specific antibodies.

The risk of rejection of the graft is assessed using a technique known as the mixed lymphocyte culture (MLC). White cells from the donor are treated to prevent them from proliferating. These are then mixed with white cells from the recipient. If the MHC antigens on the donor cells are different to those on the recipient's cells they will be recognised as foreign and the recipient's cells will be stimulated by them and proliferate. The stronger the proliferative reaction, the more likely that the graft will be rejected. However, the degree of proliferation does not necessarily correlate with the degree of matching between the donor and recipient since some antigens are much stronger stimulators than others. Thus, different donor–recipient pairs matched for a single haplotype may show distinct graft survival rates due to the immunogenicity of the non-matched antigens.

The presence of pre-formed antibodies to HLAs is detected by cross-matching. A serum sample taken from the potential recipient is mixed with lymphocytes from a random panel of donors. This usually consists of between 40 and 50 samples thereby allowing for the majority of HLAs to be represented twice. The number of cell cultures that show cytotoxicity is expressed as a percentage of the panel. If the recipient shows reactivity to 15% or more of the panel, the recipient is cross-matched against the donor. If cells bearing antigens present in the proposed graft tissue are destroyed, the transplant is unlikely to be successful.

7.1.3 REJECTION

Rejection of transplanted organs and tissues is a complex event and can present as acute, hyperacute or chronic. Each is associated with particular signs and symptoms, which are related to the underlying immunological mechanisms causing the rejection. In recent years, there is mounting evidence to suggest that infectious agents, particularly viruses, may play a role in the initiation of graft rejection.

The trigger for graft rejection is allorecognition, i.e. the detection of non-self antigens derived from the same species. T cells recognise these foreign MHC-derived antigens by two distinct pathways, either direct or indirect.

The direct pathway involves the recognition of MHC-derived antigens on the surface of donor cells, whilst the indirect pathway involves the recognition of donor MHC products, which have been processed and presented on host antigen presenting cells.

Research has shown that the relative expression of the direct or indirect pathways may depend on a number of parameters including the level of expression of MHC molecules on the donor organ and the type of molecules recognised (major or minor), the number, type and distribution of professional (bone marrow-derived) and non-professional (non-haematopoietic) antigen presenting cells in the graft, and the nature of the graft and its position in relation to lymphatic drainage and vascularisation.

In addition to antigen recognition, the process of T cell activation requires signals derived from the ligation of co-stimulatory molecules on the T cell and the antigen presenting cell. Thus, the direct pathway of antigen recognition is short-lived in transplanted organs since its antigen presenting cells are depleted within a few weeks of transplantation. The parenchymal cells of the graft are unable to stimulate the direct pathway and may have a tolerising effect as evidenced by the fact that graft-specific T cells capable of direct pathway activation decrease with time, regardless of the presence of chronic rejection. Thus, whilst the direct pathway may play a role in acute rejection, it probably does not contribute to the chronic pathway of rejection.

By contrast, the indirect pathway may be constantly active as a result of recipient antigen presenting cells circulating through the graft.

DIRECT ALLORECOGNITION

Direct allorecognition depends upon T cells recognising donor antigens in association with donor MHC molecules. However, it is an accepted paradigm of immunology that T cells only recognise antigen in association with self-MHC. One potential explanation of this paradox is that direct allorecognition is a result of allogeneic MHC molecules antigenically mimicking self-MHC.

The "high determinant density" theory suggests that the TCR on some cells has a very low affinity for allo-MHC. Normally, ligation between the T cell and the target cell would not occur. However, on graft cells, the high level of MHC expression increases the avidity of the interaction allowing TCR–peptide–MHC ligation and consequent T cell activation.

The multiple binary complex hypothesis proposes that particular peptide–allo-MHC complexes are able to stimulate specific T cells. Distinct MHC molecules may have a similar structure in the regions that are involved in TCR contact. If the allo-MHC molecules share such similarity with self-MHC, allo-MHC presentation would be possible. Since an individual MHC molecule can present a number of distinct processed antigens, a range of T cell clones specific for each of the antigens may be activated. The resulting immune response to the graft would be intense as is seen in direct recognition rejection reactions.

INDIRECT ALLORECOGNITION

The indirect pathway of allorecognition represents the usual pathway of antigen presentation that is operative for all other protein antigens. Thus, via this pathway, allogeneic MHC molecules are recognised in a truly self-MHC-restricted manner.

MECHANISMS INVOLVED IN HYPERACUTE REJECTION

Hyperacute rejection of a graft is caused by a Type II hypersensitivity response initiated by the presence of anti-ABO isohaemagglutinins or antibodies to MHC Class I antigens. When present in high enough concentration, these antibodies bind to the vascular endothelium thus initiating the fixation and activation of the complement cascade. The sequelae include activation of the clotting pathway and, if the reaction is great enough, formation of microthrombi, which block the capillaries of the graft preventing blood flow (ischaemia) and causing necrosis of the graft.

MECHANISMS INVOLVED IN ACUTE REJECTION

In the early stages post-transplantation, most of the cells invading the graft tissue are lymphocytes. However, 4 to 7 days after transplantation the tissue contains a heterogeneous collection of cells. Rejection may be mediated by direct or indirect allorecognition of the graft. Alloantigens on the graft stimulate the activation of T cells leading to the development of specific, cellular immune responses. Once activated, these cells release interleukin 2, which stimulates the proliferation and maturation of alloantigen-specific cells leading to the development of both $CD4^+$ and $CD8^+$ effector T cells. The latter circulate from the lymphoid tissue, through the vascular system, to the graft, where they cause antigen-specific damage either directly or by stimulating the release of cytotoxic antibodies. In addition, stimulated Th_1 cells produce IFNγ, which has been shown to have a variety of effects resulting in enhanced graft rejection (Table 7.1).

By contrast, stimulation of Th_2 cells leads to the production of IL-4 and IL-5, which promote the proliferation and differentiation of B cells capable of recognising graft-specific antigens. The resultant antibody causes cytolytic damage to the graft either through the activation of complement or by mediating antibody-dependent cell-mediated cytotoxicity. When the host has been primed to donor antigens before transplantation, a more rapid effect may occur, often marked by antibody-mediated vasculitis.

MECHANISMS INVOLVED IN CHRONIC REJECTION

Chronic rejection, which can occur months or even years after transplantation, is characterised by proliferation of the endothelial cells lining the blood vessels leading to a narrowing of the lumen. Some of the pathological changes may result from indirect allorecognition of the graft by host T cells. The precipitating signal for this reaction is unknown but it is likely to be caused

Table 7.1 Effect of interferon gamma in organ transplantation

Effects of gamma interferon	Consequences of effects
Gamma interferon enhances the expression of MHC Class I and Class II antigens on the cells of the graft	Increased MHC antigen expression may increase the effectiveness of graft-specific cytotoxic T cells
Gamma interferon activates macrophages both within and around the graft	Macrophage activation results in a delayed-type hypersensitivity response which gives rise to the characteristic symptoms of inflammation associated with graft rejection. In addition, the macrophages themselves may express enhanced cytotoxic activity towards the graft

by the release of interleukin 1 from monocytes and platelet-derived growth factor from platelets and endothelial cells. In the initial stages, this condition is reversible with immunosuppressive therapy. However, once the changes have become fibrotic, the condition becomes progressive leading to ischaemia and ultimately loss of function of the grafted tissue.

THE ROLE OF THE GRAFT ENDOTHELIUM IN REJECTION

Correct haemoperfusion is vital to the survival of any grafted tissue. The endothelium of the blood vessels therefore is a front-line participant in any rejection reaction. When the endothelium becomes activated, it expresses adhesion molecules and produces cytokines, which encourage the migration of the recipient's immune cells into the grafted tissue. In addition, it expresses both Class I and II MHC molecules and can potentially stimulate the direct pathway of allorecognition.

Early after activation, P and E-selectins are expressed followed later by ICAM-1 and VCAM-1. The latter is intimately associated with the recruitment of T cells during allo-induced inflammation. Extravasation and migration into the parenchyma of the graft requires cell–cell interactions involving receptor–ligand interactions including molecules such as PECAM-1 (CD31), vascular endothelium cadherin and α-, β- and γ-catenin.

Chemokines (IL-8, MCP-1) and other inflammatory mediators such as leukotrienes, eicosanoids, coagulation proteins, complement products, IL-1, IL-6, PDGF and TGFβ are secreted by the activated endothelium and mediate cell migration and activation. In particular, MCP-1, which attracts monocytes to the sight of inflammation, is thought to be key in the development of chronic rejection. Perhaps predictably, the chemokines RANTES and IP-10, which are known to be functional in T cell recruitment, and the chemokine receptors CXCR3, CCR1 and CCR3, are expressed in allografts undergoing rejection. Indeed, it has been suggested that the endothelium expresses specific chemokines and their respective receptors in order to selectively recruit specific CD4$^+$ T cell subtypes to the allograft.

The endothelium of allografts is thought to promote the indirect pathway of allorecognition by promoting the differentiation of monocytes into myeloid-derived dendritic cells. The indirect pathway is particularly important in chronic rejection. Alloantigen is processed and presented in association with self-MHC. This complex is recognised by CD4$^+$ T cells, which promote the differentiation of effector cells. It was thought that the MHC molecules released from the graft were taken up by lymph node antigen presenting cells. It is now thought that these reactions occur locally in the graft and recruited monocytes reverse transmigrate as dendritic cells into lymph nodes, their co-stimulatory capacity enhanced by the allograft endothelial cells.

7.1.4 KIDNEY TRANSPLANTATION

The transplantation of kidneys is one of the most successful operations of its kind. Contributing to this success is the option to perform related-donor grafts. The close genetic relatedness between the recipient and donor gives the transplant a greater chance of success. Indeed, studies have shown that when the recipient and donor are siblings with two matching haplotypes, the graft survival rate after 1 year is 90%. One-haplotype-matched pairs (the organ being from either a sibling or a parent) have 75–85% graft survival rate after 1 year. This rate declines to only 50–60% in zero-haplotype-matched family members unless the recipient receives some form of immunosuppressive or modulatory treatment such as transfusion therapy. Studies have shown that transfusion therapy is beneficial in related-donor transplantation where the donor and recipient share none, or only one haplotype. Obviously, this technique allows the identification of those recipients in whom transplantation is contra-indicated due to their ability to immunologically recognise the donor tissue. It has been suggested that the success of this form of therapy is due to a number of mechanisms (including clonal deletion, selection of immunologic non-responders, induction of suppressor T cells or the production of blocking or anti-idiotypic antibodies) acting individually or in concert.

Transfusion therapy usually consists of three transfusions of small amounts (100–200 ml) of donor blood given over a period of several weeks. The production of cytotoxic anti-donor antibodies (which occurs in approximately 10–30% of recipients) is carefully monitored. In most donor–recipient pairs matched for only one haplotype, anti-donor antibody production can be reduced by the use of azathioprine during the transfusions. In those individuals who do not become sensitised to the donor during this therapy, 2-year survival rates in one-haplotype-matched related-donor transplantations are 95%. Indeed, pre-transplant transfusion treatment has resulted in greatly improved survival rates in non-haplotype-matched allografts (>90% at 2 years).

PRE-SENSITISATION

Organ donation by relatives, whilst having a greater chance for success, also allows for the possibility of pre-sensitisation, making cross-matching vital. Patients who have already rejected a graft are likely to have cross-reactive antibodies. In addition, a patient undergoing rapid rejection of a primary graft (in less than 3 months) is much more likely to reject a subsequent graft. However, the use of tissue typing, cross-matching and improved immuno-suppressive therapy regimes (Table 7.2) greatly increases the success rates of related-donor transplantation.

Table 7.2 Examples of immunosuppressive therapy used post-operatively

Therapy	Effects
Cyclosporine (5–15 mg/kg/d)	Has enhanced allograft survival in recipients of both cadaveric and related-donor transplants
Cyclosporine	Has received widespread use but is nephrotoxic; doses and in vivo levels must be carefully monitored
Azathioprine	An anti-metabolite that interferes with DNA formation in proliferating cells. Often used in combination with prednisolone and cyclosporine. Potentially hepatotoxic
Cyclophosphamide	Used as a non-hepatotoxic alternative to azathioprine
Anti-lymphocyte (ALG) or anti-thymocyte globulin (ATG). Therapeutic dose: 10–20 mg/kg	Polyclonal antisera prepared in animals immunised with human lymphocytes or thymocytes (respectively). The cytolytic activity of the antibodies results in profound immunosuppression
Lymphoplasmapheresis	Used concurrently, occasionally, with immunosuppressive drugs to remove recipient lymphocytes and immunoglobulin

CADAVERIC KIDNEY TRANSPLANTATION

In some cases, an appropriate relative for organ donation cannot be found and the recipient must receive an organ from a recently deceased individual. After screening, but before transplantation, patients are "pre-conditioned". It has been found that performing pre-operative, random blood transfusion correlates with improved allograft survival. This transfusion treatment means that individuals can be identified who are capable of producing cytotoxic, blocking or anti-idiotypic antibodies, and specific or non-specific suppressor T cells. Such individuals are not suitable recipients for a transplant.

ABO-compatible recipients who are cross-match negative are subjected to further cross-match testing using additional sera to eliminate the possibility of undetected pre-sensitisation. The most well-matched recipients are selected and further criteria are taken into consideration such as the urgency of their medical condition, the length of time on the waiting list and whether they have received a previous transplant.

Once removed, the kidney must be cleaned (to remove all donor blood) and cooled (to help its preservation). This is achieved by flushing it through with a mixed electrolyte solution. It is then stored either (a) by packing in ice to maintain sub-physiological temperatures or (b) by pulsed, cold perfusion with mixed electrolyte solution. Preferably, the organ is used within 48 hours.

Rejection: Classical acute rejection of kidney transplants presents as swelling and tenderness over the allograft and decreased renal function (decreased urine volume and increased blood urea, nitrogen and creatinine levels). In addition, patients may present with elevated temperature, malaise, decreased appetite and generalised myalgia.

7.1.5 LIVER TRANSPLANTATION

Originally considered to be an immunologically privileged site, transplanted livers are now known to be susceptible to immunological responses. However, rejection reactions in liver transplant patients are clearly distinct to those observed in kidney and other whole organ transplant patients.

The most common cause of liver damage requiring transplantation is chronic active non-A, non-B, viral, hepatitis. However, liver transplantation has been performed also in individuals with primary biliary cirrhosis, hepatitis B, cirrhosis, and inborn errors of metabolism.

Post-transplantation infection is common and patient survival is related to the type of infectious agent involved. In general, bacterial infections respond well to antibiotic therapy whilst fungal or viral infections are associated with a poor prognosis.

PROCEDURE

Livers for transplantation are usually matched for blood group with the recipient. Generally, donor and recipient are not matched for MHC antigens and indeed, in recent years, evidence has accumulated to suggest that there is an inverse relationship between MHC antigen matching and graft survival.

Another factor influencing liver transplantation is the size of the donor organ, although surgical reduction in the size of donor livers and partial grafts from live donors may be used in smaller/younger recipients.

Since there are very few reports of hyperacute rejection due to pre-formed anti-donor antibodies, cross-matches are performed only post-operatively. The mechanisms underlying the apparent resistance of the liver to rejection are unknown; maybe the liver is not sensitive to pre-formed antibodies or the size of the liver itself causes the dilution of the antibody to a non-pathogenic level.

PRIMARY NON-FUNCTION AND REJECTION

Following transplantation, patients may present with a range of clinical conditions, which are collectively known as primary non-function. This is really a spectrum of diseases ranging from a total lack of function of the graft (leading to death if a second transplant is not available) to a mild, initial impairment of function that corrects within the first days or weeks following transplantation. Factors affecting the development of primary non-function are listed in Table 7.3.

Generally, liver transplants are successful; survival rates being 70–90% after 1 year and approximately 60% after 5 years. Histologically defined

Table 7.3 Factors affecting the development of primary non-function in liver transplants

Factor
The nature of the donor's injury
Problems during excision of the donor organ
The type of preservation solution used
The length of organ preservation
The immunological background of the recipient
The transplantation procedure
Factors affecting the recipient's cardiovascular system

rejection reactions that may be easily treated are seen in approximately 75% of all patients. Delayed failure of the organ usually results from chronic rejection or recurrence of the original disease.

Clinically, rejection is associated with non-specific signs and symptoms such as fever, abdominal pain, enlargement of the liver and depressed appetite. Histologically, livers undergoing rejection show a mixed cellular infiltrate with damage to the epithelium of the bile duct, central or portal veins. Serum levels of bilirubin, alkaline phosphatase and transaminases may be abnormal but are not predictive of rejection. Treatment with a range of immunosuppressive regimes, which include methylprednisolone, anti-lymphocyte globulin, or anti-CD3 monoclonal antibody help to prevent rejection and cyclosporine, post-transplantation, improves survival.

7.1.6 HEART TRANSPLANTATION

The first successful heart transplant was in 1967 and since that time the techniques have been extensively refined. Usually, donor organs are obtained from persons less than 40 years of age and without a previous history of cardiac disease. After death, the heart is maintained in optimal condition by hydration and the use of vasopressor and myotropic drugs. After removal from the body, the coronary circulation is flushed with a mixed electrolyte solution and the organ kept on ice for no more than 4 hours.

Before transplantation, the donor and recipient undergo blood group and HLA typing. Cross-matching is also performed against a random panel of lymphocytes from a number of donors. If the recipient has antibodies to more than 15% of the panel, then cross-matching with the donor must be performed before the transplantation.

REJECTION

Typically, acute rejection is seen as a mononuclear cell infiltrate, which comprises lymphocytes, lymphoblasts and monocytes. Early predictive signs of pathological changes in the vasculature of cardiac transplants include endothelial cell dysfunction, which presents as a loss of coronary endothelium vasomotor responses to acetylcholine. During the rejection reaction, endothelial cells may be activated and release cytokines that stimulate the production of enzymes capable of affecting the structure of the extracellular matrix – matrix metalloproteinases. These cytokines may also affect the endothelial function by altering the synthesis of nitric oxide. Treatment for this condition involves the use of anti-lymphocyte globulin and/or high concentrations of corticosteroids.

7.1.7 BONE MARROW TRANSPLANTATION

Owing to the limitations of the early syngeneic or allogeneic marrow transplantations (only 40% of patients may have an HLA identical donor), techniques have been developed to improve the success of marrow transplants from only partially matched family members or unrelated donors.

There are five principal diseases that are treatable by marrow transplantation. These are severe combined immunodeficiency, aplastic anaemia, leukaemia, lymphoma and certain solid tumours.

Donor marrow is obtained by multiple aspirations from the top of the hip girdle (the iliac crest). The aspirate is placed in heparinised, buffered, culture medium, filtered through fine meshes to produce a single-cell suspension and nucleated-cell counts are obtained. Blood group compatible recipients are given 2–6×10^8 nucleated cells/kg of body weight by intravenous infusion. Erythrocytes are given simultaneously. If the blood groups of the donor and recipient are not compatible, either the recipient undergoes plasmapheresis (to remove anti-A or anti-B antibodies) or the donor marrow is treated *in vitro* to remove the erythrocytes.

The immune system of most recipients must be destroyed in order to prevent rejection of the marrow and to allow the development of a new haemapoietic system. This is achieved by treating with cyclophosphamide (50–60 mg/kg, for 2 or 4 days) and by total body irradiation (7.5–15 Gy administered over 3–5 days; a single dose of radiation would damage the lungs and eyes). This combination of therapies eliminates the immune system and has an anti-neoplastic effect in most cancer patients. Obviously, patients undergoing bone marrow transplantation to combat severe combined immunodeficiency disease do not require this treatment since they lack a functioning immune system.

Success of the transplant is indicated by an increasing white cell count, raised levels of circulating monocytes (monocytosis) and the presence of mature neutrophils in the circulation between 2 and 4 weeks post-transplantation. As these parameters normalise, antibiotic therapy can be stopped and transfusions become unnecessary.

The technique is not always successful and graft-versus-host disease and infections are responsible for the 10–30% failure rate in the first 30 days following transplantation. Other causes of transplant failure include pneumonia, certain types of liver disease and recurrence of the underlying disease.

Graft-versus-host disease is caused by the presence of immunocompetent cells in an organ given to an immunocompromised host. It even occurs in patients who are HLA identical with their donors; the disease being attributed to minor differences in histocompatibility. It presents as a skin rash associated with diarrhoea and jaundice. In severe disease, the rash resembles extensive second-degree burns and watery diarrhoea is associated with malabsorption, cramps and gastrointestinal bleeding. Hyperbilirubinaemia is often seen due to inflammation of small bile ducts as a direct consequence of the disease process. Immunocompetent CD8⁺ T cells are found in tissues with high levels of HLA-DR antigens, e.g. the skin and intestine.

7.1.8 PANCREAS TRANSPLANTATION

Pancreas transplantation is used to prevent the sequelae of diabetes, which include damage to the kidneys (nephropathy), nerves (neuropathy) and retinas (retinopathy). Since the purpose of the procedure is to provide biologically responsive insulin-producing tissue, it may be performed with a whole organ, a segmental graft or dispersed islets of Langerhans. Recipients and donor organs are typed for both blood group and human leukocyte antigens and recipients undergo cross-matching.

The survival of isolated islet cells is shorter than that of any other allograft. However, animal studies have shown that syngeneic implants in the liver or under the capsule of the kidney are able to produce insulin to reverse hyperglycaemia, thus research has centred on perfecting the techniques for allograft islet transplantation. Either the adult or the foetal pancreas is used as a source of islet cells. However, the islets themselves contain dendritic cells and other antigen presenting cells, which render the tissue immunogenic. Attempts to reduce this effect have included treatment with antibodies to MHC Class II antigens, irradiation, and culturing purified islets in an oxygen-rich atmosphere.

Since Type I insulin-dependent diabetes mellitus is autoimmune in nature, patients often have autoantibodies in their serum that react with the cytoplasm or surface antigens of the cells of the islets of Langerhans. The latter are surrounded by mononuclear cells; the lymphocytes being predominantly

CD8$^+$ve. Thus, the histological picture is similar to that seen in other autoimmune diseases and in graft rejection reactions. This makes it difficult to distinguish rejection from autoimmune pathology in these patients.

Treatment to prevent rejection is of limited efficacy. Cyclosporine and corticosteroids are somewhat successful although a more potent protocol, which involves cyclosporine, azathioprine and prednisolone, may be used in appropriate patients. When evidence of rejection is observed, the patient is treated with large, intravenous doses of corticosteroids, increased oral prednisolone or a temporary course of anti-lymphocyte globulin.

7.1.9 XENOTRANSPLANTATION

In xenotransplantation, donors and recipients are of different species. Early experiments in xenotransplantation were performed in patients whose clinical condition was life-threatening and for whom no suitable human donor could be found. Amongst the earliest experiments were the transplantation of kidneys from a rhesus monkey and a chimpanzee into human recipients. Although both recipients died relatively rapidly after transplantation, other operations performed by the same group were more successful with one recipient surviving more than 6 months.

In recent years, our improved understanding of the immune response to transplanted organs, and particularly the difficulties presented by xenotransplants, has resulted in new therapies that make this technique more likely to succeed.

CHOICE OF DONOR

The pig is currently the most favoured donor animal for xenotransplants. Factors influencing this choice include the fact that pigs have large litters, a short maturation time (6 months), they are easily managed, their organ size is comparable to humans', the risk of transmitting infection is low, their reproductive cycle is well defined and the methods required for genetic manipulation are well established.

Pigs have an anatomy similar to humans and share characteristics with them such as size, haemodynamics and coronary artery distribution. One drawback is the potential for zoonotic infections, which has yet to be fully explored.

BARRIERS TO XENOTRANSPLANTATION

Although there are many physical similarities between man and pigs, there are some key differences, which are of particular concern in xenotransplantation.

The α-Gal epitopes: Early in our evolutionary history, the α-1,3-galactosyltransferase gene became inactive leading to the elimination of the expression of α-Gal epitopes (Galα1-3Galβ-4GlcNAc-R) in man. These epitopes are expressed however by common gastrointestinal bacteria which provide a constant immunological stimulus to the host. Thus, anti-Gal polyclonal antibodies comprise about 1% of the circulating natural antibodies in man. In contrast to man, pigs do express the α-Gal epitopes and these therefore present a key target for rejection of porcine xenotransplants. Current research is focusing on the elimination of the Gal epitope in pigs bred for transplantation.

Vascular biology: Maintenance of healthy organs is dependent upon a patent circulatory system. The viscosity of human blood is lower than that of pigs' and so a transplanted porcine organ will experience increased haemoperfusion when transplanted into a human. In addition, human erythrocytes are larger than porcine cells. This could affect circulation in the capillary beds and cause damage to the organ.

A further influence on circulation may derive from the fact that man is bipedal whilst pigs are quadrupeds. Posture affects both blood circulation and organ function and in an upright position, the organs are subjected to a difference in blood pressure. For example, porcine–primate lung xenotransplants successfully provide gaseous exchange but are of limited success due to severe vasoconstriction. Thus, post-lung transplantation, ventilation may become ineffective, or oedema could result in death.

Cross-matching for ABO blood groups is important to reduce the risk of hyperacute rejection. Porcine cells only express A and O group antigens. In addition, the A antigen is not expressed on the vascular endothelium but is expressed in the kidney. Clearly, the risk of rejection owing to group A antigens may be overcome by only using pigs with blood group O.

Molecular incompatibilities: The protein albumin often acts as a carrier for a range of enzymes, influencing their activities. Since porcine and human albumin share less than 65% homology, enzymes with a functional dependence on albumin may not function effectively. Enzyme function may also be affected by the fact that pigs have a higher body temperature than humans.

Factors affecting renal function such as cholesterol, calcium and phosphate levels are also different between species and could lead to complications such as electrolyte imbalance.

Other molecular compatibilities and incompatibilities between species are becoming known such as NK/T cell interactions, coagulation regulatory proteins, and effect of growth hormones on xenogeneic tissues. Thus, although we have some way to go, the potential for xenogeneic transplantation may in the not too distant future offer real hope to individuals who would otherwise have very little.

- *Determining the suitability of tissue for a particular recipient depends on tissue typing and cross-matching.*
- *This process involves ABO and HLA typing.*
- *Previous exposure to alloantigens may lead to rejection of subsequent grafts due to the formation of HLA-specific antibodies.*
- *Rejection may be acute, hyperacute or chronic.*
- *The trigger for rejection is allorecognition.*
- *Direct allorecognition depends upon T cells and the "high determinant density" and "multiple binary complex" hypotheses have been proposed to explain the process.*
- *The indirect pathway of allorecognition represents the normal pathway of antigen presentation.*
- *Hyperacute rejection of a graft is caused by a Type II hypersensitivity response.*
- *Acute rejection involves both T and B cell responses.*
- *Chronic rejection is characterised by the narrowing of blood vessels due to proliferation of endothelial cells and involves the activity of T cells.*
- *Transplantation methods and success rates directly relate to the type of organ being grafted and vary greatly from one organ to another.*
- *Xenotransplantation involves donors and recipients of distinct species.*
- *The most appropriate choice of donor for xenotransplants is the pig.*
- *Molecular and vascular differences and the possibility of zoonosis present distinct hurdles for xenotransplantation.*

7.2 THE IMMUNOLOGY OF REPRODUCTION

The aim of this section is to familiarise you with the role of the immune system in reproduction. Reproduction requires the immune system of the female host to accept what is, in essence, a foreign graft. Advances in our understanding of the processes involved has led to the development of new approaches to the treatment of spontaneous abortion and primary infertility.

7.2.1 THE DEVELOPMENT OF MATERNAL AND FOETAL TISSUES

Fertilisation occurs high in the Fallopian tube and the fertilised egg (known as the blastocyst) passes into the uterus where it implants. During this stage, most of the cells formed make up the membranes that surround the embryo providing protection and nutrition.

The wall of the **blastocyst** consists of an inner cellular layer – the **cytotrophoblast** (or cellular trophoblast) and an outer layer – the **syncytial trophoblast**. The latter destroys the epithelium and underlying stroma of the uterus allowing the blastocyst to implant. At implantation, the syncytial trophoblast stimulates an inflammatory reaction, which results in the formation of the **decidua** – a highly specialised tissue with the capacity to produce endocrine hormones. It derives from the uterine endometrium and under the influence of female hormones, proliferates. After implantation, it becomes thick, spongy and highly vascularised.

In early gestation, the trophoblast invades the maternal decidua and proliferates within it. This contact with the foetus is maintained throughout gestation; the decidua giving the foetus the ability to absorb nutriment from the mother. The decidua consists of three layers: the **decidua basalis** (in which the foetus implants); the **decidua capsularis** (which lies over the foetus); and the **decidua vera** (Figure 7.1). The decidua basalis forms the maternal part of the haemochorial placenta. Thus, the decidua provides the contact between the mother and the foetus.

The extravillous trophoblast cells of the foetus that invade the decidua express the MHC Class I gene products HLA-C, -E and -G. In addition, the decidua basalis (which is in contact with the extravillous trophoblast cells) contains large numbers of CD3$^-$, CD16$^-$ and CD56^{hi+} natural killer (NK) cells. The NK cells also express the CD94/NKG2, KIR and ILT receptors that recognised MHC Class I gene products, including HLA-E and -G. Thus, they may play a role in controlling foetal invasion of the maternal tissues. HLA-G has been associated with immune tolerance.

7.2.2 FEMALE REPRODUCTIVE IMMUNOLOGY

Half the chromosome complement of the foetus is derived from the father and molecules encoded by paternal genes theoretically could be recognised as foreign by the maternal immune system. Importantly, the maternal and foetal immune systems coexist for a period of time and so the potential exists for either to reject the other. However, the mother and foetus appear to have a symbiotic relationship. This mutual state of tolerance is critical for a healthy delivery. Several mechanisms exist that may explain this mutual acceptance. Foetal tissues may lack MHC Class I antigens (trophoblast cells) or express non-classical members of this family (extravillous trophoblast cells), the maternal immune system may be non-specifically suppressed, blocking antibodies may be produced and/or complement regulatory protein expression may be altered.

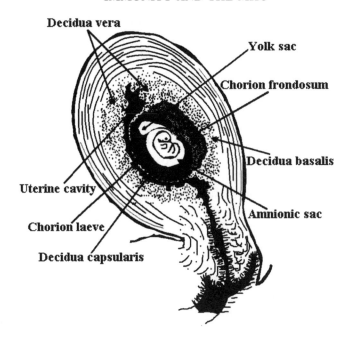

Figure 7.1   Structure of the human decidua

The first exposure of the female to paternal antigens (that may be expressed by the foetus) occurs after sexual intercourse. Although sperm bear foreign antigens, they are not recognised by the female's immune system and so are not destroyed. This may be due to non-specific suppressor factors in the semen. Indeed, high molecular weight substances found in seminal plasma have been shown to inhibit antigen-, mitogen- and alloantigen-stimulated lymphoproliferation. This inhibition may influence subsequent responses after implantation of the foetus.

7.2.3   MATERNAL–FOETAL EXCHANGE

Syncytial trophoblast cells are continuously released from the placenta and from the 18th week of gestation, can be found circulating in the mother's blood. This may allow recognition of foetal antigens by the mother's immune system and may protect the mother from the extensive and otherwise unchecked growth and invasion of the trophoblast, as occurs in choriocarcinoma.

The only class of antibody readily transferred from the mother to the foetus is IgG. This transference is probably mediated by Fc receptors on the surface of placental cells. Unless infection occurs *in utero*, the newborn cannot mount a quick, effective response to pathogenic organisms and the transplacentally acquired maternal antibody is the only protection a baby has against infection for the first 6–8 months of its life.

In certain circumstances, maternal antibody is not beneficial to the foetus, e.g. haemolytic disease of the newborn. This disease is due to incompatible blood groups in the mother and foetus. The disorder occurs primarily in blood group O mothers carrying a foetus with group A or B blood. It is thought to result from the transfer of IgG antibodies (from mother to foetus) that react with the foetal erythrocyte antigens. Although women of group A or group B have antibody to type B and type A erythrocytes respectively, these natural antibodies are usually of the IgM class and therefore do not readily cross the placenta and cannot harm the foetus.

A more important complication that affects foetal development involves the rhesus (Rh) antigens, which are expressed only on blood cells. During pregnancy, if an Rh-negative mother is carrying an Rh-positive foetus, foetal erythrocytes can cross the placenta and stimulate the production of antibodies to the Rh antigen in the maternal circulation. If untreated, in subsequent pregnancies this antibody may cross the placenta and lyse the erythrocytes of any Rh-positive foetus. Anti-rhesus antibodies may also be formed in the mother if there is transplacental haemorrhage at birth or after an abortion. Lysis of foetal red blood cells can be prevented by giving the mother anti-Rho (D) antiserum immediately after delivery of her first Rh-positive child or following an abortion. Any foetal erythrocytes present in the mother's circulation are destroyed by the passively administered antibody and are rapidly cleared. In this way they are not present long enough to sensitise the mother effectively.

7.2.4 EFFECT OF PREGNANCY ON THE MATERNAL IMMUNE RESPONSE

PERIPHERAL IMMUNITY

Pregnancy is associated with a depression in cellular immunity, which may result from a change in the number and function of T cells. Blood lymphocyte counts fall during gestation, reflected by a decrease in T cell numbers. Towards the end of pregnancy, CD4$^+$ cells decrease and CD8$^+$ cells increase. In addition, circulating NK cell numbers decline during pregnancy but their level of activity is probably unchanged. *In vitro* tests of T cell function, using mitogens and mixed lymphocyte reactions, show a decrease in lymphoproliferation during pregnancy. Serum immunoglobulin concentrations increase, but alterations of specific immunoglobulin subclasses have not been well characterised.

FOETAL–UTERINE IMMUNITY

The trophoblast, which does not express MHC Class I gene products, does express Fas ligand. This means that maternal cells at the interface between the placenta and the decidua will under go apoptosis if they bear Fas. In addition, the trophoblast expresses CD46, CD55 and CD59, all of which are complement regulatory proteins.

The local immune response is influenced by the large array of cytokines produced by both decidual and placental cells. These may contribute to the change from a Th_1-type response to a Th_2-type response. Such a switch may mean that the mother is more susceptible to infections usually regulated by Th_1-type (or cell-mediated) responses. Interestingly, a persistent Th_1-type cytokine array has been implicated in spontaneous abortion and underweight babies.

7.2.5   CYTOKINE–ENDOCRINE RELATIONSHIP IN PREGNANCY

OESTROGEN AND PROGESTERONE

During pregnancy, progesterone (released by the corpus luteum after ovulation) accumulates and induces differentiation in the endometrium thus ensuring its preparedness for implantation of the fertilised egg. It has been suggested that progesterone may induce the conversion of Th_0 cells to Th_2 cells, which may explain the observed decrease in the ratio of Th_1 to Th_2 cells at this time. However, other factors may also influence this change including prostaglandin and cytokines released by maternal or foetal cells.

Using a murine model, oestrogen (and progesterone) have been shown to increase the concentration of monocyte colony-stimulating factor (M-CSF) in the uterus. This cytokine is produced by a number of different cells including $CD3^-CD16^-CD56^{hi+}$ NK cells and stromal cells of the decidua. It induces the differentiation and proliferation of trophoblasts and appears to regulate the functions of decidual macrophages. In addition, M-CSF promotes the production of human chorionic gonadotrophin (hCG).

HUMAN CHORIONIC GONADOTROPHIN

hCG, which is secreted by trophoblast cells, helps to maintain a healthy pregnancy by preventing the apoptosis of the corpus luteum. Release of hCG is enhanced by the Th_2-type cytokines IL-4 and IL-6. Thus it has been suggested that hCG, progesterone and cytokines may form a magnifying loop whereby hCG stimulates the release of progesterone, which in turn causes the production of Th_2-type cells that release the cytokines required for enhanced hCG.

7.2.6 IMMUNITY TO INFECTION IN PREGNANCY

The pregnancy-related alteration in the immune response in infection includes changes in T cell subpopulations, neutrophil function, lymphocyte function, serum immunoglobulin concentrations, immunosuppressive serum factors, and maternal immune recognition mechanisms. The decrease in cell-mediated immunity associated with pregnancy, whilst clearly affected by the altered Th_1/Th_2 balance, is also influenced by a number of factors including the steroid hormones progesterone, oestrogen, cortisol, α-feto protein and uromodulin.

A number of infectious agents are thought to behave differently in pregnant women as a result of the altered immune response. These include viruses (e.g. cytomegalovirus (CMV), Epstein–Barr virus (EBV), influenza A virus), bacteria (e.g. *Neisseria gonorrhoeae*, *Streptococcus pneumoniae*) and fungi. Increased susceptibility to these infections may result from changes in the humoral immune response. Serum IgG decreases with advancing gestation. A decrease in the levels of IgM and IgM-bearing lymphocytes has also been reported in the first trimester, but these levels do not continue to decrease with advancing gestation. Antibody production in response to infection during pregnancy is probably unaltered. Despite this range of changes in immune reactivity, the human foetus usually remains relatively unaffected by maternal infectious diseases. However, there are some infectious agents which may have serious effects if the foetus is exposed during the early stages of its development. These include rubella, CMV, syphilis and toxoplasmosis.

In recent years, progress has been made to ensure pregnant women are aware of the potential dangers associated with certain foodstuffs such as non-pasteurised cheese. *Listeria monocytogenes* (which may be found in such cheese) tend to replicate at the maternal–placental interface and are an important cause of foetal morbidity and mortality. However, studies in animals have suggested that trophoblast cells responsive to colony-stimulating factor 1 (CSF-1) influence the maternal immune response to such bacterial infections.

7.2.7 IMMUNOCOMPETENT CELLS IN THE DECIDUA

The endometrium and decidua contain large numbers of leucocytes, the proportions of which vary during early pregnancy. T cells, $CD14^+$ macrophages and a population of $CD3^-CD16^-CD56^{++}$ large granular lymphocytes (LGL) are present. B cells are virtually absent. After the first trimester, there is a decline in the number of decidual T cells suggesting they are not important in the maintenance of pregnancy.

Large numbers of MHC Class II^+ macrophages in the early placenta provide a first line of defence to infection. However, at the time of implantation the most abundant cells (70–80% of all leukocytes in the endometrium) are the LGLs.

LARGE GRANULAR LYMPHOCYTES

Endometrial granulated lymphocytes comprise up to 70–80% of lymphocytes in the decidua during the first trimester of pregnancy. This number quickly declines after the second trimester. These lymphocytes are CD16$^-$, CD57$^-$ and CD56^{hi+} and are weakly lytic. Thus they are thought to be a type of NK cell. They contain perforin, granzyme A and T cell-restricted intracellular antigen 1 (TIA-1) which is phosphorylated by Fas-activated serine/threonine kinase before onset of DNA fragmentation.

Typically CD16$^-$CD56^{hi+} NK cells express the c-kit receptor (expressed on haematopoietic stem cells), CD2 and CD7 (expressed on T cells) and the killer inhibitory (KIR), and killer activatory (KAR), receptors (expressed on NK cells). Thus, it is thought that these cells are undifferentiated, progenitor cells able to differentiate into T cells or NK cells. During the first trimester of pregnancy, 58% of CD16$^-$CD56^{hi+} cells in the decidua express a low level of CD69 (an early activation marker). These cells also express the mRNA for TNFα, IFNγ, M-CSF, G-CSF, GM-CSF and LIF.

MACROPHAGES

Macrophages constitute approximately 14% of the immunocompetent cells in decidua. In addition to CD14, the majority of these cells express the MHC Class II antigens HLA-DR, -DP or -DQ. Enzymatically released decidual macrophages have been shown to suppress mixed lymphocyte responses and allo-reactive cytotoxic T cell activity *in vitro*. The molecule responsible for this suppression was shown to be prostaglandin E$_2$ (PGE$_2$), since the effect could be wiped out by adding anti-PGE$_2$ antibody or indomethacin to the cultures. These "suppressor" macrophages produce little to no free oxygen derivatives but produce more of the anti-inflammatory molecules IL-10 and IL-1-R antagonist. In addition, decidual macrophages have been shown to possess tryptophan catabolic enzymes, which control the activation of maternal cytotoxic T cells and prevent them attacking the placenta.

DECIDUAL ANTIGEN PRESENTING CELLS

Antigen presenting cells from the decidua have been shown to be capable of stimulating the generation of CD8$^+$ suppressor T cells specific for antigens expressed on villous chorion and foetal cells to which the APC were exposed *in vitro*. These T cells were capable of inhibiting allogeneic mixed lymphocyte reactions and the development of antigen-specific cytotoxic T cells. This suggests that, unlike a peripheral immune response, the immune response in the decidua is geared towards suppression (or tolerance) rather than to the elimination of an invader.

T LYMPHOCYTES

T cells represent about 7–8% of mononuclear cells in the decidua. About 5% of these have been shown to be $\gamma\delta$T cells but this is contentious, others suggesting $\gamma\delta$T cells form a much larger portion of the decidual T cells. In mice two populations have been identified, one producing TNFα and IFNγ and the other producing TGFβ2 and IL-10. Thus, they may also influence the Th$_1$ and Th$_2$ cells in the decidua.

Interestingly the level of expression of both CD3 and the TCR on decidual T cells is much less than that on peripheral blood T cells. They also express CD69 and HLA-DR, although expression of the latter is lower than that seen in peripheral blood. Most of the T cells in the decidua are CD45RA$^-$, CD45RO$^+$ memory T cells, with low expression of the IL-2 receptor.

NKT cells, which express the NK cells marker NK1.1 and CD3, also have been demonstrated in human decidua. Intrathymic NKT cells secrete IFNγ and IL-4 and are thought to be involved in the thymic differentiation of Th$_0$ cells into Th$_1$ or Th$_2$ cells. Thus, decidual NKT cells may influence the local Th$_1$:Th$_2$ balance.

In women undergoing natural spontaneous abortion, the percentage of HLA$^-$ DR$^+$ T cells in the decidua is increased. Since only activated T cells express HLA-DR, it is possible that these cells may play an active role in foetal rejection.

7.2.8   RECURRENT, SPONTANEOUS, ABORTION

In order for the mother to recognise and accept the foetus, it is thought that an allogeneic incompatibility is necessary at an HLA or closely linked locus. If this incompatibility is not present, the foetus may be rejected by cell-mediated or humoral reactions. Recurrent, spontaneous, abortion has been shown to be more common in couples that share certain HLA specificities.

The minor histocompatibility antigens TA1 and TLX appear to be important in preventing recognition of foetally expressed paternal antigens. If these antigens are not matched in the male and female, the pregnant female may recognise the paternal TLX as foreign thereby being stimulated to produce an immune response. This may result in the production of an antibody that prevents a response to the foreign TA1, thus preventing rejection. If mates are matched for TLX, the maternal immune system cannot recognise the paternal TLX antigen and antibody, which prevents a response to TA1 will not be produced. Thus, an immune response to TA1, may occur leading to rejection of the foetus.

7.2.9 THE IMMUNOLOGY OF MALE REPRODUCTION

Since the male immune system is not exposed to antigens from the female during intercourse, any immunological abnormalities affecting the male reproductive system are likely to be autoimmune. Autoimmune recognition of sperm antigens is frequently reported in infertile couples and in individuals who have undergone vasectomy. Normally, antibodies that recognise determinants on the sperm surface are not found in the sera of healthy males or females; their presence indicating an unusual immune response which may affect the function of the spermatozoa. In contrast to this, antibodies directed towards spermatozoan cytoplasmic antigens have been demonstrated in 90% of sera from children of both sexes before puberty. The incidence declines to about 60% and thereafter persists throughout life.

The genital tract of female rabbits has been shown to contain sperm, the head region of which is coated with antibody. The antibody was bound by a receptor found only on non-motile sperm and those that appeared to be dying. It has been suggested that this antibody may be important in the removal of spermatozoa from the female reproductive tract.

THE BLOOD-TESTIS BARRIER

During development, the male immune system may not be tolerised to sperm-specific antigens due to the fact that they are sequestered behind a blood–testis barrier. However, this same barrier may be effective enough to prevent subsequent development of autoimmune diseases affecting the sperm or testicular cells by maintaining a partition between the spermatozoa and the host immune system. Unfortunately, evidence exists to suggest that this barrier is not totally exclusive since some sperm-specific antigens have been detected in the seminiferous tubules. Reaction to these antigens may be prevented in a number of ways, e.g. suppressor cells, non-specific suppressive mechanisms, lack of antigen presentation and lack of lymphocyte trafficking through the testes.

SPERM-SPECIFIC ANTIGENS

HLA antigens have not been demonstrated on the surface of spermatozoa. Anti-sperm antibodies appear to recognise tissue-specific antigens since they react with sperm from individuals with different HLA antigens.

> *Since tolerisation to spermatozoa does not normally occur, vasectomy may lead to exposure of the immune system to sperm-associated antigens and the development of autoimmune disease. An association has been demonstrated between the expression of HLA-A28 and the development of anti-sperm antibodies in vasectomised men. These antibodies have been shown to form circulating immune complexes which, in monkeys, have been implicated in the rapid onset of atherosclerosis.*

IMMUNOLOGICALLY ACTIVE CELLS IN SEMEN

Immunologically active cells have been demonstrated in the semen of healthy men. $CD8^+$ suppressor T lymphocytes, which have been demonstrated in the epithelium of the epididymis, are thought to prevent autoimmune reactions by controlling local B cell differentiation and production of anti-sperm antibody. Alternatively, these suppressor cells may suppress local antigen processing and presentation by macrophages.

KEY POINTS FOR REVIEW

- *Reproduction requires the maternal immune system to accept what is in essence a foreign graft.*
- *The blastocyst or fertilised egg implants in the uterus.*
- *The blastocyst wall consists of the inner cytotrophoblast and the outer syncytial trophoblast, which destroys uterine tissue allowing implantation.*
- *Implantation triggers an inflammatory response that results in the formation of the decidua.*
- *The trophoblast invades the maternal decidua and proliferates, providing a contact between the maternal and foetal systems.*
- *The decidua consists of the decidua basalis, the decidua capsularis and the decidua vera.*
- *The trophoblast cells express non-classical MHC Class I molecules HLA-E and -G. NK cells in the decidua expressing KIR, ILT and CD94/NKG2 receptors that recognise these molecules may prevent uncontrolled foetal invasion of the maternal tissues.*

- *Trophoblast cells may not express classical MHC Class I molecules or only express them at very low levels, preventing maternal rejection of the foetus.*
- *Only IgG is efficiently transported across the decidua, probably via FcγR on placental cells.*
- *The maternal immune system may be primed by foetal cells in the circulation leading to the prevention of uncontrolled proliferation of foetal cells.*
- *Transfer of maternal antibodies may lead to erythroblastosis foetalis.*
- *A Rh⁺ foetus in a Rh⁻ mother may lead to maternal sensitisation such that in subsequent pregnancies the antibodies cross the placenta and destroy the erythrocytes of a Rh⁺ foetus.*
- *Pregnant women appear to be peripherally immunosuppressed to some degree. They show a decrease in circulating T and NK cells whose activity is also depressed.*
- *The trophoblast cells bear FasL and complement regulatory proteins meaning that maternal cells at the interface of the placenta and decidua may be induced to undergo apoptosis (if they bear Fas) or may undergo complement-mediated lysis.*
- *Oestrogen and progesterone can influence the immune surveillance and reactivity in both local maternal and foetal tissues.*
- *Altered immune function during pregnancy may affect maternal susceptibility to a range of microorganisms.*
- *Immune competent cells have been identified, quantitatively and qualitatively enumerated.*
- *Minor histocompatibility antigens appear to be important in preventing recognition of paternal antigens on the foetus.*
- *Immunological abnormalities affecting the male reproductive system are likely to be autoimmune in nature.*
- *The male immune system may not be tolerant to sperm-specific antigens due to their sequestration behind the "blood–testis" barrier.*
- *Semen contains immunologically active cells thought to be involved in preventing autoimmune destruction of spermatozoa.*

BIBLIOGRAPHY

Cainelli F, Vento S. (2002) Infections and solid organ transplant rejection: a cause-and-effect relationship. Lancet Infect Dis, 2; 539–549.

Carosella ED, Dausset J, Rouas-Freiss N. (1999) Immunotolerant functions of HLA-G. Cell Mol Life Sci, 55; 327–333.

Cohen PE, Nishimura K, Zhu L, Pollard JW. (1999) Macrophages: important accessory cells for reproductive function. J Leukoc Biol, 66; 765–772.

Côté I, Rogers NJ, Lechler RI. (2001) Allorecognition. Transfus Clin Biol, 8; 318–323.

Denton MD, Davis SF, Baum MA, Melter M, Reinders MEJ, Exeni A, Samsonov DV, Fang J, Ganz P, Briscoe DM. (2000) The role of the graft endothelium in transplant rejection: evidence that endothelial activation may serve as a clinical marker for the development of chronic rejection. Pediatr Transplant, 4; 252–260.

Game DS, Lechler RI. (2002) Pathways of allorecognition: implications for transplantation tolerance. Transplant Immunol, 10; 101–108.

Gaunt G, Ramin K. (2001) Immunological tolerance of the human fetus. Am J Perinatol, 18; 299–312.

Goldman M, Le Moine A, Braun M, Flamand V, Abramowicz D. (2001) A role for eosinophils in transplant rejection. Trends Immunol, 22; 248–251.

Guleria I, Pollard JW. (2000) The trophoblast is a component of the innate immune system during pregnancy. Nat Med, 6; 589–593.

Hill JA, Choi BC. (2000) Maternal immunological aspects of pregnancy success and failure. J Reprod Fertil Suppl, 55; 91–97.

Hutter H, Hammer A, Dohr G, Hunt JS. (1998) HLA expression at the maternal–fetal interface. Dev Immunol, 6; 197–204.

Illigens BM, Yamada A, Fedoseyeva EV, Anosova N, Boisgerault F, Valujskikh A, Heeger PS, Sayegh MH, Boehm B, Benichou G. (2002) The relative contribution of direct and indirect antigen recognition pathways to the alloresponse and graft rejection depends upon the nature of the transplant. Human Immunol, 63; 912–925.

Loke YW, King A. (2000) Immunology of implantation. Baillière's Best Pract Res Clin Obstet Gynaecol, 14; 827–837.

Lu L, Thomson AW. (2002) Manipulation of dendritic cells for tolerance induction in transplantation and autoimmune disease. Transplantation, 73; S19–S22.

McKenna RM, Takemoto SK, Terasaki PI. (2000) Anti-HLA antibodies after solid organ transplantation. Transplantation, 69; 319–326.

Rose AG. (2002) Understanding the pathogenesis and the pathology of hyperacute cardiac rejection. Cardiovasc Pathol, 11; 171–176.

Saito S. (2000) Cytokine network at the feto-maternal interface. J Reprod Immunol, 47; 87–103.

Thellin O, Coumans B, Zorzi W, Igout A, Heinen E. (2000) Tolerance to the foeto-placental 'graft': ten ways to support a child for nine months. Curr Opin Immunol, 12; 731–737.

Vince GS, Johnson PM. (2000) Leucocyte populations and cytokine regulation in human uteroplacental tissues. Biochem Soc Trans, 28; 191–195.

Weetman AP. (1999) The immunology of pregnancy. Thyroid, 9; 643–646.

NOW TEST YOURSELF!

1.   In certain circumstances, maternal antibody is not beneficial to the foetus, e.g. haemolytic disease of the newborn. This disease is due to incompatible blood groups in the mother and foetus. In which of the following combinations does the disease most usually occur?

(a)   A blood group O mother carrying a foetus of blood group A or B.

(b)   A blood group A mother carrying a foetus of blood group O.

(c)   A blood group B mother carrying a foetus of blood group O.

(d)   A blood group A mother carrying a foetus of blood group B.

(e)   A blood group A or B mother carrying a foetus of blood group O.

2. **An important complication which affects foetal development involves the rhesus antigens which are expressed only on blood cells. Which of the following statements is CORRECT?**

(a) *Cells from a rhesus-positive foetus may cross the placenta and stimulate the production of antibodies which lyse the mother's red cells.*

(b) *All rhesus-negative individuals have antibodies to the rhesus antigen and these may cross the placenta and lyse the red cells of a rhesus-positive foetus.*

(c) *Cells from a rhesus-positive foetus may cross the placenta, stimulating the production of anti-rhesus antibodies which, in subsequent pregnancies, may destroy the red cells of any rhesus-positive foetus.*

(d) *Anti-rhesus antibodies may be formed in the foetus if there is transplacental haemorrhage at birth.*

(e) *Lysis of foetal red blood cells may be prevented by giving the foetus anti-Rho(D) antiserum after birth.*

3. **Pregnancy has an effect on the maternal immune system. Which of the following is NOT commonly observed in pregnant women?**

(a) *Decreased cell-mediated immunity.*

(b) *Decreased systemic total lymphocyte counts.*

(c) *Decreased peripheral blood T cell numbers.*

(d) *Numbers of circulating natural killer cells decrease although their level of activity remains unchanged.*

(e) *Towards the end of gestation, $CD4^+$ cells increase in number whilst $CD8^+$ cells decrease.*

4. **Studies on the cellular constituents of human first-trimester decidua have shown that the largest population of cells are:**

(a) *Large granular lymphocytes.*

(b) *Macrophages.*

(c) *Antigen presenting cells.*

(d) *$CD4^+$ T cells.*

(e) *$CD8^+$ T cells.*

5. **Which of the following statements concerning the immunology of male reproduction is INCORRECT?**

(a) *Since the male immune system is not exposed to antigens from the female during intercourse, any immunological abnormalities affecting the male reproductive system are likely to be autoimmune.*

(b) *Immune responses to sperm antigens are frequently reported in infertile couples.*

(c) *Individuals who have undergone vasectomy often demonstrate anti-sperm antigen immune responses.*

(d) *Antibodies to sperm surface antigens are found in 90% of sera from children of both sexes.*

(e) *Antibodies to cytoplasmic sperm antigens persist through life in about 60%*
       of adults.

6.   Which of the following would NOT prevent an individual receiving a kidney transplant?

(a) *No relatives capable of being living donors.*
(b) *Cancer.*
(c) *Peptic ulcers.*
(d) *Infections which complicate the use of anaesthetics.*
(e) *Diseases or infection which affect the heart or lungs.*

7.   For patients awaiting cadaveric transplantation, pre-operative, random blood transfusion is correlated with improved allograft survival. Which of the following statements is INCORRECT?

(a) *As little as one unit of random blood may be effective in increasing transplant*
       survival.
(b) *Transfusion therapy identifies individuals who will produce cytotoxic,*
       blocking or anti-idiotypic antibodies.
(c) *Transfusion therapy identifies individuals who will produce specific or non-*
       specific suppressor T cells.
(d) *Screening for pre-sensitisation after transfusion therapy involves the use of a*
       panel of usually between 20 and 30 samples, allowing the majority of HLAs
       to be represented twice.
(e) *Transfusion therapy encourages the formation of specific antibodies which*
       are detected by repeated screening which determines the extent of pre-
       sensitisation of the recipient.

8.   Which of the following BEST DESCRIBES the types of rejection that may occur in transplant patients?

(a) *Acute.*
(b) *Acute or hyperacute.*
(c) *Hyperacute or chronic.*
(d) *Acute, hyperacute or chronic.*
(e) *Acute or chronic.*

9.   Which of the following statements is CORRECT? Direct allorecognition:

(a) *Depends upon B cells alone presenting antigens to self-reactive T cells.*
(b) *Depends upon B cells alone presenting antigens to antigen-specific T cells.*
(c) *Depends upon self-reactive T cells recognising self-antigens on antigen*
       presenting cells.
(d) *Depends upon T cells recognising donor antigens in association with self-*
       MHC.
(e) *Depends upon T cells recognising donor antigens in association with donor*
       MHC.

10. **Which of the following are NOT involved in the migration of T cells into the tissues during allo-induced inflammation?**

(a) P and E-selectin.
(b) ICAM-1.
(c) γ Catherine.
(d) Cadherin.
(e) VCAM-1.

8

OTHER DISEASES

This chapter is designed to introduce you to our understanding of the immune mechanisms involved in atherosclerosis and cancer. A strange combination? Perhaps, except in recent years our understanding of the molecular processes involved in these diseases has grown enormously and has demonstrated a clear similarity between them. Atherosclerosis is a disease affecting the large arteries of the body. It is characterised by proliferation of the smooth muscle cells of the arterial wall and the formation of a fatty streak. Evidence suggests that this characteristic lesion may be initiated by mutation of transformation of a single smooth muscle cell (SMC) (as a result of a chemical or infectious insult) leading to the clonal expansion of the cell. With extrapolation, this matches the clonal expansion hypothesis of carcinogenesis. Both diseases are characterised by tissue damage caused by the production of oxygen and nitrogen-derived free radicals as a result of oxidative stress. A wide range of other characteristics are common to both diseases, providing us with an opportunity to look at how similar alterations in the normal functioning of cells may lead to distinct diseases.

8.1 ATHEROSCLEROSIS

Coronary, peripheral and cerebral disease all result from atherosclerosis, which is a disease affecting the walls of large and medium-sized arteries. The typical pathological changes or lesions (**plaques**) associated with advanced disease were called "atheroma" (derived from the Greek word meaning a porridge-like swelling).

Immunology for Life Scientists, Second Edition. Lesley-Jane Eales.
© 2003 John Wiley & Sons, Ltd: ISBN 0 470 84523 6 (HB); 0 470 84524 4 (PB)

8.1.1 NORMAL ARTERIAL WALL

The normal arterial wall comprises three layers, the intima, the media and the adventitia. The **intima** consists of the endothelium on the basement membrane surrounded by the internal elastic lamella. The **media** comprises layers of elastic lamellae interlaced with SMC and surrounded by the external elastic lamella. The **adventitia** comprises the connective tissue sheath, lymphatics and the blood vessels supplying the arterial wall (vasa vasorum) and associated nerves. The structure of arteries varies depending upon where they are found in the body; those closer to the heart have more elastic lamellae whilst those further away are more muscular.

8.1.2 EXTRACELLULAR MATRIX

The extracellular matrix is found in all tissues of the body and provides a framework upon which tissue structure is built. Its composition varies depending upon the site in the body. It has a major influence on the homeostasis of growth factors and undergoes structural changes that influence, and are influenced by, a range of cells. In atherogenesis, structural changes in the extracellular matrix lead to instability of the plaque or lesion, which can be a major predictor of clinical outcome. The major components of the extracellular matrix are shown in Table 8.1.

8.1.3 PATHOGENESIS OF ATHEROSCLEROSIS

The processes which induce the changes in the structure of arterial walls that characterise atherosclerosis are typically inflammatory in nature. Virchow (1856) was the first to observe this and proposed the "response to injury" hypothesis to explain the disease-associated pathological changes. He suggested that injury to the endothelium (caused by an unidentified event that could be haemodynamic stress or infection) caused an inflammatory response resulting in pathology. However, the endothelium is usually only damaged in advanced lesions and so this hypothesis required modification. It is now considered that insults cause subtle changes in the endothelium leading to altered function. These changes become more pronounced, ultimately leading to rupture of the lesions, platelet activation and thombosis. This is supported by the fact that lesions are commonly (but not solely) seen in haemodynamically stressed regions of the aorta and coronary arteries. Early lesions are characterised by mild or severe thickening of the intimal layer of the blood vessel caused by

Table 8.1 Composition of the extracellular matrix

Component	Properties
Collagen	Usually found in a polymerised, fibrillar form but when exposed to certain enzymes – the matrix metalloproteinases – it becomes depolymerised and its monomeric form promotes vascular smooth muscle cell proliferation and migration
Fibronectin	Not only part of the extracellular matrix but also found in plasma. Depending on its structure, it affects the adhesion of cells to the extracellular matrix and to the endothelium
Laminin	Component of basement membranes. Promotes cell adhesion, migration, growth and differentiation
Proteoglycans	e.g. Heparan sulphate, dermatan sulphate, and chondroitin sulphate. Large molecules with a central protein linked to unbranched glycosaminoglycan (GAG) chains. Soluble components of ECM, also found as transmembrane receptors that bind growth factors and may regulate cell proliferation, differentiation, adhesion and migration. Heparan sulphate is released from cells and ECM during inflammation. Causes macrophages to release proinflammatory cytokines
Vitronectin	S-protein, serum spreading factor or epibolin. Found in blood and ECM. With fibronectin, comprises the major adhesive proteins in plasma and serum. Binds to cells through an interaction with surface receptors such as integrins $\alpha v \beta 3$ and $\alpha v \beta 5$. With the plasminogen activation system, it is involved in the non-proteolytic migration and proliferation of cells

proliferation of the smooth muscle cells. Monocytes from the blood migrate into the affected tissues and with local macrophages accumulate lipids intracellularly forming foam cells, which comprise the characteristic fatty streaks (Figure 8.1). These plaques are characterised by a fibrous cap formed from the collagen secreted by the smooth muscle cells and may have a necrotic centre filled with damaged macrophages and extracellular lipid (cholesterol). Such plaques may become ulcerated causing haemorrhage, thrombosis and calcification.

ROLE OF LIPOPROTEINS IN ATHEROSCLEROSIS

Lipoproteins, particularly low-density lipoproteins such as cholesterol, become particularly cytotoxic when oxidised. In this form, oxidised low-density lipoproteins (oxLDL) affect endothelial function and kill both smooth muscle cells and macrophages. They are taken up by scavenger receptors, the cells becoming lipid-laden foam cells. These altered lipids may be antigenic (presented by CD1) causing lesional immune reactions.

Oxidised phospholipids produced during the oxidation of lipoproteins can induce the expression of adhesion molecules such as VCAM-1 on endothelial cells, providing a direct relationship between hypercholesterolaemia and arterial wall inflammation.

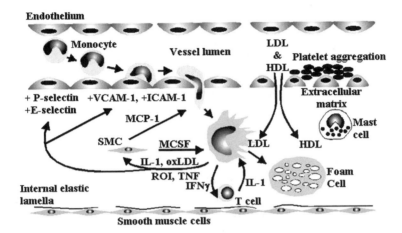

Figure 8.1   Immunopathogenesis of atherosclerosis
Low-density liproprotein (LDL) is taken up by macrophages and smooth muscle cells (SMCs) in the vessel wall leading to the formation of foam cells. Activated macrophages release damaging substances such as reactive oxygen intermediates (ROI) and tumour necrosis factor (TNF) along with other cytokines that stimulate T cells, endothelial cells and SMCs. This leads to an increase in the expression of adhesion molecules (P-selectin, E-selectin, intercellular adhesion molecule (ICAM)-1 and vascular cell adhesion molecule (VCAM)) on the endothelium and leukocytes. This leads to decreased adhesion between endothelial cells allowing monocyte and T cell migration into the vessel wall. Exposure of the extracellular matrix causes the endothelium to exhibit a pro-coagulatory activity encouraging the adhesion and activation of platelets leading to clot formation.

8.1.4   PLAQUE DEVELOPMENT

One of the earliest discernable stages in atherogenesis is characterised by altered endothelial function. The causes of these changes (exemplified by altered nitric oxide-dependent relaxation) may be legion. Indeed a large number of risk factors for atherosclerosis have been identified including smoking, obesity, diabetes, hypertension and family history.

Changes in the structure and function of the endothelium may result in altered endothelial permeability and increased leukocyte adhesion (particularly of monocytes and T cells) due to increased expression of adhesion molecules such as E-selectin, ICAM and VCAM. ICAM-1 expression may be altered not only by cytokines but also by haemodynamic stress. This may explain why hypertension is a risk factor for atherosclerosis, this raised level of ICAM-1 leading to recruitment of mononuclear cells into the wall of the artery.

As we have previously learnt, adhesion occurs in stages, initially being mediated by selectins (rolling) and subsequently (firm adhesion) by VCAM and ICAM-1. The main ligand for VCAM is the very late antigen 4 (VLA-4), which is found chiefly on monocytes and lymphocytes, thus explaining why these cells accumulate in atherosclerotic lesions.

Following adhesion, cells migrate through the endothelium into the intima. This is encouraged by the release of chemotactic factors such as C5a (complement is activated in the subendothelial layers in hypercholesterolaemic animals), and chemokines produced by intimal macrophages, smooth muscle cells and endothelial cells. One such chemokine, monocyte chemotactic protein 1 (MCP-1), is induced by complement activation and cytokines, and recruits monocytes and T cells into the lesions.

Monocytes extravasate between the endothelial cells into the media where they phagocytose oxidised lipoproteins, ultimately becoming lipid-laden foam cells. They release enzymes (e.g. matrix metalloproteinases (MMPs) and collagenases), which digest the connective tissue matrix, reactive oxygen intermediates that oxidise LDL taken up by scavenger receptors and monokines that recruit more monocytes. Smooth muscle cells migrate from the media into the intima (probably under the influence of platelet-derived growth factor), changing from a contractile to a synthetic phenotype. They rapidly proliferate, synthesising connective tissue components (collagen, elastin and mucopolysaccharide) and secreting enzymes (e.g. collagenase) that remodel the extracellular matrix. Platelets aggregate on the ulcerated surface of advanced lesions, which may rupture into the vessel lumen leading to clotting and thrombosis.

8.1.5 MONONUCLEAR CELLS IN ATHEROSCLEROSIS – MACROPHAGES AND DENDRITIC CELLS

Monocytes are recruited from the circulation into atherosclerotic plaques where they are differentiated into macrophages and eventually foam cells. Their capacity to present antigen to memory T cells and their production of reactive oxygen and nitrogen intermediates, a range of enzymes, complement components and cytokines make them key to the inflammatory process. They are able to take up modified lipoproteins via scavenger receptors on their surface, the expression of which is regulated by cytokines (Table 8.2).

Table 8.2 Scavenger receptors on macrophages and their regulation by cytokines

Receptor	Regulatory cytokines and their effects
SR-A	Expression reduced by IFNγ, TNFα, IL-6
CD36	Expression increased by IL-4
LOX-1	Expression regulated by TNFα, TGFβ

OxLDL taken up by macrophages may directly activate these cells. Components of oxLDL resemble platelet activating factor (PAF), a proinflammatory mediator capable of activating both macrophages and endothelial cells.

> *Phosphatidyl cholines (PCs) formed by the oxidative breakdown of low-density lipoproteins cause platelet aggregation via the receptor for platelet activating factor (PAFR). This is thought to be due to their structural similarity to PAF. These PAF-like lipids have been shown to influence DNA synthesis and nitric oxide production in smooth muscle cells independently of PAFR.*

Large numbers of macrophages are found in lesions and as the disease progresses these cells become lipid-laden foam cells and along with smooth muscle cells form the bulk of the lesion. Their role as antigen presenting cells may be key to the activation of T cells within the lesion leading to the release of proinflammatory cytokines, which perpetuate the pathological processes.

Another form of antigen presenting cell is also found in atherosclerotic lesions, the dendritic cell. These cells present antigen to naïve T cells and may be key to the activation of cells recruited to the atherosclerotic lesion.

8.1.6 MONONUCLEAR CELLS IN ATHEROSCLEROSIS – T CELLS

T cells in atherosclerotic lesions largely express the $\alpha\beta$TCR and other markers suggesting that they are memory cells in a state of constant activation.

Macrophages, endothelial cells and smooth muscle cells in the plaques produce osteopontin (or early T-lymphocyte activation protein-1) which induces IL-12 production by many of the lesional cells. This cytokine preferentially induces Th_1 cell differentiation, which may explain the preponderance of this subtype within the lesions. Th_1 cells produce IFNγ (amongst other cytokines), which is a key macrophage-activating cytokine and causes the secretion of phospholipase A_2, which results in the production of proinflammatory lipid mediators such as eicosanoids, lysophosphatidyl choline and PAF.

In addition to Th_1 cells, Th_2 and Th_3 cells may be found in lesions. Th_2 cells, which produce cytokines that can downregulate the activity of Th_1 cells, may be important in dampening down the inflammation associated with plaque formation. In addition, Th_3 cells are thought to be important in plaque stabilisation.

$CD8^+$ T cells are associated with apoptotic cells in atherosclerotic lesions. However, apoptosis can be caused by reactive oxygen and nitrogen intermediates produced by cytokine-activated macrophages and SMCs. Thus, both CD4$^+$ and CD8$^+$ cells may cause apoptosis in atherosclerosis.

$\gamma\delta$T cells, which are capable of recognising lipid antigens presented by CD1, have been demonstrated in atherosclerotic plaques but little is known of their role in the pathogenesis of the disease.

8.1.7 MONONUCLEAR CELLS IN ATHEROSCLEROSIS – B CELLS

Few B cells are associated with atherosclerotic lesions although accumulations may be found in the associated connective tissue. These foci of B cells may develop into perivascular lymphoid aggregates containing plasma cells and high concentrations of IgG, some of which is locally produced.

8.1.8 OTHER IMMUNE CELLS IN ATHEROSCLEROTIC PLAQUES

Mast cells, typically found in connective tissue and mucosal membranes, have been identified in atherosclerotic lesions. These cells are capable of producing a range of enzymes and are found in high numbers in ruptured plaques. They are known to produce a wide range of cytokines that may influence the activity of cells in the vicinity. In addition, their presence may indicate that they have a key role in the degradation of the extracellular matrix and locally sequestered lipoproteins.

8.1.9 CYTOKINES IN ATHEROSCLEROSIS

We have already established the importance of cytokines such as IL-12, IFNγ and PAF in atherosclerosis. However a number of others may also play key roles in the pathogenesis of this disease. TNFα and IL-1, which are found in lesions, affect smooth muscle cell proliferation, stimulate macrophages, induce the secretion of enzymes such as matrix metalloproteinase-9 and enhance the expression of adhesion molecules. In addition, IL-1 is important in T cell activation whilst TNFα may induce the apoptosis seen in atherosclerotic lesions.

IFNγ and other proinflammatory cytokines are able to induce the expression of CD40 and CD40L (CD154) on endothelial and smooth muscle cells. This key, co-stimulatory, receptor–ligand pair, is vital for T cell stimulation of antibody production. Ligation of CD40 causes expression of tissue factor on endothelial cells and can stimulate the release of proteinases from macrophages and smooth muscle cells. Upregulation of CD40 and CD154 has been demonstrated in atherosclerotic lesions.

IL-6 is also present in high concentration in atherosclerotic lesions. IL-1 secreted by macrophages stimulates smooth muscle cells to produce large amounts of IL-6. Additionally, the complement membrane attack complex may also promote IL-6 production.

The cytokines produced by Th$_2$-type cells (e.g. IL-4, IL-5 and IL-10) are present at low concentration in atherosclerotic lesions. *In vitro*, IL-4 and IL-10 have been shown to inhibit the inducible nitric oxide synthase (iNOS) and the cyclooxygenase 2 genes. Since Th$_1$ and Th$_2$ cells may negatively influence each other, the preponderance of Th$_1$ cytokines may downregulate the Th$_2$ response.

TGFβ is found in atherosclerotic plaques where it may be secreted by smooth muscle cells, macrophages or Th$_3$ cells. It promotes fibrin deposition and collagen synthesis suggesting that it may be important in cap formation. Its anti-inflammatory activity may help to stabilise the structure of advanced plaques.

8.1.10   IS ATHEROSCLEROSIS AN AUTOIMMUNE DISEASE?

We have already learnt that the immunopathology of autoimmune diseases is inflammatory in nature. The relatively recent acceptance that atherosclerosis is an inflammatory disease and the demonstration of cellular and humoral responses to specific self-antigens have led to the question of whether or not atherosclerosis is an autoimmune disease.

POTENTIAL AUTOANTIGENS

Perhaps the most obvious candidate as an autoantigen is oxidised, low-density lipoprotein. Antibodies to oxLDL have been found in the blood of patients with atherosclerosis and in atherosclerotic lesions. In addition, T cells isolated from plaques have been shown to respond to *in vitro* stimulation with oxLDL. Indeed, a quarter of all plaque-associated CD4$^+$ T cells were shown to recognise MHC Class II presented oxLDL. This demonstrates distinct cellular and humoral specific immune responses to oxLDL in patients with atherosclerosis. Furthermore, animal experiments have demonstrated that immunisation against oxLDL, or neonatal tolerance induction to it, prevents lesion progression. This suggests that the immune response to oxLDL is responsible (at least in part) for the pathology associated with the disease, indicating that it may indeed be autoimmune in nature. However, it has been suggested that antibodies recognising the phospholipids in oxLDL may be "natural antibodies" that also bind to apoptotic cells and particular bacteria. This would suggest that the driving stimulus for the anti-oxLDL response is not oxLDL itself but that this molecule merely shows cross-reactivity with the true stimulus.

Another candidate autoantigen is β_2-glycoprotein Ib (β_2-GPI), which is found on the membranes of platelets. Specific antibodies to this molecule have been found in atherosclerosis and animal studies have demonstrated that the immune response to β_2-GPI is pathogenetic.

Heat shock proteins have also been proposed as candidate autoantigens in atherosclerosis. They are associated with a number of other autoimmune and inflammatory diseases and are produced in large quantities by injured cells. In addition, macrophages exposed to oxLDL release hsp60, antibodies to which are elevated in early atherosclerosis and may predict disease progression.

Heat shock proteins are highly conserved between species, those of man and microbes being structurally and antigenically similar. Thus, it is possible that heat shock proteins produced by microbes stimulate an immune response, the antibodies being able to bind to human heat shock proteins expressed on damaged endothelial cells.

Thus, the pathology of atherosclerosis may be the result of antigen mimicry and may be associated with infection by particular microorganisms.

8.1.11 INFECTION AND ATHEROSCLEROSIS

A number of microorganisms have been associated with atherosclerosis, in particular *Chlamydia pneumoniae*. Some patients have been shown to have high levels of chlamydia-specific antibodies. Also, the organism has been identified in, and isolated from, atherosclerotic lesions. Thus there is evidence that *Chlamydia pneumoniae* plays a role in atherosclerosis but precisely what that role is, has yet to be established. These organisms produce heat shock proteins and so may provide an antigenic stimulus for the production of self-reactive anti-hsp antibodies.

Recently, animal studies have demonstrated a role for the vaccine strain of *Mycobacterium bovis* (BCG) in the development of atherosclerosis. The pathogenetic role of BCG is unclear. It may be due to the proinflammatory "adjuvant effect" of the lipoarabinomannan in the bacterial cell wall or the production of hsp65 by these organisms.

Viruses have also been implicated in the pathogenesis of atherosclerosis. Herpes viruses such as Herpes simplex type 1 and Cytomegalovirus have been demonstrated in human atherosclerotic plaques. *In vitro* studies have demonstrated that CMV can stimulate smooth muscle cell migration and expression of scavenger receptors. Thus, CMV may have a direct effect on the pathogenesis of atherosclerosis rather than influencing the immunopathogenesis of the disease.

- *Atherosclerosis has been associated with a number of risk factors including obesity, smoking, hypercholesterolaemia, hypertension, family history of heart disease.*
- *Atherosclerosis is a disease affecting the walls of large and medium-sized arteries.*
- *The normal arterial wall comprises the intima, media and adventitia.*
- *Extracellular matrix provides a framework upon which tissue structure is built and influences homeostasis of growth factors.*
- *The ECM comprises a range of chemicals with distinct structures and functions.*
- *Atherosclerosis is inflammatory in nature and involves changes in the structure of the vascular wall, infiltration by inflammatory cells and concentration of modified lipoproteins.*
- *Oxidised lipoproteins affect endothelial cell function, smooth muscle cells and macrophages.*
- *The plaque is the characteristic lesion of atherosclerosis and represents distinctive cellular and chemical changes in normal vascular morphology and biochemistry.*
- *Macrophages play a key role in atherogenesis, forming the characteristic foam cells of advanced lesions.*
- *T cells in atherosclerosis appear to be largely memory cells in a constant state of activation.*
- *Proinflammatory cytokines appear to predominate in atherosclerosis and contribute to the pathology of the disease.*
- *Oxidised low-density lipoproteins and heat shock proteins have been suggested as potential autoantigens that promote disease progression possibly due to antigen mimicry.*
- *A range of microorganisms have been associated with atherogenesis including Chlamydia spp. and viruses such as CMV.*

8.2 TUMOUR IMMUNOLOGY

The term cancer is used to describe a wide range of disease states involving nearly every type of tissue in the body. Cancer cells lose the functional and phenotypic characteristics of the tissue from which they are derived and are said to have undergone **malignant transformation** and to be de-differentiated. As the malignancy progresses, the cancer cells compete with normal ones for both physical space and nutrients. Some malignancies are capable of breaking up and spreading via the circulatory or lymphatic systems to remote sites of the body. As a result, new foci of malignant cell growth (**metastases**) are established far removed from the original tissue in which the cancer developed. This section is designed to introduce you to current ideas about the role of the immune system in cancer progression and therapy.

8.2.1 THE NATURE OF MALIGNANT DISEASE

Normally, the differentiation and proliferation of cells is largely governed by their stage of development and by the nature of the tissue from which they derive. Organs and tissues have discrete structures and defined histological make-ups within which the rate of cell death is balanced with the rate of the production of new cells. In some pathological conditions, production of a particular stimulus may lead to increased cell proliferation such that the number of new cells exceeds that of dying cells. This results in organ **hypertrophy**. When the stimulus is eliminated, cell proliferation decreases and the hypertrophy resolves. By contrast, if a cell undergoes malignant transformation (i.e. it becomes a tumour cell), it is able to replicate without any stimulus. This ability to grow unchecked allows the tumour cells to invade and disrupt local tissues, preventing their normal function and, if untreated, causing death. The poor prognosis (expected outcome) of a number of cancers is a direct result of this ability as well as their ability to metastasise and grow in distant organs. Some characteristics of malignant cells are summarised in Table 8.3.

Table 8.3   Common properties of tumour cells

Properties

Fail to respond to signals which normally regulate cell growth and tissue repair

Exhibit autonomous (self-directed, independent) growth, i.e. they do not require outside (exogenous) signals

Invade normal tissues and, unlike normal cells, their growth is not inhibited by tissue boundaries

Metastasise, i.e. they are capable of spreading into distant organs through the lymphatic, and blood, circulation and there establish new foci of growth

Exhibit phenotypic and antigenic differences from non-transformed cells in the same tissue

Are monoclonal in origin but heterogeneity may develop at the phenotypic and genetic level as the tumour grows

Table 8.4   Some examples of carcinomas and their causative agents

Agent	Outcome
Epstein–Barr virus	Burkitt's lymphoma
Papilloma virus	Cervical and anal cancers
Hepatitis B and C viruses	Liver cancer
Human herpesvirus B	Kaposi's sarcoma
HTLV-1	Lymphocytic leukaemia and lymphoma
Helicobacter pylori	Gastric cancer and lymphoma
Schistosomes	Bladder cancer
Benzene derivatives; nitrogen mustard	Damage DNA
Gamma irradiation	Induces malignancies

8.2.2   CAUSES OF MALIGNANCY

The transformation of a normal cell into a malignant one may be the result of a wide range of stimuli, the nature of which may determine whether or not the growth of the tumour can be controlled by the immune system. Transformation may occur spontaneously (as a result of gene rearrangements or random mutations), or may be induced by viral, chemical or physical **carcinogens** (cancer-promoting substances). Some examples are shown in Table 8.4.

PHYSICAL CARCINOGENS

The discovery and subsequent use of X-rays and radioactivity in the late 19th century resulted in the first examples of cancer caused by physical carcinogens. In more recent years, the most convincing evidence of radiation-induced carcinogenesis has come from studies of the survivors of the Hiroshima atomic bomb and the population who lived in the vicinity of the Chernobyl atomic energy plant. These people have presented with increased incidences of a range of tumours usually several years after the event. Ionising radiation directly damages DNA resulting in mutation, abnormal gene rearrangements and chromosomal breakage. However, the long period between exposure and appearance of the tumour suggests that another genetic event or the activation of a promoter is required for tumour development.

In recent years, there has been a distinct increase in the incidence of skin cancer, particularly in sunny countries such as Australia. Evidence suggests that this is related to increased exposure to UV light, which may cause the production of carcinogenic oxygen metabolites and pyrimidine dimers.

CHEMICAL CARCINOGENS

Tumours induced by chemical carcinogens were initially described in the 18th century when chimney sweeps were observed to have an unusually high incidence of carcinoma of the scrotum. It is believed that tar in the wrinkles of the scrotum was responsible for these tumours since the polycyclic aromatic hydrocarbons in soot and tar have been found to be a major class of carcinogens. Other aromatic hydrocarbons such as the aromatic amines have been implicated in malignancy due to the observation of a high frequency of bladder cancer among factory workers using aniline dyes.

VIRAL CARCINOGENS

Cells transformed by viral genes may be expected to express viral antigens, which may be capable of stimulating an immune response. Thus, tumours caused by **oncogenic** (tumour-causing) viruses may present an opportunity for immunological control or elimination of the tumour.

Such viruses may contain either DNA or RNA. When a potentially oncogenic virus infects a permissive cell (i.e. one which allows viral replication), infection usually results in cell lysis. However, if the same virus infects a non-permissive cell, the viral DNA may integrate into the host cell genome. The resulting transformation of the cell may result from viral DNA triggering host genes or from the abnormal splicing of viral mRNA by the host, which results in the production of novel transformation-promoting proteins.

Retroviruses contain RNA (rather than DNA) and possess genes that code for the polymerase enzyme – reverse transcriptase. This produces a DNA copy of the viral RNA that can be integrated (incorporated) into the host genome. Oncogenic retroviruses were isolated first from chicken tumours and have subsequently been shown to be responsible for a large number of cancers in many different species, e.g. the human T cell leukaemia virus (HTLV). Some cause transformation directly through the presence of oncogenes (see below) in their genomes, others activate the host's genes.

ONCOGENES

Several genes have been identified in normal cells which, when activated under appropriate conditions, lead to the malignant transformation of the cell. Some of these cellular oncogenes have been shown to have a role to play in normal growth and development. However, changes that cause permanent, active transcription of these genes are thought to cause malignant transformation of the cell (Table 8.5).

Table 8.5   Examples of some events that result in malignant transformation

Event
Mutation of a regulatory gene, which may interfere with its activity
Translocation of an oncogene next to an active cellular gene (e.g. in some B cell lymphomas translocation of an oncogene next to an immunoglobulin variable region gene has been demonstrated) resulting in its inappropriate activation
Insertion of a promoter that enhances the expression of an oncogene

Oncogenes have been shown to code for membrane receptors, autocrine growth factors and regulators of gene expression. In malignant cells, the products of these genes are increased and thus may make the malignant cells immunologically distinct from the normal cells in the surrounding tissues.

8.2.3   TUMOUR ANTIGENS

Many studies in animals have shown that tumour rejection or regression is largely dependent on cellular immune responses. In addition, with the exception of antibodies that bind to growth factor receptors, immunotherapy using tumour-specific antibodies has not been particularly successful. Thus in recent

Table 8.6   Examples of tumour antigens recognised by T cells

Type	MHC restriction	Examples
Melanoma–melanocyte differentiation antigens	Class I	MART-1, gp100; tyrosinase, melanocyte stimulating hormone receptor
Cancer testes antigens	Class I	MAGE-1, 2, 3, 12, BAGE, GAGE
Renal carcinoma antigen	Class I	RAGE
Mutated antigens	Class I	β-catenin, MUM-1, CDK-4, caspases-8
	Class II	Triosephosphate isomerase, CDC27
Non-mutated shared antigens	Class I	Carcinoembryonic antigen, α-fetoprotein, telomerase catalytic protein, Her2/neu, mdm2, MUC-1
	Class II	gp100, MAGE-1, 3, tyrosinase

years, a large amount of research has concentrated on identifying antigens on tumours capable of stimulating a cell-meditated immune response. The majority of those antigens identified so far are MHC Class I-presented, melanoma-derived, which are capable of stimulating T_{cyt} (CD8$^+$) cells. However, more recently, techniques have advanced to allow us to identify MHC Class II-presented antigens that stimulate CD4$^+$ T cells. Examples of both these types of antigen are shown in Table 8.6.

Previously, antigens have been classified as tumour-specific, tumour-associated or tumour-related. However, owing to the observation that many of the antigens found on tumours may be expressed on other tissues (albeit in "immunologically" privileged sites), this classification is rather contentious and not particularly helpful. One way to categorise antigens identified in tumours is shown in Table 8.6. Some of these will be discussed further below.

MELANOMA–MELANOCYTE DIFFERENTIATION ANTIGENS (MMDAs)

These antigens are normal, non-mutated molecules found on the pigment-producing melanocytes and on melanomas derived from such cells.

MART-1: Melanoma antigen A or melanoma antigen recognised by T cells 1 (Melan-A/MART-1) is widely expressed in primary melanomas and the metastatic growths derived from them. The immunodominant peptide comes from the transmembrane domain of Melan-A.

CANCER TESTES ANTIGENS (CTAs)

These are antigens found on a range of epithelial tumours, on placental tissues and in the testes. Although found on melanomas, these antigens are distinct from MMDAs in that the genes coding for these antigens, althought silent, are found in a wide variety of tissues.

MAGE, BAGE and GAGE: MAGE-1 (melanoma antigen) was the first human tumour antigen characterised. The gene is one of a family of at least 12 found on the long arm of chromosome 12. Although present, the genes are silent in a wide range of tissues. The exception is in the testes and placenta. In the testes the antigen is found on spermatocytes but since these cells do not express MHC Class I, MAGE-1 cannot be recognised by T_{cyt} cells.

As well as being expressed on melanomas, antigens coded for by the MAGE family of genes are found on a proportion of breast and ovarian tumours, bladder, head and neck, gastric and oesophageal carcinomas, and sarcomas.

BAGE and GAGE were identified using the same melanoma cell line as that used to identify MAGE. BAGE is predominantly expressed on melanomas but is also present in some infiltrating bladder and breast cancers. GAGE is found in melanomas, sarcomas, and head and neck cancers.

RENAL CARCINOMA ANTIGEN

The renal carcinoma antigen RAGE has been identified on a number of renal carcinoma cells. It is presented by the MHC Class I gene product HLA-B7. Like MAGE, this gene is silent in a wide range of tissues. Although expressed by retinal cells, a lack of MHC Class I antigen expression by these cells protects them from T_{cyt} attack.

NON-MUTATED SHARED ANTIGENS

These are a controversial group of antigens because they are found on a wide range of tissues. However, their expression on tumours is usually greatly increased.

Many of the Class II restricted antigens in this group are epitopes from MMDAs or CTAs.

Carcinoembryonic antigen: Carcinoembryonic antigen (CEA) is a glycoprotein found on foetal gut cells and on colorectal tumours (tumours affecting the colon and rectum). However, serum levels of CEA are also raised in patients with colitis (itis – inflammation; inflammation of the colon), pancreatitis and pancreatic, lung and breast cancer. Thus, although elevated serum CEA levels may not be indicative of cancer of the colon, measurement of these levels during treatment has been shown to be a prognostic marker for tumour progression and response to treatment.

α-fetoprotein: Alpha-fetoprotein is a glycoprotein (70 kDa) expressed mainly by the yolk sac and liver of the foetus. Serum levels decline in the final weeks before birth and, shortly thereafter, have completely disappeared. Thus, the detection of this antigen in adults with liver cancer was thought to be diagnostic of this condition. However, with the development of highly sensitive assays, it has been demonstrated that low levels of α-fetoprotein may be found in normal adult sera, in patients with acute hepatitis and in pregnant women.

Her2/neu: Her2/neu is a transmembrane growth factor receptor found in normal and malignant breast epithelial cells. Phosphorylation of the receptor-associated intracellular tyrosine kinase results in intracellular signalling and activation of genes involved in cell growth. Thus, the gene coding for Her2 is an oncogene, amplification or overexpression of which is linked with poor prognosis in breast cancer. It is transactivated by heterodimerisation with other family members (such as the epidermal growth factor receptor – EGFR), resulting in enhanced tumour cell motility, protease secretion and invasion, and also altered cell cycle regulation, DNA repair and apoptosis.

MUTATED ANTIGENS

These are normal proteins found on a wide range of cells that have undergone translation errors or mutations leading to abnormal proteins with unique epitopes.

β-catenin: The most common form of union between cells is the adherens junction, which influences tissue structure, cell movement and proliferation. These junctions involve the interaction between the surface membrane-exposed domains of cadherin receptors on neighbouring cells. Intracellularly, these cadherins bind to *β*-catenin or plakoglobin (*γ*-catenin), which are linked to the actin cytoskeleton via *α*-catenin. This association between the cadherins, catenins and the cytoskeleton is vital for the stabilisation of the junction and for normal cell physiology.

In tumour cells there are often major changes in cytoskeletal organisation, cell–cell adhesion and adhesion-dependent signalling, which may contribute to the invasiveness and metastasis of the tumour. These changes may result from the decreased expression of, or mutations in, the genes coding for cadherins or catenins. Indeed, several pro-oncogenic factors including ras, epidermal growth factor (EGF), Her2 and MUC-1 release *β*-catenin from the cadherin–catenin–cytoskeletal complex. By contrast, anti-oncogenic factors such as TGF*β*, retinoic acid and vitamin D have been shown to inhibit nuclear *β*-catenin-dependent signalling.

In colorectal cancer, *β*-catenin associates in the nucleus with the T cell factor (TCF)/lymphoid enhancer factor (LEF) transcription factors resulting in the production of several molecules important in the development of the tumour such as c-myc, cyclin D1, cyclooxygenase (COX)-2, matrix metalloproteinase (MMP)-7 and urokinase-type plasminogen activator receptor.

8.2.4 TUMOUR SUPPRESSOR GENE – ONCOGENE NETWORKS

Cell proliferation is a strictly regulated process governed by signals dependent upon extracellular growth factors, cell size and DNA integrity.

Most cells in the body are terminally differentiated. However, stem cells in the bone marrow are capable of proliferation and are in the resting G_0 stage of the cell cycle. Upon stimulation, these cells can enter the cell cycle but once the signal is removed they return to a resting state.

Most neoplastic cells demonstrate dysregulation of the cell cycle to a greater or lesser extent resulting in a large increase in cells. It is thought that accumulated genetic changes result in more cells entering the growth phase of the cell cycle, the daughter cells demonstrating increased viability rather than the tumour cells having a shorter growth cycle. Thus, events that control the transition from quiescence to cell growth are more likely to be important in

Table 8.7 Examples of oncogenes and tumour suppressor genes associated with cancer

Gene/molecule	Oncogene/TSG	Function	Disease association
p53	Tumour suppressor gene	Short-lived in normal cells. Regulates response to stress and damage partly by activation of genes involved in cell cycle control, DNA repair and apoptosis	
mdm2	Oncogene	Induced by p53 and promotes the nuclear degradation of p53	Overexpression is found in high-grade, metastatic malignancies, e.g. sarcomas, leukaemias, breast and prostate cancer
p19 ARF	Tumour suppressor gene	Regulates mdm2 degradation of p53 by blocking the nuclear to cytoplasmic movement of mdm2	
PTEN	Tumor suppressor protein	Dephosphorylates PIP3. Inhibits activation of PI3-kinase and Akt signal pathway, blocking nuclear entry of mdm2	Mutated in large proportion of high-grade gliomas and tumours of the prostate, breast and lung

tumorigenesis than those that regulate the rate of cell division. The products of oncogenes (growth promoting) and tumour suppressor genes regulate these events (Table 8.7).

p53 is a tumour suppressor antigen. From this it might be logical to suggest that overexpression of p53 might be beneficial, inhibiting tumour growth. However, the situation is more complex than that! Cells grow as a result of growth factors binding to their cell surface receptors and setting up signalling cascades within the cell. Recently, it has been demonstrated that movement of the mdm2 oncoprotein from the cytoplasm to the nucleus occurs as a result of its phosphorylation caused by receptor ligation and activation of the phosphoinositide 3 (PI3)–kinase–Akt signalling pathway. Once in the nucleus, mdm2 downregulates p53 protein expression. By contrast, the PTEN tumour suppressor protein inhibits the activation of Akt, preventing the phosphorylation of mdm2 and its movement to the nucleus. This enhances p53 expression.

When first expressed, p53 induces mdm2, affording the cell the opportunity to repair cell and nuclear damage. However, p53 subsequently induces PTEN expression, resulting in the death of mutated or irrevocably damaged cells.

Thus, as we can see, there is a complex network of tumour suppressors, growth signalling pathways and oncoproteins that are essential for maintenance of normal cell and tissue function. During the progression of cancer, it is possible that the loss or mutation of one of these elements may undermine the function of another.

8.2.5 TUMOUR IMMUNOLOGY

The immune system, at least theoretically, has the potential to control the outgrowth of malignant cells. However, the regulation of tumour cell growth is proving more complex and many tumours appear to possess the ability to evade or overcome the potentially lethal immune response.

Clearly, the ability of particular tumour cells to stimulate antigen-specific effector mechanisms such as antibody-mediated cellular cytotoxicity and T cell-mediated cytolysis will depend upon their antigenicity. These mechanisms are likely to be most effective against highly immunogenic tumours (e.g. those induced by oncogenic viruses) whilst non-specific effector responses (e.g. NK cell activity) are likely to be of greater importance with less immunogenic tumours.

It is thought that the initial appearance of transformed cells may be controlled by non-specific effector mechanisms and that failure of these to eliminate the malignancy results in the stimulation (at some later stage of development) of tumour-specific immune responses. This is supported by observations of the regression of metastatic lesions after the removal of primary tumours and of the spontaneous regression of tumours.

INNATE IMMUNITY

Cells and chemicals involved in innate immunity may play a role in the early regulation of growth of malignantly transformed cells.

Natural antibodies: Recently, it has been suggested that "natural" antibodies may limit tumour cell growth. These are antibodies secreted by B cells, which have not been specifically activated by antigen and may be $CD5^+$ or $CD5^-$ and $CD45Ra^{lo}$. Natural antibodies recognise certain viral and bacterial antigens and are involved in the removal of altered self-antigens. Early in malignant transformation, altered self-antigens may be expressed on the surface of the cells. It has been proposed that natural antibodies may help to eliminate these transformed cells in the early stage of development when the tumour load is minimal.

Natural killer cells: Many studies have reported the presence of NK cells in a wide range of tumours. They usually only form a small proportion of mononuclear cells present and their relevance to tumour regression is still unclear. Our understanding of the anti-tumour activity of NK cells has largely derived from observations made of their activity *in vitro*, but they may provide an initial defence against tumours at both primary and metastatic sites. NK cell lysis depends upon the target cell not expressing certain MHC Class I gene products. Some oncogenic viruses have been shown to downregulate surface MHC antigen expression in their target cells, which may mean NK cells have a role to play in the early stages of tumour development induced by these viruses.

Macrophages: Macrophages (and neutrophils) upon activation by bacterial products *in vitro* may be demonstrated to have cytolytic activity towards tumour cells. However, in order to exhibit cytotoxic activity, tissue macrophages must be activated by cytokines such as gamma interferon, tumour necrosis factor, IL-4 and granulocyte–macrophage colony-stimulating factor. Antigen-stimulated T cells produce these cytokines and so the ability of macrophages to affect tumour cell growth may depend upon antigen-specific T cell activity.

The mechanisms by which macrophages recognise and destroy tumour cells in the absence of antibody are not fully understood and evidence for this activity *in vivo* is limited. Attachment is energy-dependent and brought about by trypsin-sensitive membrane receptors. Lysis may result from the intercellular transfer of lysosomal products, the production of superoxide, the release of neutral proteases or secretion of tumour necrosis factor; the effective mechanism being influenced by the cytokines which activate the macrophage.

Although it has been demonstrated that tumour-associated macrophages can destroy cancer cells, in some instances a symbiotic relationship appears to exist between the tumour cells and macrophages, each providing growth factors for the other. Tumour cells appear to be capable of blocking the activity of macrophages and may even promote their survival. The macrophages respond to environmental changes such as hypoxia and provide growth factors and cytokines that promote angiogenesis. Clearly, a better understanding of this relationship is key to our understanding of the immune regulation of tumorigenesis.

INFLAMMATION AND THE DEVELOPMENT OF CANCER

The association between inflammation and cancer has been recognised for many years. One clearly established example is the correlation between inflammatory bowel disease and colorectal cancer. The mechanisms behind this association are unclear. The "landscape theory" suggests that abnormal cells from stromal tissues, influenced by factors in the local environment, cause susceptibility to malignant transformation in epithelial cells. These environmental factors include those that favour genomic changes (resulting in the loss of tumour suppressor function or activation of oncogenes) or enhanced growth, thus providing transformed cells the opportunity to proliferate.

The association between *H. pylori* infection and gastric cancer is another example where inflammation is clearly related to tumour development. *H. pylori* causes mucosal inflammation and can persist as a chronic inflammatory response associated with the release of reactive oxygen intermediates and tissue cell proliferation. This can result in DNA damage and the outgrowth of transformed cells, increasing the risk of cancer.

Inflammation has been associated with cancer caused by a range of infectious agents as well as with cervical cancer, ovarian cancer, oesophageal adenocarcinoma, mesothelioma and bronchial lung cancer.

Inflammation involves cycles of tissue damage and repair, which can include damage to DNA. Resulting mutations may affect the function of tumour suppressor or oncogene products. In addition, the process of repair involves promotion of cellular replication providing the opportunity for clonal expansion of transformed cells.

SPECIFIC IMMUNITY

T cells: In tumour-bearing patients, the T cell response may cause direct killing of tumour cells and activate other components of the immune system capable of exerting control over tumour cell growth. Immunity to tumours involves both CD4$^+$ve, Class II-restricted and Class I-restricted, CD8$^+$ve, T cells. The former are largely Th cells that secrete lymphokines, which activate other effector cells (e.g. T_{cyt} and B cells) and enhance inflammatory responses. The CD8$^+$ T cells are mostly cytotoxic, causing direct lysis of tumour cells. However, these cells are capable also of producing lymphokines.

Since tumour cells generally express Class I rather than Class II MHC molecules, Th cells are unable to recognise the transformed cells themselves and must rely on antigen presenting cells to present tumour-derived antigens. This may be a further role for macrophages in the development of an anti-tumour response. Once stimulated by antigen, Th cells secrete lymphokines that activate T_{cyt} cells, macrophages, NK cells (Th$_1$ cells) and B cells (Th$_2$ cells). Th$_1$ cells and activated macrophages also produce TNF, which may be directly lytic to tumour cells.

In contrast to Th cells, T_{cyt} cells are able to directly recognise and kill tumour targets by disrupting the membrane and nucleus of the latter.

B cells and antibodies: Occasionally it has proven possible to identify tumour-reactive antibodies in the serum of patients. This suggests that antibodies may play a role in the immune response to tumours. This is also supported by the fact that B cell lines producing antibodies to tumour-associated antigens have been derived from the draining lymph nodes of human tumours. Such tumour-reactive B cells may also play an important role in the processing and presentation of tumour antigens to Th cells.

Table 8.8 Non-beneficial effects of anti-tumour antibody production

Nature of antibody	Effect
Blocking antibodies	These may mask antigenic determinants, preventing the recognition of the tumour cells by T_{cyt} cells
Soluble immune complexes	These may form between anti-tumour antibodies and shed tumour antigen – these suppress T_{cyt} and NK cell activity *in vitro*

Antibodies may cause tumour cell lysis either by fixing complement to the tumour cell membrane (resulting in the formation of the membrane attack complex and the ultimate loss of the osmotic and biochemical integrity of the cell) or by antibody-dependent cellular cytotoxicity (ADCC) mediated by natural killer (NK) cells, killer cells, macrophages or granulocytes. *In vitro*, the latter has been shown to be a more efficient method of cell lysis than complement-mediated cytotoxicity since it requires fewer antibody molecules per cell to cause cytolysis. Despite this theoretically positive outcome, the production of anti-tumour antibodies may not be beneficial in all instances (Table 8.8).

TUMOUR CELL EVASION OF THE IMMUNE RESPONSE

Tumours have been shown to possess the capability to avoid detection or destruction by the immune system (Table 8.9).

The poor, or ineffective, immune response that occurs with particular tumours may be due to selective pressures within the tumour itself causing a reduction in (or loss of) expression of a tumour antigen, which might be capable of stimulating a good immune response (immunoselection). Such cells would not stimulate an antigen-specific response and thus would be unlikely to be recognised and destroyed. In other words, these tumour cells possess a selective advantage, which allows them to form the dominant population; the resulting tumour being relatively resistant to immune attack.

Table 8.9 Mechanisms of tumour cell evasion of the immune response

Mechanism
Immunoselection
Antigenic modulation
Production of suppressor factors

Antigenic modulation (which is typically caused by antibodies) occurs when the immune response to a tumour antigen causes the loss of expression of that antigen. This process is similar to immunoselection except that when the immune response is "switched off", the antigen will be re-expressed.

Antibodies have been implicated in other ways. Patients with progressive tumours have been shown to have circulating blocking factors in their serum that inhibit tumour-specific, cell-mediated cytotoxicity and antibody-dependent, cellular cytotoxicity. Such blocking or masking factors have been shown to be antibodies. However, it is likely that other molecules may mediate a similar effect. Certainly, circulating antigen or antigen–antibody complexes, when in excess, may block antigen-specific receptors and may alter the immune response by redirecting effector cells to non-tumour sites.

Some tumour cells themselves can release soluble suppressor factors, which directly or indirectly inhibit the normal immune response. Such factors may activate certain cells of the immune system causing them to produce cytokines or other factors, which may prevent the development of effective anti-tumour responses. Indeed, macrophages from individuals with progressive tumours are immunosuppressive, an effect that appears to be mediated through the production of prostaglandins.

8.2.6 CANCER BIOTHERAPY

In the last few decades, cancer therapy has advanced considerably. Many cancers are now completely curable either by chemotherapy or by a combination of surgery and chemotherapy. Unfortunately, many others remain difficult to control, let alone cure. Modern treatments for cancers include the use of tumour vaccines, biological response modifiers, chemo- and radio-therapy, adoptive cellular immunotherapy and affinity column apheresis.

ANTI-TUMOUR VACCINES

The production of anti-tumour vaccines has relied to a great extent on the technology used to develop vaccines against infectious agents. The immunogen is usually cells derived from the patient's own tumour. However, in some cases, cells from a similar but allogenic tumour are used to prepare the vaccine. Prior to inoculation, the cells are treated to prevent division and may be modified by the use of enzymes, chemicals or radiation to increase the expression of tumour-specific antigens. Alternatively, tumour-specific antigens are isolated from the cells and inoculated often with an adjuvant such as BCG, to enhance the response to the antigens.

Although the technique is well established, many tumour-specific vaccines have not affected the tumour load. This may be due to a number of factors including immune defects in tumour-bearing patients, tumour vaccines only stimulate weak responses resulting in immunoselection.

Recently, a technique has been developed which entails cancer patients being inoculated with their own tumour cells, which have been transfected *in vitro* with genes that code for immunoregulatory molecules such as IL-2 and TNFα. The theory proposes that these transfected cells will stimulate the immune response and lead to the activation of tumour-specific T cell-mediated immunity. The transfection procedure has proved to be difficult in some instances but results suggest that this technique may prove beneficial for certain cancers.

In recent years, viruses have been used as vectors and transfected with genes coding for antigens expressed on particular tumours. However, a trial of one such vaccine (vaccinia virus transfected with chorioembryonic antigen) did not show any clinical improvement in the test group.

ANTI-IDIOTYPIC ANTIBODIES

Monoclonal antibodies specific for tumour antigens have been used to stimulate the production of anti-idiotypic antibodies. Some of the latter may be able to stimulate a strong anti-tumour immune response when inoculated in the tumour-bearing patient. Thus, the anti-idiotypes must be screened for those that possess this capability before being used in a clinical setting. Although this technique is potentially very attractive, it is limited by the need to develop the anti-idiotypes in animals (which may be recognised as foreign by the patient and rapidly cleared). In addition, the ability of a strong humoral response to affect tumorigenesis has not been clearly established. However, the humanised, anti-Her2 monoclonal antibody Hercepten has been shown to have beneficial effects in patients with chemotherapy-resistant breast cancer.

BIOLOGICAL RESPONSE MODIFIERS (BRM)

One of the first biological response modifiers used in the treatment of cancer was alpha interferon (IFNα; Table 8.10). It probably exerts its effects directly on the tumour cells (possibly by inducing their re-differentiation) rather than by boosting the immune response.

Indeed, an analogue of vitamin A (transretinoic acid) has been shown to have a similar effect to IFNα in acute promyelocytic leukaemia. It appears to induce the re-differentiation of the cancer cells by inhibiting the release of growth factors from activated immune cells.

Table 8.10   Therapeutic effects of IFNα in cancer patients
Effect
Induces prolonged remission in chronic, progressive, hairy cell leukaemia
Induces remission in particular lymphomas and chronic myelogenous leukaemia
Slows the progression of certain solid tumours, e.g. melanoma

High dose recombinant IL-2 either alone or in combination with chemotherapy has been used to treat a number of patients. Results in patients with breast cancer suggest that IL-2 (and IFNγ) may improve outcome but only when used in combination with more conventional therapy.

KEY POINTS FOR REVIEW

- *If a cell undergoes malignant transformation, it is able to replicate without any stimulus.*
- *Such tumour cells invade and disrupt local tissues, preventing their normal function.*
- *Although tumour cells may derive from any tissue and may be caused by a range of stimuli, many share a range of common properties.*
- *Malignancy may be caused by physical, chemical or viral carcinogens and oncogenes.*
- *More recently, a range of tumour-specific antigens have been identified that may be recognised by T cells. These include melanoma–melanocyte differentiation antigens, cancer testes antigens, renal carcinoma antigens, non-mutated shared antigens and mutated antigens.*
- *Most neoplastic cells show dysregulation of the cell cycle and events that control transition from quiescence to cell growth are important in tumourigenesis. These events are regulated by the products of oncogenes and tumour suppressor genes.*
- *Elements of both the innate and specific immune responses influence tumour development and metastasis. Different leukocytes have been identified within tumours and their roles are being/have been elucidated.*
- *Tumours may escape destruction by the immune response in a number of ways including immunoselection, antigenic modulation or production of suppressor factors.*
- *Treatment of cancer depends upon the nature of the tissue from which the cells are derived, the location, the patient, and on the presence of metastases.*

- *Modern treatments for cancer include the use of tumour vaccines, biological response modifiers, chemo- and radiotherapy, adoptive cellular immunotherapy and affinity column apheresis.*

BIBLIOGRAPHY

al-Sarireh B, Eremin O. (2000) Tumour-associated macrophages (TAMS): disordered function, immune suppression and progressive tumour growth. J R Coll Surg Edinb, 45; 1–16.

Basse PH, Whiteside TL, Chambers W, Herberman RB. (2001) Therapeutic activity of NK cells against tumors. Int Rev Immunol, 20; 439–501.

Bingle L, Brown NJ, Lewis CE. (2002) The role of tumour-associated macrophages in tumour progression: implications for new anticancer therapies. J Pathol, 196; 254–265.

Bohn J. (1999) Are natural antibodies involved in tumour defence? Immunol Lett, 69: 317–320.

Bremers AJ, Parmiani G. (2000) Immunology and immunotherapy of human cancer: present concepts and clinical developments. Crit Rev Oncol Hematol, 34; 1–25.

Buckminster Farrow B, Evers B. (2002) Inflammation and the development of pancreatic cancer. Surg Oncol, 10; 153–169.

Conacci-Sorrell M, Zhurinsky J, Ben-Ze'ev A. (2002) The cadherin–catenin adhesion system in signaling and cancer. J Clin Invest, 109; 987–991.

Coulie PG. (1997) Human tumour antigens recognized by T cells: new perspectives for anti-cancer vaccines? Mol Med Today, 3; 261–268.

Donner DB, Mayo LD. (2002) The PTEN, Mdm2, p53 tumor suppressor–oncoprotein network. Trends Biochem Sci, 27; 462–467.

Eccles SA. (2001) The role of c-erbB-2/HER2/neu in breast cancer progression and metastasis. J Mammary Gland Biol Neoplasia, 6; 393–406.

Hadden JW. (1999) The immunology and immunotherapy of breast cancer: an update. Int J Immunopharmacol, 21; 79–101.

Hansson GK. (2001) Immune mechanisms in atherosclerosis. Arterioscler Thromb Vasc Biol, 21; 1876–1890.

Hansson GK. (2001) Regulation of immune mechanisms in atherosclerosis. Ann N Y Acad Sci, 947; 157–165.

Ho A, Dowdy SF. (2002) Regulation of G1 cell-cycle progression by oncogenes and tumor suppressor genes. Curr Opin Genet Devel, 12; 47–52.

Kita T, Kume N, Minami M, Hayashida K, Murayama T, Sano H, Moriwaki H, Kataoka H, Nishi E, Horiuchi H, Arai H, Yokode M. (2001) Role of oxidized LDL in atherosclerosis. Ann N Y Acad Sci, 947; 199–205.

Lohrisch C, Piccart M. (2001) An overview of HER2. Semin Oncol, 28; S3–S11.

Ludewig B, Zinkernagel RM, Hengartner H. (2002) Arterial inflammation and atherosclerosis. Trends Cardiovasc Med, 12; 154–159.

Marx N. (2002) Peroxisome proliferator-activated receptor gamma and atherosclerosis. Curr Hypertens Rep, 4; 71–77.

Mayr M, Kiechl S, Willeit J, Wick G, Qingbo Xu Q. (2000) Infections, immunity, and atherosclerosis. Associations of antibodies to *Chlamydia pneumoniae*, *Helicobacter pylori*, and cytomegalovirus with immune reactions to heat shock protein 60 and carotid or femoral atherosclerosis. Circulation, 102; 833–839.

Ngeh J, Anand V, Gupta S. (2002) Chlamydia pneumoniae and atherosclerosis – what we know and what we don't. Clin Microbiol Infect, 8; 2–13.

O'Byrne KJ, Dalgleish AG. (2001) Chronic immune activation and inflammation as the cause of malignancy. Br J Cancer, 85; 473–483.

Pittet MJ, Zippelius A, Valmori D, Speiser DE, Cerottini JC, Romero P. (2002) Melan-A/MART-1-specific CD8 T cells: from thymus to tumor. Trends Immunol, 23; 325–328.

Rosenberg SA. (2001) Progress in human tumour immunology and immunotherapy. Nature, 411; 380–384.

Ross JS, Stagliano NE, Donovan MJ, Breitbart RE, Ginsburg GS. (2001) Atherosclerosis and cancer: common molecular pathways of disease development and progression. Ann N Y Acad Sci, 947; 271–292.

Shacter E, Weitzman SA. (2002) Chronic inflammation and cancer. Oncology (Huntingt), 16; 217–226.

Sharpless NE, DePinho RA. (2002) p53: good cop/bad cop. Cell, 110; 9–12.

Teh BT, Larsson C, Nordenskjold M. (1999) Tumor suppressor genes (TSG). Anticancer Res, 19; 4715–4728.

Tokumura A, Sumida T, Toujima M, Kogure K, Fukuzawa K. (2000) Platelet-activating factor (PAF)-like oxidized phospholipids: relevance to atherosclerosis. Biofactors, 13; 29–33.

Tsongalis GJ, Ried A Jr. (2001) HER2: the neu prognostic marker for breast cancer. Crit Rev Clin Lab Sci, 38; 167–182.

Wick G, Perschinka H, Millonig G. (2001) Atherosclerosis as an autoimmune disease: an update. Trends Immunol, 22; 665–669.

Wong NA, Pignatelli M. (2002) Beta-catenin – a linchpin in colorectal carcinogenesis? Am J Pathol, 160; 389–401.

NOW TEST YOURSELF!

1. **The differentiation and proliferation of cells is largely governed by their stage of development. Which of the following statements related to malignant disease is INCORRECT?**

(a) *In some pathological conditions, the rate of production of new cells exceeds that of dying cells.*

(b) *Organ hypertrophy results from the overproduction of new cells in a tissue.*

(c) *Cells that are able to replicate without any stimulus have undergone malignant transformation.*

(d) *Tumour cells invade and disrupt local tissues and the immune response to this invasion prevents the normal function of the tissues and organs, preventing normal function and ultimately causing death.*

(e) *A tumour cell is one which has undergone malignant transformation.*

2. **Which of the following IS a common property of tumour cells?**

(a) *Tumour cells respond to regulatory signals which normally regulate cell growth and tissue repair.*

(b) Tumour cells exhibit autonomous growth.
(c) Tumour cells invade tissues but their growth is inhibited by tissue boundaries.
(d) Tumour cells exhibit the same phenotype as non-transformed cells in the
     same tissue.
(e) Tumour cells are polyclonal in origin and heterogeneity increases at the
     phenotypic and genetic level as the tumour grows.

3.   Which of the following may NOT induce transformation of a cell?
(a) Radioactivity.
(b) Gene rearrangement.
(c) Oncogenic viruses.
(d) UV light.
(e) Aniline dyes.

4.   Which of the following processes involved in the production of transformed
cells is NOT caused directly by ionising radiation?
(a) Damage to DNA.
(b) Mutation at the level of DNA.
(c) Abnormal gene rearrangements.
(d) Chromosomal breakage.
(e) Promoter activation.

5.   Which of the following statements concerning oncogenes is INCORRECT?
(a) In malignant cells, the products of oncogenes are increased but do not make
     the cells immunologically distinct from normal cells that also express these
     genes.
(b) Malignant transformation of a cell may result from the translocation of an
     oncogene next to an active cellular gene, resulting in its inappropriate
     activation.
(c) Oncogenes may code for membrane receptors.
(d) Oncogenes may code for molecules that regulate gene expression.
(e) Cellular oncogenes play a role in the normal growth and development of a
     cell.

6.   Which of the following is NOT a component of the extracellular matrix?
(a) Dermatan sulphate.
(b) Fibronectin.
(c) Collagen.
(d) Vibronectin.
(e) Heparan sulphate.

7.   Which of the following statements is CORRECT?
(a) Macrophages express the scavenger receptor SR-A, expression of which is
     induced by IL-4.

(b) *Expression of the scavenger receptor CD36 is increased by IL-6.*
(c) *Expression of the LOX-1 receptor is regulated by TNFα and TGFβ.*
(d) *SR-A expression is increased by IFNγ.*
(e) *CD36 expression is decreased by IL-4.*

8.   Which of the following statements is INCORRECT?
(a) *The majority of T cells in atherosclerotic lesions are quiescent and have markers characteristic of naïve cells.*
(b) *The majority of T cells in atherosclerotic lesions express the αβTCR.*
(c) *A large proportion of T cells in atherosclerotic lesions are Th₁ cells.*
(d) *γδT cells have been demonstrated in atherosclerotic lesions.*
(e) *Plaques contain Th₁, Th₂ and Th₃ cells, the latter being important in plaque stabilisation.*

9.   Cytokines are important in atherogenesis. Which of the following is only found in low concentrations in atherosclerotic plaques?
(a) *TNFα.*
(b) *IL-1.*
(c) *IL-6.*
(d) *TGFβ.*
(e) *IL-10.*

10.   Which of the following has NOT been identified as a risk factor for atherosclerosis?
(a) *Smoking.*
(b) *Obesity.*
(c) *Family history of heart disease.*
(d) *Low blood pressure.*
(e) *Hypertension.*

ANSWERS TO "NOW TEST YOURSELF!"

1. Cells and Tissues of the Immune System

Q1
(a) The discrete microenvironments in lymphoid tissues have distinct lymphocyte subsets and stromal cells.
(b) Stromal cells are non-specialised cells.
(c) Tertiary lymphoid tissues contain few lymphocytes but during an inflammatory reaction they are invaded by specific memory cells.
(d) Trafficking refers to the movement of lymphocytes around lymphoid tissue.
(e) **This is the answer required.**

Q2
(a) The appendix is part of the gut-associated mucosal tissue, which is considered to be part of the human bursa equivalent.
(b) Peyer's patches are part of the gut-associated mucosal tissue, which is considered to be part of the human bursa equivalent.
(c) During gestation, the liver forms part of the human bursa equivalent.
(d) Following birth, the bone marrow forms part of the human bursa equivalent.
(e) **This is the answer required.**

Q3
(a) Lymph is the extracellular fluid, which bathes the tissues and is derived from the blood.
(b) Lymph nodes are discrete aggregates of lymphoid tissue found at the junction of the major lymphatic vessels.
(c) **This is the answer required.**
(d) The lymph node provides the perfect environment for an antigen-specific immune response.

Immunology for Life Scientists, Second Edition. Lesley-Jane Eales.
© 2003 John Wiley & Sons, Ltd: ISBN 0 470 84523 6 (HB); 0 470 84524 4 (PB)

(e)   The thoracic duct is a major lymphatic vessel that provides a route for lymph to return to the blood circulation in the region of the vena cava.

Q4
(a)   Lymph nodes are found at the junction of major lymphatic vessels.
(b)   Lymph nodes range between 1 and 25 mm in diameter.
(c)   The resting lymph node has three main areas, the cortex, medulla and paracortical areas.
(d)   The cells within it are supported by a fine meshwork known as a reticulum.
(e)   **This is the answer required.**

Q5
(a)   **This is the answer required.**
(b)   The erythroid red pulp acts as a filter for damaged or aged red cells.
(c)   The white pulp consists of concentrations of lymphoid cells.
(d)   The lymphoid follicles of the spleen show a similar spatial arrangement of cells to those in lymph nodes.
(e)   The spleen is partitioned by fibrous septae and is enclosed by a capsule.

Q6
(a)   Neutrophils are not the only myeloid cells.
(b)   Mast cells derive from a distinct but unidentified progenitor cell.
(c)   Lymphocytes are mononuclear leukocytes and do not derive from the common myeloid progenitor.
(d)   Mast cells are polymorphs but derive from a distinct progenitor cell.
(e)   **This is the answer required.**

Q7
(a)   Monocytes and macrophages are not the only phagocytes.
(b)   Lymphocytes are not capable of phagocytosis.
(c)   Other polymorphs are capable of phagocytosis.
(d)   Basophils are not thought to be capable of phagocytosis.
(e)   **This is the answer required.**

Q8
(a)   B lymphocytes are not capable of phagocytosis.
(b)   **This is the answer required.**
(c)   B cells do not express CD3.
(d)   B cells are not the only mononuclear cells which can produce cytokines.
(e)   B cells are not the only mononuclear cells which can produce cytokines.

Q9
(a)   **This is the answer required.**
(b)   Some fungal infections require the help of other cells to bring about their elimination.

(c) Viruses usually require more precise effector mechanisms for elimination.
(d) Some bacteria are able to avoid being killed by neutrophils.
(e) Other granulocytes are more efficient in eliminating parasitic infections.

Q10
(a) T lymphocytes are conditioned by the thymus.
(b) B lymphocytes are conditioned by the bone marrow.
(c) Antibody production is not a characteristic of T cells.
(d) **This is the answer required.**
(e) T cells produce a variety of cytokines.

2.   Antigens and their Receptors
Q1
(a) **This is the answer required.**
(b) An antigen cannot necessarily induce an immune response.
(c) All immunogens are antigens but not all antigens are immunogens.
(d) Immunogens can stimulate an immune response.
(e) An immunogen does not only react with antigen-specific receptors on T cells and B cells.

Q2
(a) **This is the answer required.**
(b) T cells do not have membrane-bound immunoglobulin.
(c) B cells do not express CD3.
(d) All the receptor molecules on a single B cell recognise the same antigenic determinant.
(e) T cells can only bind altered or processed antigen, whilst B cells bind unmodified antigens.

Q3
(a) Antigens show a wide range of chemical composition.
(b) Antigens may comprise a single antigenic determinant or many, such as a bacterium.
(c) **This is the answer required.**
(d) Complex antigens comprise a number of antigenic determinants, each made up of a small cluster of amino acids or sugar residues.
(e) Antigens may be recognised by the immune system in either soluble or particulate form.

Q4
(a) The more foreign an immunogen, the greater its immunogenicity.
(b) Larger molecules are usually better immunogens than smaller molecules.
(c) **This is the answer required.**

(d) *Too large or too small a dose of an antigen may prevent it being an immunogen.*

(e) *More complex chemicals and particular amino acids make the molecule a more potent immunogen.*

Q5

(a) *The immune system distinguishes between self and non-self.*

(b) **This is the answer required.**

(c) *The more foreign a substance, the more immunogenic it will be.*

(d) *Potent immunogens require a molecular mass of 100 kDa or more.*

(e) *Larger, carrier molecules when attached to a small, non-immunogenic molecule may stimulate an immune response to that molecule which acts as an antigenic epitope of the carrier.*

Q6

(a) *The HLAs expressed on an individual's cells are distinct for that person and therefore will appear foreign if introduced into a distinct host. Thus they will act as immunogens.*

(b) *The tissue type of an individual is composed of their human leukocyte antigens.*

(c) *The MHC comprises a large number of separate genes, the products of which are the human leukocyte antigens.*

(d) *There are three classes of MHC genes.*

(e) **This is the answer required.**

Q7

(a) *The expression of MHC Class I gene products is widely distributed on tissues throughout the body.*

(b) **This is the answer required.**

(c) *Expression of MHC Class I products on tissue cells means that they may be recognised as foreign when introduced into a different host and thus must be matched as closely as possible during transplantation.*

(d) *Different MHC gene products are coded for by different regions within the Class I genome.*

(e) *The genes comprising the different regions of the Class I genome are known as A1, A2, B1, B2, etc.*

Q8

(a) *MHC Class I molecules do not have two chains encoded by the MHC.*

(b) *Beta-2 microglobulin is not covalently linked to the polypeptide chain.*

(c) **This is the answer required.**

(d) *The polypeptide chain does not have four domains.*

(e) *Beta-2 microglobulin is not encoded by the MHC and is not membrane bound.*

Q9

(a) Human B cells all express MHC Class II molecules whilst T cells only express them when activated.

(b) Products of the MHC Class II molecules are HLA-DR, HLA-DP and HLA-DQ.

(c) Both the alpha and beta chains are coded for by genes of the MHC.

(d) **This is the answer required.**

(e) Class II molecules only comprise four regions, two of which are extracellular.

Q10

(a) The alpha and beta glycoprotein chains comprise two extracellular domains the first of which in each molecule forms the antigen-binding cleft of the molecule.

(b) The structure created by the alpha-1 and beta-1 domains is composed of eight beta strands and two alpha helices, the resulting cleft being similar to that created by the domains of the Class I molecule.

(c) Class II antigen polymorphism is expressed in the antigen-binding cleft which influences the peptide-binding capabilities of the molecule.

(d) The nature of the antigen-binding cleft in Class II molecules allows a range of antigens to bind; this is distinct to the exquisite specificity of antibody molecules.

(e) **This is the answer required.**

Q11

(a) Antibodies have a four-chain basic structure comprising two heavy and two light chains bound together by disulphide bonds.

(b) **This is the answer required.**

(c) The heavy chains are identified by these Greek letters.

(d) Human light chains are antigenically distinct and are either kappa or lambda.

(e) An antibody molecule contains either kappa or lambda chains, not both.

Q12

(a) Heavy chain variable region products may associate with heavy chain constant region products.

(b) Light chain variable region products may associate with light chain constant region products.

(c) Kappa chain variable region products may associate with kappa chain constant region products.

(d) Lambda chain variable region products may associate with lambda chain constant region products.

(e) **This is the answer required.**

Q13

(a) *VL and VH region products are defined by the relatively conserved regions of the molecules.*

(b) **This is the answer required.**

(c) *The selectivity of the antigen-binding site of an antibody is dependent in part on the hypervariable regions of the antibody.*

(d) *Heavy chains have four hypervariable regions, light chains one less.*

(e) *V region products are classified as either V kappa, V lambda or VH according to structural differences.*

Q14

(a) *IgD comprises less than 1% of serum immunoglobulin.*

(b) **This is the answer required.**

(c) *The biological role of IgD is largely unknown but the molecule is thought to be involved in antigen-triggered lymphocyte differentiation.*

(d) *IgD has a tendency to undergo spontaneous proteolysis.*

(e) *IgD is more sensitive to proteolytic cleavage than many other antibody molecules and is easily destroyed by heat.*

Q15

(a) *Gamma/delta T cells appear to perform MHC-unrestricted cellular cytotoxicity.*

(b) *The MHC-unrestricted cellular cytotoxicity exhibited by gamma/delta T cells is more like that shown by natural killer cells than cytotoxic T cells.*

(c) *The gamma/delta receptor may recognise antigens associated with non-classical MHC molecules.*

(d) *The proportion of mature T cells expressing gamma/delta receptors depends upon the state of activation of the immune system and the nature of the activating antigen.*

(e) **This is the answer required.**

Q16

(a) *The TCR alpha chain gene locus comprises a single constant region gene.*

(b) **This is the answer required.**

(c) *The extracellular part of the constant region, which includes a short connecting peptide, is coded for by two exons.*

(d) *The third exon codes for the transmembrane region and intracellular cytoplasmic tail.*

(e) *The TCR alpha chain gene locus comprises a group of J alpha and V alpha genes.*

Q17

(a) *The genome which codes for the TCR beta chain contains a duplicated set of one C beta and D region gene and several J region genes.*

(b) *This is the answer required.*

(c) The transmembrane region is encoded by part of the third exon.

(d) The cytoplasmic tail is coded for by the fourth exon.

(e) The V beta region comprises about 20 genes in the mouse and 50–100 genes in the human.

Q18

(a) *This is the answer required.*

(b) Single base changes are produced in the VH and VL regions by somatic mutation.

(c) The affinity of an antibody for its antigen is increased through somatic mutation.

(d) Maturation of an antibody response is thought to be the result of a number of events, including an increase in the affinity of antibody for its antigen.

(e) B cells proliferating in limiting antigen concentration have undergone somatic mutation and have mIg with a high affinity for the stimulating antigen.

Q19

(a) Conserved sequences of either seven or nine bases are found flanking the V, D and J gene segments.

(b) A spacer of either 12 or 23 bases separates the V, D and J gene flanking regions.

(c) *This is the answer required.*

(d) Although VH–D and D–JH joins may occur, rearrangement of VH region genes to non-rearranged D region genes rarely occurs suggesting that other mechanisms also control VDJ rearrangement.

(e) RAG-1 and RAG-2 products are thought to take part in the processes which result in recombination by forming a vital part of the recombinase enzyme complex.

Q20

(a) The antigen-binding region is formed by the VH and VL regions, and the association of different rearranged heavy and light chain regions gives rise to combinatorial diversity.

(b) Some VH and VL combinations prevent the association of functional H and L chains.

(c) During maturation, L chain gene rearrangement only ceases once a fully assembled, functional protein is produced.

(d) *This is the answer required.*

(e) The insertion of additional nucleotides correlates with the level of activity of an enzyme called terminal deoxynucleotide transferase (TdT) and the type of nucleotide inserted reflects the preference of this enzyme for guanosine nucleotides.

3. The Innate Immune Response

Q1
- (a) C1 is made up of C1q, C1r and C1s.
- (b) **This is the answer required.**
- (c) Activation of C1 leads to the exposure of active enzymatic sites in the other molecules comprising C1.
- (d) C1 is a pentameric molecule comprising three different components.
- (e) C4 is cleaved by the activated C1 molecule.

Q2
- (a) C4 has three chains, the largest of which is the alpha chain.
- (b) C4 has an alpha chain which is cleaved by C1s, causing the release of a small fragment called C4a.
- (c) **This is the answer required.**
- (d) C4b requires the presence of magnesium ions to interact with and bind C2.
- (e) C4b2a forms the C3 convertase of the classical pathway.

Q3
- (a) C3 of the alternative pathway exists as the native form or the hydrolysed form.
- (b) **This is the answer required.**
- (c) Factor B is cleaved in the presence of Factor D, a serine protease, to Bb.
- (d) C3bBb forms the alternative pathway C3 convertase.
- (e) Another serum protein, properdin, stabilises the alternative pathway C5 convertase.

Q4
- (a) C5 is not the first to interact with the lipids present in the membrane surrounding the immunogen.
- (b) C6 is not the first to interact with the lipids present in the membrane surrounding the immunogen.
- (c) **This is the answer required.**
- (d) C8 is not the first to interact with the lipids present in the membrane surrounding the immunogen.
- (e) C9 is not the first to interact with the lipids present in the membrane surrounding the immunogen.

Q5
- (a) Antibody must be bound to antigen to effectively activate either pathway the classical or alternative.
- (b) Organisms which are easily handled by other mechanisms do not require complement activation and only stimulate low levels of specific antibody.
- (c) C1INH binds to the active sites of C1s and C1r, thus inhibiting their activity.
- (d) **This is the answer required.**

(e) iC3b which does not play a role in the complement cascade but promotes phagocytosis is formed by the cleavage of the alpha chain of hydrolysed C3 or C3b by Factor I in the presence of Factor H.

Q6
(a) Opsonisation occurs before ingestion.
(b) Tissue macrophages are relatively inefficient at killing ingested micro-organisms.
(c) Neutrophils are the most efficient of the professional phagocytes.
(d) **This is the answer required.**
(e) Eosinophils are phagocytic and geared to killing extracellular pathogens.

Q7
(a) Phagocytosis of a particle is enhanced if it is coated with an opsonin.
(b) Activation of complement leads to the deposition of C3b on the activator surface which enhances phagocytosis by neutrophils and macrophages by binding to the C3b receptors on their surface.
(c) Neutrophils and macrophages (amongst other cells) have receptors which bind to the Fc portion of IgG, thus enhancing phagocytosis of particles coated with this antibody.
(d) **This is the answer required.**
(e) Complement fragment receptors are inactive and require further signals before they can stimulate phagocytosis.

Q8
(a) The metabolic burst is characterised by a rapid, marked increase in the consumption of oxygen by the cell.
(b) The oxygen metabolites produced as a result of the oxidative burst are toxic.
(c) The enzymes involved form the nicotinamide adenine diphosphate oxidase.
(d) The superoxide anion has two unpaired electrons.
(e) **This is the answer required.**

Q9
(a) **This is the answer required.**
(b) Defensins are usually cationic with molecular masses between 3 and 4 kDa.
(c) The richest source of defensins in humans is the granules of neutrophils.
(d) Human defensins have a triple-stranded structure which dimerises in crystalline form.
(e) Defensins exhibit antimicrobial activity.

Q10
(a) The cardinal signs of inflammation do include heat, redness and pain but this is not a complete answer.

(b) The cardinal signs of inflammation do include heat, redness, pain and swelling but this is not a complete answer.

(c) The cardinal signs of inflammation do include heat, pain, swelling and loss of function but this is not a complete answer.

(d) The cardinal signs of inflammation do include heat, redness, pain and loss of function but this is not a complete answer.

(e) **This is the answer required.**

Q11

(a) Both specific and non-specific immune responses may be involved in the inflammatory process.

(b) **This is the answer required.**

(c) The fibrinolytic system is involved in the inflammatory process.

(d) The clotting system is involved in the inflammatory process.

(e) The complement cascade is involved in the inflammatory process.

Q12

(a) Kinins are basic peptides.

(b) Kinins are small peptides.

(c) Kallikreins are arginine esterases.

(d) Kinins do not prevent vasodilation.

(e) **This is the answer required.**

Q13

(a) Chemokines are structurally related.

(b) Chemokines stimulate migration and activation of a variety of cells.

(c) **This is the answer required.**

(d) Neutrophils predominate due to their larger number in the circulation.

(e) Chemokines are a large family of structurally and functionally related molecules.

Q14

(a) Factor Xa is part of the common coagulation pathway.

(b) Plasminogen is part of the fibrinolytic system.

(c) **This is the answer required.**

(d) Thrombin is part of the common coagulation pathway.

(e) Tissue Factor VII is part of the extrinsic coagulation pathway.

Q15

(a) Factor XII may be activated by surface exposed collagen.

(b) **This is the answer required.**

(c) Tissue Factor VII may activate Factor X.

(d) Plasmin does degrade cross-linked fibrin.

(e) Thrombin does convert fibrinogen to fibrin.

4. The Adaptive Immune Response

Q1
(a) *IL-12 is produced by B cells, monocytes/macrophages and B lymphoblastoid cells.*
(b) *Production of IL-12 is stimulated by a variety of microorganisms and lipopolysaccharide.*
(c) *IL-12 helps to promote responses, which are responsible for clearing infections caused by intracellular pathogens.*
(d) *IL-12 stimulates T and NK cells to produce interferon gamma.*
(e) **This is the answer required.**

Q2
(a) **This is the answer required.**
(b) *IL-1 binds to its receptors expressed on T cells and provides a signal that enhances those generated by the initial interaction with antigen.*
(c) *IL-2 production and receptor expression by T cells results from the signals produced by the early activation events.*
(d) *IL-2 stimulates T cell proliferation and differentiation into effector and memory cells. It may act on the cell that produced it, or on other appropriate cells in the vicinity.*
(e) *IL-1 is released by antigen presenting cells after presenting antigen to T cells.*

Q3
(a) *Human and murine T helper cells are thought to be either Th_0, Th_1 or Th_2 cells.*
(b) **This is the answer required.**
(c) *Th_1 cells produce cytokines, which stimulate those responses associated with delayed-type hypersensitivity reactions and that may be classified as cell-mediated immunity.*
(d) *Th_2 cells produce cytokines, which stimulate those responses associated with immediate hypersensitivity reactions that are largely humorally mediated.*
(e) *The predominant type of immune response is thought to be determined by the balance of cytokines produced by the different types of T helper cells.*

Q4
(a) *GM-CSF is produced by activated lymphocytes, macrophages, fibroblasts and endothelial cells.*
(b) *The disulphide bonding in GM-CSF is vital for its biological activity.*
(c) *Eosinophil colony formation is stimulated by high concentrations of GM-CSF.*
(d) *GM-CSF is bound by neutrophils, eosinophils and monocytes.*
(e) **This is the answer required.**

Q5

(a) IL-2 is mainly secreted by Th_0 and Th_1 cells.

(b) IL-4 stimulates both Th_1 and Th_2 cells, but at later stages only Th_2 cells continue to respond to both IL-2 and IL-4, whilst Th_1 cells respond only to IL-2.

(c) **This is the answer required.**

(d) It is thought that IL-10 – a Th_2 cytokine – inhibits the production of IL-12 and thus prevents the development of a Th_1-type response.

(e) GM-CSF and TNF are produced by both Th_1 and Th_2 cells but are produced in greater quantities by Th_1 cells.

Q6

(a) Antigen-specific antibody is produced only after a lag phase following exposure to antigen.

(b) **This is the answer required.**

(c) IgG production occurs quite a long time after exposure to antigen, reaches a plateau and then declines.

(d) The secondary response to antigen is characterised by an initial, small IgM response.

(e) The secondary IgG response is quicker and larger in formation and much slower in decline than the primary response.

Q7

(a) The B cell response to an antigenic challenge results in the production of antigen-specific antibody.

(b) The B cell response to an antigenic challenge depends on whether or not the host has previously seen the antigen.

(c) The secondary B cell response is much more rapid and much greater than the primary response.

(d) **This is the answer required.**

(e) Cellular maturation, differentiation and activation are necessary prerequisites for antibody class switching and affinity maturation.

Q8

(a) B cells mature in the bone marrow and are released into the blood as mature cells.

(b) **This is the answer required.**

(c) Class switching which occurs during maturation involves the rearrangement (and ultimate expression) of immunoglobulin heavy and light chain genes.

(d) Class switching occurs as the immune response matures and results in a change from IgM production to either IgG, IgA or IgE production.

(e) Maturation of the immune response is characterised at the genetic level by the rearrangement of a V region gene from a mu chain gene to a gamma, alpha or epsilon chain gene.

Q9

(a) B cells are stimulated to express surface antigens which enables them to migrate to distinct microenvironments.
(b) Primary follicles in the secondary lymphoid tissues harbour B cells as well as some T cells and follicular dendritic cells.
(c) Germinal centres develop in the primary follicles after antigenic stimulation.
(d) Interdigitating cells, follicular dendritic cells and macrophages are found in different areas of the secondary lymphoid tissues and are thought to play different roles in the various stages of B cell responses.
(e) **This is the answer required.**

Q10

(a) Memory B cells do not require macrophages and dendritic cells to present antigen to T cells.
(b) **This is the answer required.**
(c) Memory B cells do require T cell-derived cytokines for their activation.
(d) Endocytosis occurs at relatively high levels of antigen.
(e) Memory B cells do require interaction with T cells for activation.

Q11

(a) Clonal deletion is one of the mechanisms involved in the regulation of self-tolerance.
(b) Clonal abortion is one of the mechanisms involved in the regulation of self-tolerance.
(c) Clonal anergy is one of the mechanisms involved in the regulation of self-tolerance.
(d) Idiotypic networks are involved in the regulation of self-tolerance.
(e) **This is the answer required.**

Q12

(a) **This is the answer required.**
(b) Adult splenic B cells take longer than a few hours to tolerise with a T-dependent antigen.
(c) Adult splenic B cells take longer than 1 day to tolerise with a T-dependent antigen.
(d) Mature bone marrow B cells take longer than 10 days to tolerise with a T-dependent antigen.
(e) Splenic or thymic T cells take longer than a few minutes to tolerise with a T-dependent antigen.

Q13

(a) *Different cell types show distinct reactions to different levels of antigen. Thus a dose that may tolerise T cells, may not tolerise B cells.*

(b) *Generally, an antigen must be present continually to maintain tolerance.*

(c) *Depending upon the site at which an antigen is introduced into the body, the host may or may not become tolerised. Different routes of administration mean that the antigen is processed by different types of antigen presenting cells and is presented to different populations of T cells.*

(d) **This is the answer required.**

(e) *If the antigen is simple and has only a single determinant, tolerance is easily developed. It is more difficult to develop tolerance to more complex antigens with a large number of determinants, since lack of tolerance to a single determinant may allow recognition of the antigen and immunity.*

Q14

(a) **This is the answer required.**

(b) *Intraepithelial lymphocytes are found above the basement membrane distributed amongst the epithelial cells.*

(c) *Intraepithelial lymphocytes are phenotypically heterogeneous.*

(d) *T cells found amongst the intraepithelial lymphocytes are typically $CD3^+$, $CD2^+$ and $CD8^+$.*

(e) *The intraepithelial lymphocytes along with the lamina propria lymphocytes comprise the diffuse mucosal lymphoid tissue.*

Q15

(a) *The mucosal immune response is characterised by an antigen-specific IgA response.*

(b) *The B cells which home to the mucosae typically produce IgA.*

(c) *T cells and other cells in the mucosae may influence the production of IgA by B cells.*

(d) **This is the answer required.**

(e) *T cells influence B cell differentiation by the secretion of certain cytokines and thus the secretion of IgA by mucosal tissues may reflect the selective distribution of these T cells in such tissues.*

5. Abnormalities of the Immune System

Q1

(a) *Paul Richet first coined the term anaphylaxis and its early use was to describe the damage resulting in some individuals as a result of a protective response to a particular antigen.*

(b) *Hypersensitivity is an extreme response to antigen which results in tissue damage.*

(c) **This is the answer required.**

(d) The clinical signs and symptoms of allergy result from a hypersensitivity response.
(e) The outcome of the response to an antigen on second exposure was initially called allergy.

Q2

(a) **This is the answer required.**
(b) A Type I hypersensitivity response does not involve specific antibody-recognising cell surface antigens.
(c) A Type I hypersensitivity response does not involve specific antibody-forming circulating immune complexes with soluble antigen.
(d) Antigen-specific T cells do not cause the signs and symptoms of Type I hypersensitivity reactions.
(e) The formation of giant cells, which occurs when macrophages and fibroblasts proliferate during a hypersensitivity response is not typical of Type I responses.

Q3

(a) IgE is not involved in a Type III hypersensitivity response.
(b) A Type III hypersensitivity response does not involve specific antibody-recognising cell surface antigens.
(c) **This is the answer required.**
(d) Antigen-specific T cells do not cause the signs and symptoms of Type III hypersensitivity reactions.
(e) The formation of giant cells which occurs when macrophages and fibroblasts proliferate during a hypersensitivity response is not typical of Type III responses.

Q4

(a) IgE is not involved in a Type II hypersensitivity response.
(b) **This is the answer required.**
(c) A Type II hypersensitivity response does not involve specific antibody-forming circulating immune complexes with soluble antigen.
(d) Antigen-specific T cells do not cause the signs and symptoms of Type II hypersensitivity reactions.
(e) The formation of giant cells, which occurs when macrophages and fibroblasts proliferate during a hypersensitivity response is not typical of Type II responses.

Q5

(a) Th_1 cells do not regulate the switch to IgE production.
(b) IL-4 favours a class switch from IgM to IgE.
(c) The signals that favour the development of Th_2 cells are delivered via the T cell antigen receptor.
(d) Complexes that bind the TCR with high avidity tend to favour the development of a Th_1-type response.
(e) **This is the answer required.**

Q6
(a) Recognition of self is vital during an immune response.
(b) T cells only recognise and respond to antigen when it is processed and presented in association with self-MHC gene products.
(c) Breakdown of self-tolerance results in autoimmune disease.
(d) **This is the answer required.**
(e) Self-tolerance occurs early in foetal development.

Q7
(a) The MHC and antigen receptor genes control the magnitude and type of immune response.
(b) Associations have been established between the expression of certain MHC and immunoglobulin allotypic genes and the development of autoimmune diseases.
(c) Seropositive rheumatoid arthritis has been associated with the expression of HLA-DR4.
(d) HLA-DR2 is an MHC Class II gene.
(e) **This is the answer required.**

Q8
(a) Autoimmune disease more usually presents in women than in men.
(b) Sex hormones clearly influence the occurrence of autoimmune disease.
(c) **This is the answer required.**
(d) Androgen levels show an inverse correlation with disease activity in autoimmune disease.
(e) Oestrogen levels positively correlate with disease activity in autoimmune disease.

Q9
(a) REGA stands for remnant epitope generates autoantigen.
(b) The REGA model proposes that disease is triggered by an agent which induces the production of disease-enhancing cytokines.
(c) Disease-enhancing cytokines stimulate the production of other cytokines, including chemokines for monocytes and neutrophils.
(d) **This is the answer required.**
(e) Activated metalloproteinases cause the production of peptides from myelin basic protein in multiple sclerosis.

Q10
(a) Witebsky's postulates require the presence of autoantibody or a CMI response directed against a self-antigen.
(b) Autoimmune diseases may be classified as either organ-specific or non-organ-specific.
(c) **This is the answer required.**

(d) An antigen that is expressed in many tissues and which is recognised by an immunologically active cell will cause a non-organ-specific disease.

(e) Autoimmune diseases, which are directed at an antigen expressed in a specific tissue result in organ-specific disease. An example of this is diabetes myelitis.

Q11

(a) **This is the answer required.**

(b) Abnormalities that arise during development may be a cause of primary immunodeficiency.

(c) Genetic abnormalities may be a cause of primary immunodeficiency.

(d) Abnormalities inherited from one or both parents may be a cause of primary immunodeficiency.

(e) Abnormalities that arise congenitally may be a cause of primary immunodeficiency.

Q12

(a) **This is the answer required.**

(b) Patients with immunodeficiency commonly present with skin rashes.

(c) Patients with immunodeficiency commonly present with diarrhoea.

(d) Patients with immunodeficiency may present with the signs and symptoms of autoimmune disease.

(e) Patients with immunodeficiency commonly present with chronic infections.

Q13

(a) The most common primary immunodeficiency disease is IgA deficiency.

(b) Clinically, IgA presents as a heterogeneous group of disorders.

(c) The degree to which B cell development is affected in IgA deficiency determines the extent of the clinical complexity of the disease.

(d) **This is the answer required.**

(e) Somatic rearrangement leading to recombination of the switch region preceding the mu gene and the switch region preceding the alpha gene appears to be abnormal in persons with IgA deficiency.

Q14

(a) Infants are protected by maternal antibodies in the first few months of life and so XLA does not present until 7–9 months of age.

(b) The majority of affected individuals are male.

(c) XLA-infected individuals are affected by recurrent bacterial infections only.

(d) **This is the answer required.**

(e) Affected individuals have normal levels of T cells.

Q15

(a) *Patients with XLA have been reported to have fewer pre-B cells entering the S-phase of the cell cycle.*

(b) *Pre-B cells from patients with XLA have been reported to show poor survival rates.*

(c) *Patients with XLA have been reported to have low levels of circulating immature B cells.*

(d) **This is the answer required.**

(e) *Patients with XLA show an inverted ratio of pro- and pre-B cells in their bone marrow.*

6.   Infection, Immunity, Immunopathogenesis

Q1

(a) *Th cells produce cytokines, which influence the class of antibody that is produced in response to a bacterial infection.*

(b) **This is the answer required.**

(c) *Th₁ cells produce tumour necrosis factor and interferon gamma, which stimulate macrophages and natural killer cells that are important in the control of intracellular infections.*

(d) *The response to virus infection may be divided into stages according to the cytokines produced, i.e.: (1) IFN-alpha/beta and IFN-gamma/IL-12; (2) IL-2, IFN-gamma, IL-4/IL-10.*

(e) *Th₂ cells and the cytokines they produce are vital to recovery from infection in trypanosomiasis.*

Q2

(a) *Endotoxins form part of the outer layer of the bacterial cell wall.*

(b) *Endotoxin is a phospholipid–polysaccharide–protein complex.*

(c) *Endotoxin is associated with Gram-negative bacteria such as Escherichia spp., Shigella spp., Salmonella spp. and Neisseria spp.*

(d) **This is the answer required.**

(e) *Endotoxin is an important virulence factor and changes in the O-specific polysaccharide may result in major changes in virulence.*

Q3

(a) *Adhesion molecules do promote cell-to-cell adhesion.*

(b) *Adhesion molecules may be used by microbes to facilitate attachment to host cells.*

(c) *Adhesion molecules may be used by microbes to facilitate invasion.*

(d) *Adhesion molecules mediate attachment of parasitised red blood cells to brain endothelium in cerebral malaria.*

(e) **This is the answer required.**

Q4

(a) ***This is the answer required.***

(b) *Heat shock proteins exhibit a very high level of conservation between species.*

(c) *Heat shock protein synthesis increases as a result of cellular stress.*

(d) *Peptides derived from heat shock proteins are recognised by T cells expressing the $\gamma\delta$ TCR.*

(e) *Heat shock proteins are a group of molecules found both in eukaryotes and prokaryotes.*

Q5

(a) ***This is the answer required.***

(b) *Polyarteritis nodosa is associated with the hepatitis B virus.*

(c) *Polyarteritis nodosa is caused by virus-containing immune complexes which activate complement, leading to chronic inflammation.*

(d) *Chorea is caused by antibodies to streptococcal antigens that react with neurons in the caudate and subthalamic nuclei of the brain.*

(e) *Rheumatic fever is associated with throat infection with group A Streptococcus sp., antibodies which cross-react with patients' heart muscles or valves, causing myocarditis.*

Q6

(a) *Type II hypersensitivity reactions may be the cause of some of the liver necrosis seen in hepatitis B and yellow fever.*

(b) *The haemolysis seen in malaria is caused in part by a Type II hypersensitivity response.*

(c) ***This is the answer required.***

(d) *The Arthus response, which is seen as a consequence of some infections is the result of a Type III hypersensitivity response.*

(e) *IgA-containing immune complexes are relatively harmless, being filtered out in the liver and excreted in the bile.*

Q7

(a) *The fate of immune complexes in the body is governed by their size and the relative proportions of antibody and antigen.*

(b) *Monocytes/macrophages have Fc and complement receptors, which enable rapid clearance of antigen that is coated with an excess of antibody.*

(c) *Equivalent concentrations of antibody and antigen result in the formation of large lattices.*

(d) *Large lattices enable the cross-linking of Fc and complement receptors on phagocytic cells, thus promoting their clearance.*

(e) ***This is the answer required.***

Q8

(a) *Infection with Mycobacterium spp. is associated with granuloma formation.*

(b) *Infection with Actinomycete spp. is associated with granuloma formation.*

(c) Infection with Chlamydia spp. is associated with granuloma formation.
(d) Infection with Treponema pallidum is associated with granuloma formation.
(e) **This is the answer required.**

Q9

(a) Chagas' disease is caused by Trypanosoma cruzi.
(b) **This is the answer required.**
(c) The organisms spread throughout the body during an acute infection.
(d) Chronic disease emerges years later, involving the heart and digestive tract.
(e) Chagas' disease is transmitted by blood-sucking insects.

Q10

(a) Superantigens stimulate both CD4$^+$ and CD8$^+$ T cells.
(b) Superantigens also stimulate T cells which express the $\gamma\delta$ TCR.
(c) **This is the answer required.**
(d) The variable region of the beta chain of the TCR provides the attachment site for superantigens.
(e) The exotoxins of Staphylococcus aureus and Streptococcus pyogenes are superantigens.

7.   Immunity and the MHC

Q1

(a) **This is the answer required.**
(b) A blood group A mother carrying a foetus of blood group O is not usually at risk.
(c) A blood group B mother carrying a foetus of blood group O is not usually at risk.
(d) A blood group A mother carrying a foetus of blood group B is not usually at risk.
(e) A blood group A or B mother carrying a foetus of blood group O is not usually at risk.

Q2

(a) The antibodies elicited by foetal rhesus-positive cells do not lyse the maternal red cells.
(b) Not all rhesus-negative individuals have antibodies to the rhesus antigen.
(c) **This is the answer required.**
(d) Anti-rhesus antibodies may be formed in the mother if there is transplacental haemorrhage at birth.
(e) Lysis of foetal red blood cells may be prevented by giving the mother anti-Rho(D) antiserum after the birth of her first rhesus-positive baby or following an abortion.

Q3
(a) Cell-mediated immunity is commonly depressed in pregnant women.
(b) The total lymphocyte count in the peripheral blood is often decreased in pregnant women.
(c) T cell numbers in the peripheral blood often decrease during gestation.
(d) Pregnant women show decreased levels of circulating natural killer cells but their overall level of activity is unchanged.
(e) **This is the answer required.**

Q4
(a) **This is the answer required.**
(b) Macrophages constitute approximately 14% of the immunocompetent cells in the decidua.
(c) Antigen presenting cells comprise only a minor proportion of the immunocompetent cells in the decidua.
(d) $CD4^+$ T cells comprise only a minor proportion of the immunocompetent cells in the decidua.
(e) $CD8^+$ T cells comprise only a minor proportion of the immunocompetent cells in the decidua.

Q5
(a) The majority of abnormalities affecting male reproduction are usually autoimmune in nature.
(b) The male of infertile couples often demonstrates immune responses to his own sperm antigens.
(c) Men having undergone vasectomy may demonstrate immune responses to their own sperm antigens.
(d) **This is the answer required.**
(e) Antibodies to sperm cytoplasmic antigens have been demonstrated in about 60% of sera from adults.

Q6
(a) **This is the answer required.**
(b) Pre-existing cancer in a patient is a contraindication for renal transplantation.
(c) Potential renal transplant recipients must not have peptic ulcers.
(d) Infections that would complicate the use of anaesthetics preclude the sufferer from being a renal transplant recipient.
(e) Patients must not have pre-existing heart or lung disease or infections affecting these organs.

Q7
(a) Transplant success may be increased by pre-operative transfusion therapy with as little as a single unit of random blood.

(b) *Individuals capable of producing cytotoxic, blocking or anti-idiotypic antibodies are identified by transfusion therapy.*

(c) *Individuals capable of producing specific or non-specific suppressor T cells are identified by transfusion therapy.*

(d) **This is the answer required.**

(e) *Pre-sensitisation of the recipient is determined by repeated screening after transfusion therapy.*

Q8

(a) *Rejection is not just acute.*

(b) *Rejection is not just acute or hyperacute.*

(c) *Rejection is not just hyperacute or chronic.*

(d) **This is the answer required.**

(e) *Rejection is not just acute or chronic.*

Q9

(a) *Allorecognition involves other antigen presenting cells and would only involve self-reactive T cells if the graft antigens were cross-reactive with those of the host.*

(b) *Allorecognition involves other antigen presenting cells.*

(c) *Allorecognition does not involve self-recognition.*

(d) *Allorecognition does not involve the recognition of donor antigens in association with self-MHC.*

(e) **This is the answer required.**

Q10

(a) *P and E-selectin are involved in T cell–endothelial cell interactions.*

(b) *ICAM-1 is involved in T cell–endothelial interactions.*

(c) **This is the answer required.**

(d) *Cadherin is expressed on the vascular endothelium.*

(e) *VCAM-1 is expressed on the endothelium.*

8.   Other Diseases

Q1

(a) *The over-production of new cells in a tissue may result in a pathological condition.*

(b) *When the production of new cells exceeds the rate of cell death in a tissue, organ hypertrophy results.*

(c) *Malignant transformation of a cell results in its continuous replication without external stimulus.*

(d) **This is the answer required.**

(e) *Malignant transformation gives rise to tumour cells.*

Q2

(a) *Tumour cells do not respond to regulatory signals that normally regulate cell growth and tissue repair.*

(b) **This is the answer required.**

(c) *Tumour cells invade tissues but their growth is not inhibited by tissue boundaries.*

(d) *Tumour cells exhibit phenotypic and antigenic differences from non-transformed cells in the same tissue.*

(e) *Tumour cells are monoclonal in origin but heterogeneity may develop at the phenotypic and genetic level as the tumour grows.*

Q3

(a) *Transformation may be induced by radioactivity.*

(b) **This is the answer required.**

(c) *Transformation may be induced by viral carcinogens.*

(d) *Transformation may be induced by UV light.*

(e) *Transformation may be induced by chemical carcinogens.*

Q4

(a) *Ionising radiation is thought to directly damage DNA.*

(b) *Ionising radiation is thought to cause mutation of DNA.*

(c) *Ionising radiation is thought to cause abnormal gene rearrangements.*

(d) *Ionising radiation is thought to cause chromosomal breakage.*

(e) **This is the answer required.**

Q5

(a) **This is the answer required.**

(b) *The inappropriate activation of cellular genes may be caused by the translocation of an oncogene and may result in malignant transformation of the cell.*

(c) *Cellular receptors expressed on membranes may be coded for by oncogenes.*

(d) *Molecules that regulate gene expression may be coded for by oncogenes.*

(e) *Some cellular oncogenes have been shown to have a role to play in normal growth and development.*

Q6

(a) *Dermatan sulphate is a proteoglycan in the ECM.*

(b) *Fibronectin is part of the ECM and also found in plasma.*

(c) *Collagen is usually found polymerised in the ECM.*

(d) **This is the answer required.**

(e) *Heparan sulphate is a proteoglycan found in the ECM.*

Q7

(a) *SR-A expression is not affected by IL-4.*

(b) CD36 expression is not affected by IL-6.
(c) **This is the answer required.**
(d) SR-A expression is not increased by IFNγ.
(e) CD36 expression is not decreased by IL-4.

Q8

(a) **This is the answer required.**
(b) The majority of T cells in atherosclerotic lesions express the $\alpha\beta$TCR.
(c) A large proportion of T cells in atherosclerotic lesions are Th$_1$ cells.
(d) $\gamma\delta$T cells have been demonstrated in atherosclerotic lesions.
(e) Plaques contain Th$_1$, Th$_2$ and Th$_3$ cells, the latter being important in plaque stabilisation.

Q9

(a) TNFα is found in high concentrations in atherosclerotic lesions.
(b) IL-1 is found in high concentrations in atherosclerotic lesions.
(c) IL-6 is found in high concentrations in atherosclerotic lesions.
(d) TGFβ is found in high concentrations in atherosclerotic lesions.
(e) **This is the answer required.**

Q10

(a) Smoking is a risk factor for atherosclerosis.
(b) Obesity is a risk factor for atherosclerosis.
(c) Family history of heart disease is a risk factor for atherosclerosis.
(d) **This is the answer required.**
(e) Hypertension is a risk factor for atherosclerosis.

INDEX

Page numbers in *italics* refer to tables.

Immunology for Life Scientists, Second Edition. Lesley-Jane Eales.
© 2003 John Wiley & Sons, Ltd: ISBN 0 470 84523 6 (HB); 0 470 84524 4 (PB)